AF690383

THE DAUGHTERS OF CHARITY, CATHOLIC HOSPITALS, AND THE EXPANSION OF AMERICAN HEALTHCARE

THE DAUGHTERS OF CHARITY,

CATHOLIC HOSPITALS, AND THE EXPANSION OF AMERICAN HEALTHCARE

CARL F. AMERINGER

University of Notre Dame Press

Notre Dame, Indiana

Published by the University of Notre Dame Press
Notre Dame, Indiana 46556
undpress.nd.edu
All Rights Reserved

Copyright © 2026 by Carl F. Ameringer

Published in the United States of America

Library of Congress Control Number: 2026938691

ISBN: 978-0-268-21138-7 (Hardback)
ISBN: 978-0-268-21144-8 (WebPDF)
ISBN: 978-0-268-21142-4 (Epub3)

GPSR Compliance Inquiries:
Lightning Source France, 1 Av. Johannes Gutenberg, 78310 Maurepas, France
compliance@lightningsource.fr | Phone: +33 1 30 49 23 42

For Ellie, Liara, Henry, and Zoe

CONTENTS

FIGURES

TABLES

PREFACE

I had a vague understanding of this project's future direction when I first entered the Daughters' archives in Emmitsburg, Maryland, on July 16, 2018. The provincial archivist, Scott Keefer, greeted me with a bemused look on his face. I was not the typical researcher. I had no grounding in church history or women religious, nor did I know any of the scholars in these areas. My background was in health policy, health law, and health administration as a teacher, writer, and practitioner.

I did have some important questions in mind when I began my research, however. I wanted to know how Catholic sisterhoods came to own such a large share of US hospitals. What features did Catholic sisterhoods possess that made them successful owners and operators? What particular aspects of the American landscape aided their efforts? I also sought to determine the extent to which sisterhoods influenced the progress and development of American healthcare. What role did they play? What did they contribute to the formation of the US healthcare industry, and how significant was this contribution? What effect, if any, did they have on the nation's health policy?

There were many different paths, of course, that researchers could take in attempting to answer these questions, depending on their background, interests, proclivities, and resources. What I did not know on the day I entered the Daughters' archives was the approach that I would pursue. It did not take me long to discover that I had come across a rare opportunity, that writing about the Daughters' incredible journey over two centuries offered a means to informatively address these questions.

Given the type of questions I was asking, this was an ambitious undertaking. I knew that my learning curve would be steep and that I would need much help and assistance. I received it. Scott Keefer and his great staff at the archives (Bonnie Weatherly, Selin James, Mary Anne Weatherly, and Nic Henle) were highly accommodating. Scott promptly answered my queries, made recommendations, and helped me gain access to important materials. In addition to Scott, I received enormous support from Sister Betty Ann McNeil, DC. Sister Betty Ann schooled me in the church's lexicon and literature, advanced my understanding of the Daughters' distinct heritage, suggested new lines of inquiry, furnished ideas for additional research, and corrected several errors in the draft chapters.

There are many others I want to thank for their assistance. Belinda Davis arranged important interviews; Betty Crosby sent me several important documents from the archives at the Catholic Health Association; and Bonnie Weatherly helped me with the endnotes. James Mohr, William Kurtz, and Michael Hucles provided expertise and recommendations on certain topics and chapters. Particular insight also came from four anonymous reviewers. I greatly appreciate their time and suggestions. Rachel Kindler, acquisitions editor for Notre Dame Press, substantially helped me to tighten and focus the manuscript for publication. Andrew White astutely corrected several of my errors during the editing process.

My wife, Suzanne, deserves my heartfelt thanks for her devotion and support. My daughters, Caroline and Katie, and their husbands, Dave and Phil, were a strong presence and provided needed help when requested.

ABBREVIATIONS

ACA	Affordable Care Act
AMA	American Medical Association
APSL	Archives Province of Saint Louise
CCMC	Committee on the Costs of Medical Care
CHA	Catholic Hospital/Health Association
CM	Congregation of the Mission
CSC	Sisters of Holy Cross
DAR	Daughters of the American Revolution
DC	Daughters of Charity of St. Vincent de Paul
DCNHS	Daughters of Charity National Health System
NCEA	National Catholic Education Association
NCWC	National Catholic Welfare Conference
OMI	Oblates of Mary Immaculate
PJP	public juridic person
PSS	Society of Priests of Saint Sulpice
RSM	Sisters of Mercy
SFC	Sister Formation Conference
SJ	Society of Jesus
SSJ	Sisters of St. Joseph
SSM	Sisters of St. Mary
USCCB	US Conference of Catholic Bishops
USSC	United States Sanitary Commission

FEATURED HOSPITALS

Hospital	*Location*	*Dates*
Baltimore Infirmary*	Baltimore, MD	1823–1879
DePaul**	St. Louis, MO	1828–1994
Charity*	New Orleans, LA	1834–1996
Sisters of Charity	Buffalo, NY	1848–1998
St. Mary's	Milwaukee, WI	1848–1999
City Hospital*	Mobile, AL	1852–1854, 1895–1958
Providence	Mobile, AL	1855–1999
DePaul	Norfolk, VA	1855–1996
St. Mary's	Rochester, NY	1857–1997
St. Joseph's*	Philadelphia, PA	1859–1947
Hôtel Dieu	New Orleans, LA	1859–1992
Providence	Washington, DC	1861–1999
St. Agnes	Baltimore, MD	1862–1999
Carney	Boston, MA	1863–1997
St. Joseph's	Chicago, IL	1869–2000

* Under management contract or lease

** First named Mullanphy Hospital (1828), then DePaul Hospital (1930)

INTRODUCTION

Catholic sisters were a powerful force in the making of the US healthcare industry. But until an influential group of mostly women historians began to write about the contributions of Catholic sisters at the end of the twentieth century, few scholarly accounts extolled their significance.[1] Standard textbooks and journal articles proclaimed the roles of doctors, philanthropists, politicians, businessmen, and reformers while largely neglecting the sisters' importance.[2] Yet it was Catholic sisters[3]—not doctors, priests, or bishops—who founded and established the vast majority of Catholic hospitals, which in 2020 amounted to over 15 percent of all US hospitals.[4]

For several reasons, this book focuses on one group of Catholic sisters, the Daughters of Charity (the "Daughters"). While several Catholic communities deserve consideration for their contributions to nursing and hospital administration (and some have received it), few can match the scale and scope of the Daughters' undertaking. The Daughters began their healthcare ministry in 1823 at the Baltimore Infirmary (today's University of Maryland Hospital), and in 1828, they founded the nation's first hospital west of the Mississippi River, known as Mullanphy (later DePaul) Hospital. Both events preceded by years and decades the arrival of other nursing sisterhoods. Donning their large white-winged cornettes, the Daughters mended the wounds of soldiers in the Civil, Spanish-American, and First World Wars. They provided food, clothing, and care to poor immigrants who came to the United States from Ireland, Germany, and other countries.

And they served America's sick poor during severe epidemics, including cholera, typhus, typhoid, and yellow fever. Before the end of the nineteenth century, the Daughters' geographic reach extended from Boston to Los Angeles, from Buffalo to New Orleans, and from Baltimore to St. Louis. In 1986, the Daughters formed the largest private, nonprofit hospital chain in the country, the Daughters of Charity National Health System, consisting of forty hospitals and three nursing homes in seventeen states and the District of Columbia.[5]

Throughout their two-hundred-year history, the Daughters operated at the cutting edge of US healthcare delivery. They contributed to the development of nursing as a profession through uniform preparation, supervised training, and a written code of conduct that stressed the fair and ethical treatment of all patients. They pioneered health administration by stressing order, discipline, accountability, efficiency, and sanitation. They extended healthcare services beyond the inpatient setting through outpatient clinics, community health centers, and alliances with local and regional public health facilities. And they honed hospital finance and delivery, the integration of hospitals and related institutions, and the creation of specialized facilities for the elderly, the mentally ill, and women and children.

All these efforts, all that the Daughters did, were for one overriding purpose—the provision of healthcare to poor people. This was their mission; this was their heritage. This book shows how they accomplished their objective, how they delivered healthcare services to the sick poor and, in the process, spurred the rise of Catholic hospitals while expanding healthcare across America.

FRENCH BEGINNINGS

Founded in France in the early 1600s by Vincent de Paul (canonized as a saint in 1737) and Louise de Marillac (canonized as a saint in 1934), the Daughters represented a "new form of religious life"—"active" and "uncloistered"—which meant that they did not live in convents apart from secular society. Instead, they lived and worked among those they taught or cared for, in schools, hospitals, homes, and apartments.[6] After overcoming early opposition from the French clergy to their "active spirituality," the Daughters attained substantial geographic reach and mobility during the seventeenth and eighteenth centuries.

The Daughters were not the first community of Catholic women to work outside the cloister. Both the Ursulines, founded in Italy in 1535 for the education of girls, and the Visitation nuns, founded in France in 1610, had active ministries. But during the Counter-Reformation, the Catholic Church's response to the emergence and growth of Protestantism, local bishops called for their enclosure. Meeting at various times between 1545 and 1563, the Council of Trent, the impetus behind the Counter-Reformation, issued several decrees condemning Protestant beliefs and clarifying Catholic doctrines. The council called for a "return to the past," to "tradition." There was to be no middle ground, no "intermediate state between the wholly secular and the wholly religious," the council instructed. The cloister was one such "tradition."[7]

Yet the Daughters avoided the cloister in the early 1600s and the council's restrictions on religious women because of the vision, organizational skills, and political wherewithal of their founders, Vincent de Paul and Louise de Marillac. Vincent was among a group of "better educated" priests that the Catholic Church assigned to local parishes during the second wave of the Counter-Reformation. The first wave was a period of intense religious conflict. It ended in 1598 with the Edict of Nantes, which granted religious freedom to France's Protestant minority, known as the Huguenots. The second wave, starting around 1600, marked a period of church revitalization, a Catholic reformation. During the second wave, the church pursued clerical reform and religious instruction for the laity.[8]

As a young priest in the early 1600s, Vincent de Paul spread the Gospel among peasant farmers. During mass in the town of Châtillon-les-Dombes in southeastern France, Vincent learned that a nearby family was sick and suffering. On his way to provide aid, Vincent encountered several women undertaking the same journey. These women were "badly organized," he observed; the food they carried would spoil before the family could fully recover. Vincent encouraged the women to coordinate their activities, showed them how to work together, and taught them how to sustain their efforts so that they could assist other sick persons.

Vincent's work at Châtillon augured the founding of the first Confraternity of Charity in 1617, a parish-based group of laywomen. Following Châtillon, several more confraternities appeared "throughout France—a network of grassroots organizational initiatives that channeled individual good will into effective service of the poor."[9] Hospital work became the central focus of the Paris-based confraternity known as the Ladies of Charity (the "Ladies"). The Paris confraternity, historian Colin Jones noted, "included a future queen, a princess, three duchesses, two baronesses, two countesses, four marquises, and a host of other women from the best robe and sword families."[10] Because many of the Ladies came from the upper classes of French society, including the nobility, they were ill-suited for caring, cooking, and cleaning in the homes and hospitals where most of the sick poor resided. Rather than enter the homes and hospitals of the underclasses, the Ladies often sent their servants to do the work for them. Though largely limited to Paris, this arrangement raised concerns about servants' supervision and training and the quality of care they provided to sick people.[11]

The Daughters, mostly peasant women from rural areas, became the solution to the problem. Chiefly responsible for organizing the Daughters, Louise de Marillac, a widow of noble birth who was under Vincent's spiritual guidance, traveled to several confraternities outside Paris in August 1629 to survey and report on their progress. During her travels, Louise observed that there were many "good country women," as she described them, who were willing to help the Ladies, but they lacked education and discipline. If they were to care for the sick, they would require direction, organization, and training.[12] Known as the "first Daughter," Marguerite Naseau, whom Louise trained and mentored, became the model for other Daughters to follow. Meeting Marguerite in 1629 while on a mission, Vincent observed her overriding "grace" and resourcefulness.[13] Several other young "country women and village girls" soon joined the undertaking.[14]

Vincent, Louise, and the Ladies reached an understanding: The Ladies would provide financial support and social connections while the Daughters would furnish nursing care to poor persons in homes and hospitals. But if the Daughters were to walk in the streets of towns and cities, they had to evade the local bishops. Should the bishops believe the Daughters were a religious order, they would enforce the cloister. Vincent devised a strategy. He advised the Daughters not to use words, phrases, rituals, or behaviors associated with formal religious orders. Rather than call themselves "women religious," he cautioned them to say that they were poor Daughters given to acts of charity; rather than take perpetual vows of poverty, obedience, and chastity, he told them to take vows for one year only, which would allow them to leave when the year was over; rather than reside in convents and wear the habit of cloistered nuns, he counseled them to live in rented rooms and hospitals, and to dress in plain attire.[15] They would have to be above reproach in order to avoid unwanted scrutiny. "It is most important for you to be more virtuous than religious," Vincent told them.[16]

The burden fell on Louise to impose discipline. "Holy obedience [will] regulate all our desires and actions," she instructed her first group of Daughters.[17] Though stern, Louise was practical. In her own life, she followed a tight regimen that included, among other things, time for prayer, time for meditation, time for meals, and time for devotions.[18] Such routines, and many others, would appear in the rules (the "Rule")[19] that Vincent, Louise, and their successors eventually drafted for the Daughters. Before the Rule became official, Louise led by example, instilling the belief that caring for the sick poor took precedence over all other matters.

Louise was adamant that the Daughters account for the poor's belongings. When attending the sick in homes and hospitals, they were to secure all clothing and money, to make a written account or inventory, and to list each item separately.[20] In addition, Louise took Vincent's admonitions concerning living arrangements and attire seriously. The Daughters were to live in simple quarters—in Louise's words, "to choose a lodging suitable for poor girls."[21] Initially, the Daughters wore a simple headdress. Years later, in 1685, they adopted the white-winged cornette.[22]

Though Vincent's precautions and Louise's strict discipline succeeded in avoiding confrontation with the local clergy, the Daughters required formal recognition from church prelates and French authorities if they were to sustain their community into the future. In 1646, Vincent gained support from the archbishop of Paris, Jean-François-Paul de Gondi, to establish the Daughters as a "confraternity."[23] But Gondi's approval did not extend beyond his diocese or jurisdiction. In order to avoid clerical interference in dioceses outside Paris, the Daughters had to find a substitute for the local bishop, a male superior from a religious order, and the pope had to agree to it.[24]

Vincent was reluctant to challenge the bishops, but Louise persuaded him that priests from the Congregation of the Mission, which Vincent founded in 1625, should serve as the Daughters' spiritual advisors.[25] Called Vincentians or Lazarists, members of the Congregation of the Mission established ministries, seminaries, and parishes in France and other countries.[26] On January 18, 1655, with the queen's backing, Cardinal de Retz, Gondi's successor, proclaimed that the Daughters would be subject to "the care and guidance" of the Congregation of the Mission. In 1668, after more legal wrangling, political lobbying, and persuasion, the pope's legate, Cardinal de Vendôme, approved the exemption.[27]

Papal protection afforded the Daughters an uncommon degree of independence.[28] Though the Daughters needed a local bishop's approval to establish a mission in his diocese (something he likely invited them to do in the first place), the bishop lacked the authority to interfere after they entered. This did not prevent him from trying and even occasionally succeeding, but it did make it more difficult for him to enforce his decisions. "When the [mother superior] wanted to say 'no' to a bishop," historians Carol Coburn and Martha Smith have written, "she could ultimately withdraw her sisters from his diocese or use communication with Rome (which took weeks, months, and sometimes years for an answer) as a method to stonewall or ultimately refuse a demanding bishop."[29]

This unique arrangement allowed the Daughters to operate from a central location or "motherhouse" rather than from separate houses or convents in the dioceses they entered.[30] Having a central location fostered coordination and uniformity. From the motherhouse, the mother superior and her provincial council supervised the training of novices, the founding of missions, the selection of "sister servants" who managed particular missions, and the coordination of personnel and other resources. Operating from a central location greatly enhanced the Daughters' mission to the sick poor and suffering throughout succeeding generations.

THE MISSION

Theologically, the central focus of Vincentian ministry is Christological—serving Jesus Christ through the corporal and spiritual care of poor persons. The events at Châtillon-les-Dombes in 1617 established the precedent. "God gave me this thought," Vincent wrote: "Could these good women not be brought together and persuaded to offer themselves to God to serve the sick poor?"[31] Vincent believed that the poor were the focus of Christ's teachings, that by serving the poor, he and his followers were imitating the life of Jesus. Contemplation and prayer were important, Vincent preached, but finding God called for an "active" life. "Leave God for God" was one of Vincent's more notable quotations.[32]

Though the Daughters originally worked for the Ladies, they gradually gained their own identity and started their own missions as their numbers steadily increased under Louise's guidance and direction.[33] In 1633, there were only twelve Daughters; by 1658, there were approximately eight hundred.[34] While healthcare remained their priority, the Daughters also started an orphanage for abandoned children in 1638, a school for poor girls in 1641, and a hospice for the elderly in 1653. In 1640, they began serving galley convicts, taking them food and clothing.[35]

Sending the Daughters to hospitals was not Vincent and Louise's original intention (they preferred the home setting), but hospitals became the "new trend" in the mid-1600s.[36] Hospital administrators from several towns and cities approached the Daughters, seeking their assistance. In 1640, city officials engaged the Daughters to render care at Hôtel-Dieu, the Hospital of Saint-Jean, in Angers. Because the Daughters lacked "juridical status" when they went to Angers (they had yet to become an established entity under church law and civil authority), Louise wrote and signed the contract with the hospital in the capacity of "directress of the Daughters of Charity, Servants of the Sick Poor of the Hospitals and Parishes." The terms of the contract set the precedent for future engagements and provided the framework for the Daughters' Rule, which Vincent and Louise had yet to fashion.[37]

Until the Daughters had their own Rule, they could not gain formal church recognition. "The rule was the community's charter," historian Elizabeth Rapley has written: "Its general statements on poverty, prayer, chastity, humility, obedience, and fraternal correction formed a framework. . . . Every event in the community's life was subject to regulation, from the admission of novices to the burial of the dead."[38] Vincent, however, was reluctant to publish rules and distribute them freely because church prelates associated rules with religious orders. Consequently, the Daughters had no formal Rule in 1640 when they entered the hospital at Angers. Though Vincent and Louise never completed the Rule in their lifetimes (both future saints died in 1660), the contract with the hospital in Angers contained many of the important features. Louise continued to enhance and revise the Rule's provisions, as did Vincent's successors. In 1672, the Rule become official.[39]

The 1672 Rule remained in effect for over three hundred years until the Vatican in 1983 approved a new version. Caring for the sick poor was to be the Daughters' overriding mission. Article 1 of chapter VII of the 1672 Rule was explicit—the Daughters' "principal employment [is] to serve the sick poor," and, in doing so, "they shall acquit themselves . . . with all possible care and attention, considering that it is not so much to them as to Jesus Christ that they render service."[40]

ELIZABETH ANN SETON AND THE SISTERS OF CHARITY OF ST. JOSEPH'S

In addition to the Daughters, several other Catholic communities of active women appeared during the seventeenth and eighteenth centuries. But the French Revolution (1789–1799) suspended further activity. The Catholic Church came under attack, priests and nuns were martyred, and members of several clerical orders—Vincentians, Sulpicians, Jesuits, and others—fled to other countries. In the early 1800s, the political and social turmoil diminished, and the founding of religious communities devoted to charitable work resumed in many places, including the United States, Ireland, and Germany.[41] Elizabeth Ann Seton founded one of them, a new religious community for Catholic sisters in America.

Born in 1774, Elizabeth Seton's father was New York physician Richard Bayley, a Revolutionary War surgeon. At age nineteen, Elizabeth married William Magee Seton. Neither Elizabeth nor William was Catholic. Beginning in 1798, a series of tragedies struck the Seton family—the death of William's father, the bankruptcy of the import business that William managed, and finally William's death in 1803 from tuberculosis, a disease that Elizabeth would also contract and which would plague her for much of her life.[42]

Widowed, destitute, and the mother of five children, Elizabeth Seton sought spiritual guidance. In 1803, she began a correspondence with John Carroll, America's first Catholic bishop and later archbishop. Carroll supported Seton during her time of healing and discernment, leading to her religious conversion. In 1805, she entered the Catholic Church in New York, and in 1808, at the invitation of Father William DuBourg, PSS (DuBourg would later serve as bishop of Louisiana and Florida), Seton and her daughters sailed for Baltimore. Once in Baltimore, Seton took up residence near St. Mary's Seminary, where DuBourg was president, and opened a boarding school for Catholic girls, undertaking their religious instruction.[43]

Learning of the Daughters of Charity from DuBourg, Seton "expressed a fervent wish" to establish a religious community of like-minded women and made a one-year vow to pursue the endeavor.[44] Drawn by her warm personality and religious conviction, a small group of women from New York, Philadelphia, and Baltimore gathered around Seton. Samuel Cooper, a former sea captain who was studying for the priesthood at St. Mary's Seminary in Baltimore when he met Seton, observed her conviction and determination. Hoping to entice Seton and her followers to open a school for poor children in Emmitsburg, Maryland, near Mount St. Mary's Seminary and College, Cooper approached DuBourg with an offer of money. DuBourg favored the enterprise, but others, including Carroll, wanted Seton to remain in Baltimore and continue her teaching. After much thought and contemplation, Seton decided to move to Emmitsburg.[45]

On June 21, 1809, Seton and four of her followers left Baltimore, arriving in Emmitsburg on June 22. A second group led by Rose White, who would become Seton's assistant and successor, joined them several weeks later. Emmitsburg was a promising location for the fledgling community. One year before Seton arrived there, Father John Dubois, PSS (Dubois would later become bishop of the New York diocese), established Mount St. Mary's Seminary. Dubois vacated his cabin at Mount St. Mary's so that Seton's little band of women and children would have a place to stay while repairs were made to a farmhouse on the property purchased for them with Samuel Cooper's money. The repairs completed, the group moved into the farmhouse, which they called the "Stone House," on July 30, 1809. The next day, July 31, 1809, marked the beginning of Seton's community, the Sisters of Charity of St. Joseph's.[46]

DuBourg, Dubois, and many other Catholic priests in Emmitsburg and Baltimore were Sulpicians, the name derived from the seminary of Saint-Sulpice where they originated in Paris. Escaping the turmoil of the French Revolution, the Sulpicians had come to Maryland, established in 1634 as a haven for persecuted Catholics. Though the Sulpicians had recommended that Seton model her community on the French Daughters, there was no Vincentian priest to guide the effort. Carroll appointed DuBourg as Seton's first ecclesiastical superior, but DuBourg resigned soon after, and Father John Baptiste David, PSS, another Sulpician, replaced him. Seton and David were incompatible, however. In 1811, David left for Kentucky, and Dubois, a more suitable match for Seton, became the

Sisters' ecclesiastical superior. A strong proponent of the Daughters' Rule and mission, Dubois helped Seton achieve her objective. Obtaining a copy of the Daughters' Rule and translating it into English, Dubois prepared an American version for the Sisters.[47]

The American Rule that Seton and Dubois fashioned stated that "St. Vincent de Paul" was "their chief patron & founder" and that "their institute is the same as that of the [Daughters]." Seton and Dubois made some minor revisions. One of the modifications recognized the importance of teaching as well as nursing. The American adaptation also clarified the relationship between the Sisters and the Daughters, stating that the Sisters "will have no connexion [Dubois's spelling] whatever with the Company or government of the said [Daughters], or any European country, except that of mutual charity & friendly correspondence."[48] Having fled France during the Revolution because of attacks on Sulpician priests, Dubois feared European entanglements. On January 17, 1812, the Sisters voted in favor of the revised version of the Daughters' Rule, and Bishop Carroll approved it. The Sisters selected Emmitsburg as their motherhouse and made Seton their mother superior.[49]

Because the Sisters were not part of the International Company of Daughters (that would come later), important questions remained about their governing structure and their relationship with the church hierarchy. Clerical interference in the Sisters' internal affairs was a possibility, and Seton sought to dispel it.[50] Carroll's choice of Dubois as their ecclesiastical superior allayed Seton's immediate concerns, but it did not address the larger issue of Sulpician oversight moving forward. Seton wanted assurances from Carroll that Sulpician leaders in France would not interfere in community governance. Carroll did his best to mollify her, writing, "The idea of any other connection than that of charity . . . is abandoned between the daughters and the society of St. Sulpice; I mean that their interests, administration, and government are not to be the same, or at least under the same control. This removes many inconveniences for you and for Messrs. of St. Sulpice."[51]

Such assurances notwithstanding, neither Carroll nor the Sulpicians could fully protect the Sisters. Carroll was the first US bishop; there would be others as America's population and frontier expanded. Under the circumstances, the Sisters' situation remained tenuous until the Vincentians replaced the Sulpicians as their ecclesiastical superiors and they joined the Daughters, who operated with papal approbation.

THE 1850 UNION

The inevitable confrontation between the Sisters and an American bishop occurred in New York City in the late 1840s. New York's presiding bishop was John Joseph Hughes. Born in Ireland in 1797, Hughes had experienced heavy-handed English rule, including restrictions on property ownership, Catholic education, choice of profession, and form of burial. Emigrating with his family to America in 1817, Hughes found work as a gardener at Mount St. Mary's, where he met Elizabeth Seton. With Seton's support, Hughes entered Mount St. Mary's Seminary in 1820 and studied for the priesthood. After his ordination in 1826, he served as a parish priest in Philadelphia, where he gained notice for his stand against anti-Catholicism. Hughes became bishop (and later archbishop) of the New York diocese following the death of John Dubois in 1842.[52]

The Sisters ran an orphanage in New York City before Hughes was appointed bishop. Just as the French Daughters had a central motherhouse that organized their affairs, so did the Sisters, and Hughes did not like it. In a letter dated December 5, 1842, to another bishop, Hughes wrote, "I think the numbers of the Sisters of Charity who are far removed from their centre, the Mother House, would seem to call for a modification in their system."[53] Four more years passed, however, before the decisive confrontation occurred between Hughes and the Sisters. By then, the Sisters were caring for infants and children at three orphanages, four academies, and four parochial schools in the city.[54]

Hughes's rift with the Sisters arose from his efforts to find suitable homes for orphaned children. The Sisters' Rule prohibited them from caring for male children over seven, however, and Hughes wanted them to make an exception.[55] When they refused, Hughes persisted. Unless the Sisters agreed to accept boys, he threatened to form a separate community with himself as their superior.[56] A heated exchange ensued between Hughes and Father Louis Regis Deloul, PSS, the Sisters' ecclesiastical superior. Mother Etienne Hall met with Hughes in order to reconcile the situation, but no resolution was forthcoming. The Sisters serving in New York were given a choice. They could stay and form a separate community with Hughes as their ecclesiastical superior, or they could return to Emmitsburg. Following a month of prayer and contemplation, thirty-three Sisters chose to remain, while twenty-nine Sisters decided to return to Emmitsburg. Those who stayed formed the Sisters of Charity of Saint Vincent de Paul of New York. They elected Sister Mary Angela Hughes, Hughes's sister, as their mother superior. In 1849, the New York community founded St. Vincent's Hospital, the first Catholic hospital in New York City.[57]

Not long after his fiery exchange with Hughes, Deloul initiated an "affiliation" or "union" between the Sisters and the French Daughters. Fearing that other bishops might follow Hughes's lead, Deloul believed that an affiliation with the Daughters would offer pontifical protection. With Mother Hall's concurrence, Deloul contacted the Vincentian superior general in Paris, Father Jean-Baptist Etienne, CM, seeking his support for the undertaking. Etienne responded favorably and in October 1849 dispatched his emissary, Father Mariano Maller, CM, to Emmitsburg to canvass the Sisters. Hearing no objections from those Sisters residing "within two-days' journey" of Emmitsburg (a condition of the Sisters' Rule), Maller recommended the affiliation. At the end of March 1850, the French Daughters agreed to move forward, and on November 1 the union became official when the Sulpicians relinquished their title as "guardians of the Constitutions of the [US] Community" and the Vincentians replaced them.[58] Announcing the decision in a circular letter addressed to the Sisters, Etienne stated, "You are grafted on the tree planted by the Holy Founder." Explaining what he meant by "grafted," Etienne added, "Your union with the Mother House requires that you become Daughters of Charity absolutely."[59]

The union surprised the Sisters working at distant locations, however, including those in Buffalo, New Orleans, Milwaukee, Cincinnati, Detroit, and St. Louis. Because Maller's inquiries had been limited to those located "within two-days' journey" of Emmitsburg, many Sisters had no input. "All was in turmoil" was the report back from Buffalo.[60] Mother Seton would never have approved of this was the outcry from Cincinnati.[61] On March 25, 1852, the Sisters working in Cincinnati established a separate community under the auspices of John Baptist Purcell, the local bishop. They called their community the "Sisters of Charity of Cincinnati."[62] Three other communities that recognized Elizabeth Seton as their foundress also emerged—the Sisters of Charity of St. Vincent de Paul, Halifax, Nova Scotia; the Sisters of Charity of St. Elizabeth, Convent Station, New Jersey; and the Sisters of Charity of Seton Hill, Greensburg, Pennsylvania.

After the 1850 merger between the Sisters and the French Daughters, the motherhouse relocated to Paris, and Emmitsburg became the "Central House" of the newly formed US Province. The Daughter in charge of the Central House in Emmitsburg (as in other provinces) received the title "visitatrix." Her male counterpart, a priest from the Congregation of the Mission, became the "director" of the US Province.[63] Ultimate decision-making authority lodged at the Paris motherhouse, but most decisions affecting the American-based Daughters emanated from Emmitsburg.[64]

While the French Daughters' rules and constitution provided a strong foundation, the American Daughters' trajectory differed from that of their French sisters largely because the United States was different—socially, politically, and economically. Unlike the French Daughters, the American Daughters could own hospitals, giving them important economic and political advantages in a nation that was in its early stages of development. There was no dominant infrastructure in the United States as in France or most other European countries, no established traditions, laws, governments, or institutions to deter their activities. Though prejudice against Catholics and normative constraints on women impeded their efforts, hospital ownership mitigated these barriers. In their dealings with bishops, doctors, and government officials, ownership provided significant leverage. The question was not whether the Daughters could participate in the struggle to shape and define healthcare delivery in America. Rather, the question was how and to what extent they would do so.

CHAPTER OUTLINE

This book chronicles the Daughters' service to America's sick poor from 1823 to 2012, from the year they assumed management of their first hospital, the Baltimore Infirmary, to the year they tendered control of their hospitals to Ascension, a Catholic lay-sponsored entity. During their almost two-hundred-year history in the United States, the Daughters contributed to the making of America's healthcare industry. Their contributions were lasting and substantial. They included innovations in nursing and hospital administration, the founding of several of the nation's first voluntary (private, nonprofit) hospitals, the organization and management of mobile units during wars and epidemics, the promotion of outpatient clinics for the medically indigent, the desegregation of medical staff in Southern hospitals, and the formation of a large hospital network.

Chapters 1, 2, and 3 span the first one hundred years of the Daughters' service. This was a period of population growth and mobility; of immigration from North and Central Europe, particularly Ireland and Germany; of geographic expansion from east to west and north to south; and of emerging communities and institutions (schools, churches, and hospitals) in towns and cities. For the Daughters, this was a period of acclimation and opportunity—acclimation to America's diverse laws, cultures, and conditions, and the opportunity to help shape US healthcare delivery, to foster its growth and development, and to influence its configuration and trajectory.

Chapter 1 shows how the Daughters began their healthcare apostolate, how US law and public policy aided their quest for hospital ownership and autonomy, and how their French heritage in nursing and hospital administration guided their efforts. Chapter 2 examines America's burgeoning political, social, and cultural landscape, with attention to the effects of immigration, epidemics, and anti-Catholicism on the location, funding, and management of the Daughters' hospitals. Finally, chapter 3 explores the Daughters' service in three wars (the Civil War, the Spanish-American War, and World War I), their deployment to US Army encampments, and their organization and management of temporary hospitals for sick and wounded soldiers.

Chapters 4, 5, 6, and 7 cover the Daughters' work in healthcare over the course of the twentieth century. The pivotal event separating the nineteenth from the twentieth century was the discovery of germ theory. After the introduction of germ theory in the late 1800s, hospitals underwent a major transformation from long-term care facilities for chronically ill poor persons to short-term, acute-care facilities for all. For physicians, this was a time of far-reaching success in the treatment of diseases; in the education, training, and certification of medical students and doctors; and in the standardization and accreditation of hospitals. But many of the benefits of medical science did not extend to racial minorities and those in the lower classes. Racial prejudice and lack of funds for the indigent created widespread health disparities.

Several important events occurring in the 1960s—the civil rights movement, the women's rights movement, the enactment of the Medicare and Medicaid programs, and the postconciliar reforms emanating from the Second Vatican Council—altered the traditional social, economic, and religious framework. Freed from ecclesiastical constraints on many of their activities, Catholic sisters became more engaged in the public forum. For those sisterhoods who owned hospitals, the final decades of the twentieth century marked an important shift in focus related to the environmental changes taking place in the 1960s and their rapidly diminishing numbers that such changes precipitated. They turned over local management at many of their hospitals to laypersons in order to conserve dwindling resources; they coordinated their activities at the regional and national levels, forming a large, multihospital system; they assumed leadership positions in professional and political organizations; and they ultimately withdrew from their facilities.

Chapter 4 examines the Daughters' responses to the transformation of healthcare delivery following the discovery of germ theory, from the shift to acute-care hospitals to the organization of the medical profession and hospital associations. Chapter 5 covers the Daughters' emergence as policy entrepreneurs and the reforms they fostered in the healthcare industry during a period of significant social and economic turmoil in the 1960s, 1970s, and 1980s. Chapter 6 reviews the Daughters' efforts in the 1990s to expand access to care for poor persons against the backdrop of religious and political tensions over the availability of reproductive services (contraception, sterilization, and abortion). Finally, chapter 7 recounts the end of the Daughters' healthcare ministry, the sale and transfer of their hospitals, and the current state of their US community.

ONE

THE HOSPITAL, A PLACE THEY COULD CALL THEIR OWN

The Daughters' service to America's sick poor was the product of their combined heritage from the Daughters of Charity in France and the Sisters of Charity of St. Joseph's in America. Though the French Daughters commenced the healthcare ministry, the Americans took it to a new and higher level when they established a network of hospitals across the country. This chapter explains how the Sisters and, after 1850, the American Daughters built on their French heritage in nursing and hospital administration to accomplish their objectives, and how US law and public policy supported their endeavors. It also catalogues their pioneering efforts to replace community almshouses, mostly overcrowded facilities where the poor often languished, with more specialized hospitals for the chronically sick, pregnant women, children, and those suffering from mental illness.

FRENCH FORMULATION AND AMERICAN ADAPTATION

The Sisters of Charity of St. Joseph's were the beneficiaries of the Daughters' careful planning and labors. Though the Sisters retained the French Daughters' commitment to serving the sick poor and even expanded it to include mentally ill persons, they made education a "secondary aim" of their undertaking.[1] When Elizabeth Seton died from tuberculosis at age forty-six on January 4, 1821, the Sisters had yet to found and manage any hospitals. Seton's primary interest was teaching, and many today believe that the parish free school she founded, St. Joseph's Academy, on February 2, 1810, launched the parochial school system in America.[2] Soon after her death, the Sisters began their healthcare apostolate when they signed a contract in 1823 to manage the Baltimore Infirmary. Five years later, they founded their first hospital in St. Louis.

The Baltimore Infirmary

The Sisters' first invitation to manage a hospital came in 1822 from the faculty of the Maryland College of Medicine, located in Baltimore. The faculty wanted the Daughters to manage an infirmary they had established as a place for treating patients and instructing medical students. The Sisters' male superior, Father John Dubois, PSS, handled the initial arrangements.[3] "I can hardly express the joy they felt," Dubois wrote in his May 10, 1822, letter accepting the invitation on behalf of the Sisters. "It is truly now that they feel they are true Sisters of Charity."[4]

The Sisters' enthusiasm for the venture did not prevent them from making several demands that Dubois dutifully presented to the infirmary's board of managers. In return for their services, the Sisters required exclusive control over the day-to-day management of the facility, including the ability to hire and fire workers, to supervise patient admissions, and to account for operational expenses. Dubois stressed, moreover, that the Sisters' Rule had to take precedence over all other matters. "They must be at liberty to follow the rules of their institution, which so far from interfering with their duties as nurses of the Sick, will enable them to fulfill them with greater facility," he told the board of managers.[5]

Eager to proceed, the infirmary's doctors and its board of managers offered no resistance. "We will be able to place the whole direction of the institution under the management of the Sisters," the infirmary's chief physician, Granville Pattison, wrote to Mother Rose White on October 11. The "infirmary will be completed and ready for the reception of patients by the 20th of this month," Pattison added. He asked White to send the Sister who would be in charge of the mission "immediately upon the receipt of [this] letter." "Our object in wishing to have her immediately," he wrote, "is to advise with her as to the arrangement of your routine, etc. and likewise to decide what number of Sisters would be required to perform the duties of the establishment."[6]

Though the mission got off to a good start, the Sisters soon faced difficulties controlling the medical students who lived at the infirmary. The students stayed out long after the infirmary's ten o'clock curfew. Because the sister superior kept the key to the front door in her room, they often banged on the door in the middle of the night, waking the patients and the Sisters. In his January 1824 letter to the board of managers, Dubois questioned the need for the students' "services." "The Sisters can easily . . . do everything the young men have to do—dressing wounds, bleeding, administering medicines . . . ," he asserted. Emphasizing his point, Dubois further wrote that "in Europe, our Sisters have no young students to do that."[7] Dubois's reference to "our [European] Sisters," coupled with the parallel provisions in the French and US management contracts, indicated that even though it was several years before the 1850 union, the Sisters closely patterned their Baltimore undertaking on that of the French Daughters.

While the difficulties with the medical students eventually subsided, other problems occasionally surfaced to test the terms of the agreement. Still, the Sisters and later the Daughters persevered, remaining at the infirmary until 1879, when they left after "repeated difficulties." In 1880, another Catholic community, the Sisters of Mercy, took charge of the facility, staying nine years. Before the Sisters of Mercy came to America in 1848, the Sisters of Charity of St. Joseph's were the only sizeable community of Catholic women with experience in hospital administration.[8]

Mullanphy Hospital, St. Louis

The Sisters' hospital in St. Louis was their second undertaking. The person who invited the Sisters to St. Louis was Bishop Joseph Rosati, CM. Rosati had trained at an Italian seminary under the auspices of the Congregation of the Mission. Upon completing his studies, Rosati entered the priesthood in 1811. Following missionary work among the rural poor near Naples, Italy, he joined the inaugural group of Vincentians traveling to North America. Reaching Baltimore on July 26, 1816, Rosati and the others in his party made their way inland to Ohio, Indiana, and Kentucky, performing missionary work among Native Americans and frontier settlers. On October 2, 1818, Rosati arrived in the Barrens settlement (today's Perryville, Missouri), where he took charge of building St. Mary's Seminary, the house of the Congregation of the Mission in North America. On October 15, 1820, Rosati became superior of the American Vincentians, and on March 20, 1827, less than twenty months before the Sisters' arrival, Pope Gregory XVI appointed him the first bishop of St. Louis.[9]

The main impetus behind the St. Louis hospital was John Mullanphy, a local businessman and philanthropist who made his money trading in cotton and real estate. A devout Catholic, Mullanphy donated land and money for the hospital and other charitable ventures, including convents, a church, and an orphanage.[10] Mullanphy believed, as did Rosati, that the project could not succeed unless the Sisters were willing to take charge of the hospital. On June 23, 1828, Rosati wrote to Father Simon Bruté, PSS, a teacher at Mount St. Mary's College in Emmitsburg, asking him to persuade the Sisters to undertake the long journey.[11] "If we do not get the Sisters of Emmitsburg," Rosati told Bruté, "this establishment will fail, for I see too many difficulties to obtain any from France, and those of Kentucky [referring to another sisterhood] do not understand hospitals."[12]

Rosati's invitation was persuasive, but before embarking for St. Louis, the Sisters insisted that they have complete charge of the new hospital with the right to hire and fire staff, and to oversee patient care. These terms were almost identical to those at the Baltimore Infirmary. Rosati was eager to accommodate them. "Mr. Mullanphy has made over everything to me and I have given *carte blanche* to the Sisters," he told Mother Augustine Decount. "They will have the advantage of not being under any control than that of the Bishop of St. Louis, who will never be in the way of their doing what they think proper conformably to their customs and their rules," he stated.[13]

The Sisters' mission to St. Louis began with a perilous journey. On October 15, 1828, the Sister in charge of the venture, Francis Xavier Love, and three others departed Emmitsburg. After spending their first night in Frederick Town, Maryland, they made their way over the Allegheny Mountains, down the Ohio River, and across Indiana and Illinois to St. Louis, taking three weeks to reach their destination. Sister Xavier's letters to Decount described in great detail the risks, challenges, and experiences the Sisters faced on their long journey—the dangerous route by stagecoach through the Allegheny Mountains, the cumbersome travel by boat on the Ohio River, the querulous traveling companions who questioned their religion, the poor persons who lived in the wilderness in ramshackle cabins, and the black slaves "chained together, half-naked, shivering with cold,—men, women, and children."[14]

When the Sisters arrived in St. Louis, there was no one to greet them. Rosati was in New Orleans, and the hospital they had been promised was not ready. In a letter to Decount, Rosati regretted that "I was not in St. Louis at the arrival of our good Sisters." By way of explanation, he wrote, "Until there be a Bishop in New Orleans, I shall have very little time to reside in St. Louis or any other place, being continuously traveling."[15] As bishop of St. Louis and leader of North America's Vincentian community, Rosati had much to do and few to help him. Numerous towns and settlements appeared along the Mississippi River and its tributaries in the 1820s, and Rosati attempted to visit them, find suitable priests, and raise money for the building of new churches.[16] In addition, he covered the diocese of New Orleans as well as St. Louis when the Sisters made their journey. The former bishop of New Orleans had resigned in 1826, and a new one had yet to be appointed.

A small log cabin, built with Mullanphy's money, served as the original St. Louis hospital. The log cabin comprised three rooms, including a kitchen

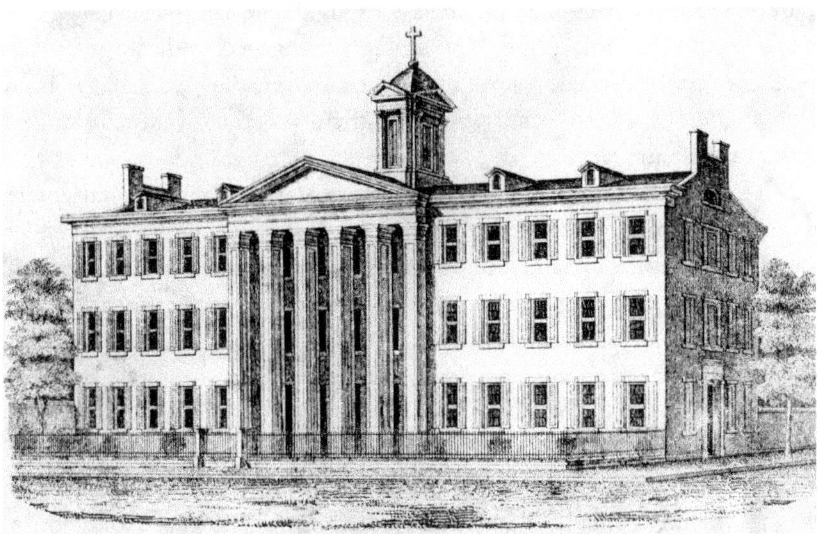

Figure 1.1. Mullanphy Hospital (later DePaul Hospital), 1832.

where the Sisters lived and slept. Four more Sisters arrived in 1831. In late September 1832, the Sisters moved into a larger structure, a three-story brick building near the log cabin, which the Sisters named Mullanphy Hospital.[17] At the end of October 1832, only one month after they opened the new facility, a cholera epidemic swept St. Louis. Cholera-stricken patients flocked to the old log cabin and the new brick building. By the end of November, the epidemic had abated. Honoring the Sisters for opening their hospital to all cholera patients, Mayor William Carr Lane designated Mullanphy Hospital the "official City Hospital of St. Louis." Until the city constructed its own hospital in 1846, the Sisters' hospital served the city's entire population.[18]

CONTRACT MANAGEMENT OR CORPORATE OWNERSHIP

The Daughters' early experiences in hospital administration illustrate some of the differences between contract management and corporate ownership. In the case of the Baltimore Infirmary, the Sisters entered into a contract with the infirmary's board of managers. As managers but not owners, the Sisters experienced problems with the infirmary's medical students, apparently an unruly group prone to staying out past curfew. Based on Father Dubois's January 1824 letter, there is a strong likelihood that, had the Sisters owned the infirmary, they would not have engaged medical students to perform certain procedures. As owners, moreover, they would have been able to directly address the "repeated difficulties" that eventually caused them to leave the facility.

The French Daughters had a long history of working in hospitals under a formal contract. In 1640, city officials engaged the Daughters to render care at the Hospital of Saint-Jean in Angers, the Daughters' first French hospital. Because the Daughters lacked "juridical status" at the time (they had yet to become an established entity under church and civil authority), Louise de Marillac wrote and signed the contract with the hospital's board of directors. Before the start of the French Revolution in 1789, hospital boards typically comprised the local elite—prosperous merchants, municipal officials, members of the nobility, and the local clergy. Their chief responsibility was the facility's financial stability. According to historian Colin Jones, "They sanctioned expenditures, made bulk purchases of supplies, invested donations and benefactions, drew legal contracts, passed leases, conserved the hospital's archives, drew up the annual accounts, introduced hospital rules and regulations, and so on."[19]

Hospital boards from small towns and large cities eagerly sought the Daughters' services following their initial engagement in Angers. At the time of the French Revolution, the Daughters had contracts with almost two hundred hospitals.[20] Their widespread appeal gave them significant leverage in contract negotiations. They had the right to fire and hire staff, to manage the hospital's daily affairs, and to refuse to work "alongside other domestics or members of other communities."[21] Most contracts, moreover, prohibited the admission or care of "any fee-paying" or "rich persons," gave the Daughters control over hospital pharmacies and dispensaries, and allowed them to run schools for poor girls within the hospital setting. In addition, they could negotiate the cost of their services, including wages, food, accommodations, pensions, and funeral expenses.[22]

While the Daughters continued to run hospitals once the worst excesses of the French Revolution receded (their services were too important and there were no viable alternatives), the political changes arising from the revolution and Napoleon Bonaparte's succession demonstrated the fragility of hospital contracts. The new regime replaced the hospital boards with "hospital commissions" comprising handpicked government officials who curtailed some of the Daughters' administrative authority, including the ability to hire and fire workers.[23] This was the state of affairs when the Sisters took charge of the Baltimore Infirmary.

From the beginning, the Sisters exercised greater control over Mullanphy Hospital than the Baltimore Infirmary. Though Mullanphy conveyed the land for the hospital to Rosati, the bishop treated the hospital as if the Sisters owned it.[24] Still, the Sisters' legal claim to the hospital was tenuous until the Missouri legislature, by an act of January 25, 1843, issued a corporate charter to "the St. Louis Hospital Association," which was under the sole auspices of the Sisters.[25] On February 20, 1843, the Sisters executed bylaws making the "Superior of the Hospital . . . the President of the 'St. Louis Hospital Association,' with full power to make what arrangements or contracts she may see proper, for the reception of patients, either Sick or Insane, sent by their friends or by the Public Authorities, either of the City or County of St. Louis."[26]

Private incorporation of hospitals, including those the Sisters and later the Daughters founded, was trailblazing. The opportunity for mapping the future course of healthcare delivery not only in St. Louis but across the United States was palpable. The Sisters could transact business on equal terms with men, resist outside interference, promote their own identity, and govern their hospitals' internal affairs, all with the government's help and approval. Such leeway and authority were unimaginable in France and many other European countries. The source of this leeway and authority was US jurisprudence.

THE PROTECTION OF PRIVATE PROPERTY: *DARTMOUTH COLLEGE V. WOODWARD* (1819)

In colonial America, the corporate landscape was unsettled. Granting corporate charters to certain groups or associations smacked of privilege, akin to the issuance of a royal charter from the king of France or England. Opposition to the incorporation of churches was particularly intense in the State of Virginia, where the Anglican Church had received a corporate charter. Once the United States achieved independence from England, Virginia refused to acknowledge the church's existence and proceeded to confiscate some of its property. Virginia's resistance to religious incorporation did not stop with the Anglican (renamed Episcopal) Church, however. It spilled over to the Catholic Church in Richmond when Virginia's courts denied a bequest to the church from one of its deceased members on the grounds that it lacked corporate status.[27]

Most states did not follow Virginia. South Carolina, New York, New Jersey, Delaware, and Pennsylvania passed laws in the late 1700s giving churches the authority to incorporate. In 1816, the Maryland legislature issued a corporate charter to the "Sisters of Charity of St. Joseph" for the purpose of promoting "works of piety, charity and usefulness, and especially for the care of the sick, the succor of aged, infirm, and necessitous persons, and the education of young females."[28] Maryland's grant of a corporate charter to the Sisters was conditional, as were many corporate charters that state legislatures provided. The legislature could seek to revoke or alter the charter at some point in the future if the Sisters failed to implement the agreement in the manner that the state desired. During the French Revolution, the new regime abolished all corporate charters. Could this happen in America? In 1819, the US Supreme Court answered no in the case of *Trustees of Dartmouth College v. Woodward*.[29] Corporations had perpetual existence and virtual sovereignty over their own affairs, the Supreme Court decided.

The issue the Supreme Court addressed in *Dartmouth College* involved the constitutionality of certain statutory changes that New Hampshire's legislature made to the college's royal charter. In 1816, the state legislature passed several acts replacing the college's president, increasing the number of college trustees from twelve to twenty-one, and establishing a governor-appointed board of overseers with the authority to check the trustees' decisions. Rather than accede to the state's demands, Dartmouth's trustees took legal action and, after losing in the state courts, appealed to the US Supreme Court, where they received a favorable ruling. On February 2, 1819, the Supreme Court held that the statutory changes were unconstitutional, that they violated the Contracts Clause of the US Constitution.

The significance of the case for the Sisters and later the Daughters was the Supreme Court's determination that Dartmouth College was a private institution that, in the words of Chief Justice John Marshall, could "manage [its] own affairs" and "hold property" in perpetuity. That Dartmouth's principal purpose was education did not change the outcome. While "education [was] an object of national concern, and a proper subject of legislation," it was not solely a government function. The ruling encompassed hospitals and other charitable corporations. "Almost all eleemosynary corporations, those which are created for the promotion of religion, of charity or of education, are of the same character. The law of this case is the law of all," the Supreme Court decided.[30]

The Supreme Court's decision in *Dartmouth College* afforded all corporations the freedom to pursue lawful initiatives absent government interference. Yet state legislatures could refuse to grant charters in the first place, a common occurrence. About twenty years after the ruling in *Dartmouth College*, the pattern changed, however. States began to enact general incorporation laws that allowed private entities to incorporate without pursuing special legislative action. By 1860, a majority of states had general incorporation laws for businesses, and by 1875, almost all states had them.[31] For the Daughters, corporate status was very important. As corporate owners of their hospitals, they gained equal standing with men in business transactions. Legal incorporation after *Dartmouth College*, moreover, meant that their hospitals could survive future political turmoil.[32]

The French Daughters were not so fortunate. Lack of an autonomous nonprofit sector in France meant that sweeping political change could alter or terminate their relationship with the hospitals they managed. This is what happened. The regime that emerged during the French Revolution repressed religious congregations and confiscated church property, putting the state in control of health and social welfare. Though the Catholic Church regained some of its former status in the early 1800s and the French Daughters reentered hospitals, the anticlericalism that the revolution fomented made their situation uncertain.[33] In 1870, Catholic sisterhoods administered about one-half of all French hospitals and hospices, but the fall of Napoleon III in the Franco-Prussian War and the reemergence of French secularism put an end to their activities.[34] Between 1880 and 1905, the French parliament passed a series of laws that hampered the role of Catholic sisterhoods in French schools and hospitals.[35] The 1901 Law on Associations was particularly constraining. Under the 1901 act, all "religious congregations," including religious hospitals, had to apply for legal status, "a rather long and restrictive procedure," which French economist Edith Archambault notes "was sparingly granted."[36]

The timing of the US Supreme Court's decision in *Dartmouth College* was auspicious. Because the decision came only a few decades after the country's founding and just a few years before the opening of their St. Louis hospital, the Sisters were among the first to exploit the opportunity that *Dartmouth College* gave them, to carve out a niche for Catholic hospitals. Insulated to a great extent from external forces, their hospitals were able to withstand anti-Catholic prejudice, social hostility, and political conflict. As law professor Mark McGarvie has argued, "The real importance of the *Dartmouth College* case [was] not simply the delineation of private and public, but the perpetuation of the alternative visions of American society by the legal recognition of public and private spheres."[37]

The Supreme Court's holding that corporations had perpetual existence, that they had "immortality," even "individuality," empowered those who founded them. "As government got out of the business of [supervision]," law professor Liam O'Melinn indicated, "it handed that business over to corporate management. The law had turned the corporation into a polity with power over its own affairs."[38] Free to manage all aspects of patient care, the Sisters assumed control of nursing, staffing, and the selection and oversight of physicians. They did not have to give medical students access to their facilities; they did not have to answer to a male-dominated board of directors; and they did not have to provide hospital privileges to doctors who disagreed with their practices. As corporate owners, moreover, the Sisters could use, manage, construct, and decorate their hospitals as they desired, consistent with their rules, beliefs, and values. They could live in them; they could adorn them with statues of saints and crosses; they could incorporate chapels; they could decorate rooms, wards, and hallways with religious symbols; and they could wear their religious attire.[39]

From the founding of the community in Emmitsburg, Maryland, in 1809 to the end of the Civil War in 1865, the Sisters and then the Daughters established fourteen general hospitals that they owned outright and entered into contracts with four others.[40] Clearly, corporate ownership became their modus operandi.

THE FRENCH NURSING HERITAGE

Though hospital ownership provided many benefits, it also presented several new challenges. The Sisters had to raise funds and manage finances, secure expert medical care, obtain food and supplies, and arrange for their own accommodations. Efforts to raise money were particularly difficult because there were few wealthy Catholics in America in the early 1800s, and most Protestants lacked sympathy for struggling Irish immigrants. Philanthropic donations of property or money typically brought the Sisters to a particular town or city, such as St. Louis, but finding the resources to keep their hospitals going once they had started was a continuing problem. There were few organizations of Catholic women in America in the early to mid-1800s. Most Catholic hospitals had no endowment and little if any government backing. The Sisters typically had to fend for themselves when they entered a new community. Bishops who had enticed them to come usually provided some help, but many were short of funds to sustain their operations. Poor and desperate, they often had to beg for money to purchase food, clothing, furniture, and medical supplies.[41]

The Sisters' French nursing heritage provided a foundation for overcoming some of these challenges. There were rules (adherence to the "vows" of poverty, chastity, obedience, and service to the sick poor and to the "virtues" of humility, simplicity, and charity) and daily regimens (specific times for rising, praying, attending Mass, eating, working, reflecting, listening, conversing, and recreating) that each member of the community had to follow. There was also the motherhouse model, which offered a central location for the training of novices, the supervision of missions, and the dispersal of resources. In addition, there was the French Daughters' governing framework, which promoted uniformity, obedience, discipline, and the flexibility needed to adapt to disparate conditions.[42]

The French Daughters' Rule comprised *Common Rules*, which addressed general items, and *Particular Rules*, which addressed specific matters.[43] In the case of hospitals such as the one at Angers, the *Particular Rules* provided a blueprint for institutional administration. The blueprint established boundaries and protocols for doctors, nurses, and administrators; ordered relationships between Daughters and patients; fixed daily routines and caregiving activities; and included certain technical skills in the handling of diseases.[44] In addition, the French Daughters prepared principles or "instructions" for the care of the sick poor, which the Sisters adopted and inserted into a handwritten, pocket-sized booklet they carried with them.[45] The first part of the booklet was a French translation, while the second part was an addendum that Sister Mary Xavier Clark authored.[46] Clark served in Emmitsburg as "mistress of novices" from 1818 to 1829 and from 1845 to 1855.[47]

Clark completed her part of the booklet on or about October 26, 1846, almost four years prior to the union between the Sisters and the Daughters. Titled "Instruction on the Care of the Sick," the booklet contained seventeen points, most of them concerning nursing practice in the hospital setting. "Never speak in a loud tone of voice to [the] poor sick," Clark admonished. "A few words said in a mild but firm tone . . . will do a great deal more good," she instructed. "The countenance of a Sister whilst waiting on the poor sick should be mild but grave; and each word should be accompanied with prudence and piety." Clark made her novices responsible for knowing "what quality and quantity of nourishment they ought to give to each patient," for properly "preparing" and "cooking" the food, and for fixing the patient's "bed and pillows." She also held them accountable for preparing the "remedies" or medications "prescribed by the physician"; for knowing "the weights, measures, and the signs which . . . physicians . . . use in writing their prescriptions"; for making sure that "the ingredients" were "mixed" in "very clean" and proper "vessels"; and for seeing that the "remedies" were administered in a timely fashion.[48]

The belief that the sick poor should receive equal treatment was important to the French Daughters. In keeping with their tradition, Clark commanded that charity "be extended to all. . . . It should never be because we like this one more than that one." Seeking to protect her fellow Sisters from accusations that they treated Catholics better than Protestants, charges that Protestant ministers were making against them, Clark wrote that "the Sister must be very prudent." Upon learning that a patient is Protestant, she "should say nothing more, but give him all the temporal assistance he needs, [and] must not say a word about the [C]atholic religion because some of these poor creatures are very bitter against our holy religion." In order to avoid blame for the shoddy work and unequal treatment of caregivers outside the community, Clark admonished the Sisters "not [to] depend" on others. "Such persons," she claimed, "love money more than conscience, and have always their favorites; they would without scruple, give the best of everything to those they like, and neglect the others."[49]

Clark's seventeen points provided few substantive additions to the manner of treating sick patients in Europe since the 1600s.[50] Imparting technical knowledge was not her intention. As mistress of novices, Clark sought to inculcate certain basic principles. She left the details of patient care to "sister servants," the designation given to those who led a particular mission.[51] Sister servants' responsibilities were wide-ranging; the trust placed in them by the community was considerable. Sister servants "will see that everything in the [hospital] wards is in the best order, neat & clean," Clark instructed. "When a Sister is first entrusted with the care of the wards . . . she should consult her Sr. Servant about everything, and never think that she herself is experienced enough, & has sufficient judgment to guide herself."[52] But there was much more that sister servants had to do than provide good nursing skills and see that hospital wards were neat and tidy. Those who succeeded, those who stood out, possessed the combined skills and talents of good administrators, fundraisers, mentors, caregivers, entrepreneurs, and social workers.

Matilda Coskery, DC, was the prototypical sister servant. Remarking on Coskery's death in 1870, Mother Euphemia Blenkinsop, DC, wrote that "there was about her an irresistible charm, which gained the affection and commanded the esteem of all who had intercourse with her." "Her kind and compassionate heart," Blenkinsop related, "would find a balm to soothe, if not to heal, the crushed and wounded spirit." When it came to the care of sick patients, Coskery had few equals. "She was looked upon as an oracle. Physicians consulted her about their patients as if she were an old professor." Those assigned to her felt protected. "She watched over her young Sisters with the solicitude of a mother, never giving them offices that would expose them to danger, treating all with that cordiality, sincerity and affection." Not only Catholics, but also Protestants, praised her abilities. "Many influential Protestants had recourse to her in their troubles with unbounded confidence and regarded her, as one of the most extraordinary persons they had ever known," Blenkinsop stated.[53]

Sometime in the late 1840s (the actual date is unknown), Coskery produced a seventy-six-page tract titled *Advices Concerning the Sick*.[54] *Advices* appears to have been compiled for at least three reasons: first as an instructional manual for new nurses, second as a resource for sister servants who rotated assignments, and third as a polemic for the humane treatment of the mentally ill. The compassionate treatment of "insane persons" was Coskery's central purpose. She advocated the curative power of "moral therapy." First implemented by the French Daughters at Les Petites Maisons in Paris in the early 1600s, refined by French doctors in the late 1700s, and promoted by American physicians in the early to mid-1800s, moral therapy emphasized "kindness to patients," a "homelike" environment, and "meaningful activity."[55] To Coskery, "kindness" stood out. "*Kindness* is the *main remedy*, because this method treats them as if they were *sane*," she wrote in *Advices* (emphasis in original). "This excites to self-respect, for the poor patient feels there is something wrong with him, but seeing he is treated like others . . . he begins to think he is not out of his mind, or that if he has been so, he must be better now, since he is considered & respected like others."[56]

Most of what Coskery wrote in *Advices* applied to the hospital setting, where nurses and doctors had to work together if patients were to recover.[57] Questions concerning who did what, when, and how typically arose in hospitals, not in homes, dispensaries, or doctors' offices. Physicians had a big advantage when it came to dealing with nurses in most US hospitals. They were often males from the middle and upper classes, and they vehemently resisted encroachments on their turf and status. Disorganized female nurses from the middle and lower classes could not easily confront organized groups of doctors.[58] The Daughters,[59] on the other hand, presented a united front when conflicts occurred with physicians over task performance. They had certain rules, procedures, and standards they followed, many of them inherited from their French sisters.[60] They were not hired nurses, moreover; they were nurse managers. Much of their work took place in hospitals they owned or managed. If physicians wanted to treat patients in their hospitals, they needed their permission. Under the circumstances, the Daughters exercised significant leverage in their dealings with doctors.[61]

There were several tasks or areas the Daughters claimed for nursing. These included patient admissions, recordkeeping, and planning.[62] The nurses' duties in these areas largely stemmed from their managerial authority. Coskery provided several examples. She wrote that it was the nurse's responsibility to take the patient's history upon admission, to make sure that beds were available "so that the poor sick may not be kept waiting," to examine and clean the patient's mouth to prevent the transmission of diseases, to establish "a particular plan of treatment" for each patient, to move a patient to another room if their illness was long-lasting, and to prevent a patient from "relapsing" during recovery.[63]

Notably, Coskery called for the Daughters to intercede when physicians' methods seemed extreme or counterproductive. Though nurses should follow doctors' orders in most instances, there were some exceptions. When the doctor was unavailable, "*experienced*" nurses could "withhold medicines" when they "observe[d] acts contrary to the designs or wishes of the [physician]," Coskery stated (emphasis in original).[64] And when a patient responded adversely to a "remedy" the doctor ordered, nurses could "suspend" or moderate "the medicine" to avoid serious "injury."[65] Coskery did not maintain that the Daughters were medical practitioners. But she did view them as sophisticated caregivers who exercised independent judgment. She characterized the Daughters' responsibilities in terms of their duties as nurses. They had a "duty" to do whatever they could to heal the sick poor who entered their hospitals, she contended.

Coskery's view of a nurse's "duty" when applied to the hospital setting was far more expansive than what courts, or most anyone else for that matter, contemplated in the mid-1800s.[66] As indicated in *Advices*, nurses had responsibilities to patients separate and apart from physicians. These were in the nature of professional responsibilities, not ordinary caregiving activities such as cleaning or washing patients. "The office of 'Nurse' is one of awful responsibility if its duties be properly considered," Coskery wrote in *Advices*.[67] "Life and Death is [in] the hands of the nurses, more than in the Physicians," she asserted.[68]

Clearly, Coskery's nurses were not "physicians' servants," nor were they in any way comparable to the typical nurse hired in the mid-1800s to care for patients in homes or hospitals. Coskery's concept of duty applied to a professional nurse, one with sophisticated skills derived from years of experience and training. Because the Daughters possessed professional nursing skills and bore a strong duty to their patients, they typically refused to work beside other nurses in hospitals they owned or managed.

FROM ALMSHOUSES TO HOSPITALS AND MORE SPECIALIZED FACILITIES

For much of the nineteenth century, the city or county almshouse was one of the few places available for the sick poor who had no one to care for them. Most Americans did not believe that the "worthy" poor, that is, hardworking individuals, should enter almshouses. Almshouses, they claimed, were for the "unworthy" poor, the incorrigible, the drunk, and the lazy. Those with means, any means at all, stayed at home rather than suffer the scorn that came from being an almshouse "inmate." In the words of medical historian Charles Rosenberg, "Admission to an almshouse ward—even for unavoidable illness or injury—was a confession of failure."[69] Many private hospitals, medical dispensaries, or ladies' benevolent societies did not want to care for such individuals.[70]

In addition to the stigma attached to them, almshouses combined several different types or classes of persons in a single location—dependent women and children, the elderly, the chronically ill, the mentally insane, and the sick poor. As a result, many almshouses were dreadfully overcrowded. Referring to Philadelphia's almshouse in a speech he gave in 1873, psychiatrist Isaac Ray noted that at certain times of the year approximately 3,600 to 4,000 persons occupied the building. Such people, Ray said, "constitute one seething mass of infirmity, disease, vice and insanity."[71] Diseases, such as dysentery and typhoid, were prevalent. Epidemics, such as cholera and yellow fever, killed many almshouse inmates.

Pursuing their goal of caring for the sick poor, the Daughters founded hospitals and other institutions that were a big improvement over almshouses. Their hospitals had trained and experienced women, unlike most almshouses in which so-called nurses (anyone could be a nurse) were often uneducated males or other inmates. Their hospitals had experienced nurse managers, unlike almshouses in which male superintendents (and their matron wives) with no clinical training ran the facility. And their hospitals were clean and orderly, unlike almshouses, which typically were dirty and unruly.[72] The Sisters' work in Philadelphia and other cities before 1850 and then the Daughters' work in Buffalo and other cities after 1850 exemplified the transition from almshouses to hospitals and more specialized facilities.

Philadelphia, 1832 to 1833

In early 1832, Americans closely followed the advance of the cholera epidemic that was sweeping Europe. US newspapers published accounts from France, England, and Ireland on a daily basis.[73] A ship arriving in Quebec on June 8, 1832, with 133 Irish emigrants on board may have been the first to bring cholera to North America. Within days of reaching Quebec, several newspapers alerted the public. "It has become our painful duty," one such newspaper imparted, "to announce that this dreadful scourge of Asia and of Europe, has at length reached the shores of America, and is now raging at Quebec and Montreal."[74] Making its way from Canada, cholera traveled in boats along the St. Lawrence River, reaching Vermont and upstate New York around June 11. After arriving in New York City on June 26, the disease spread up and down the Atlantic seaboard, striking Philadelphia on July 5, Baltimore on August 4, Boston on August 5, and Charleston, South Carolina, in late October.[75] Fear turned to panic. Almost half of New York City's population, or about one hundred thousand people, fled, many by way of Cornelius Vanderbilt's steamboats.[76] For those who stayed behind, abandonment was a strong possibility.

When cholera struck Philadelphia, the Sisters had recently begun their healthcare apostolate—serving the sick poor at the Baltimore Infirmary and the hospital they founded in St. Louis. Though relatively new to nursing, the Sisters were rapidly gaining administrative and organizational experience, not only in hospitals but also in orphanages. When the first cholera cases appeared in Philadelphia in early July 1832, several Sisters were in the city running two orphanages. At Elizabeth Seton's direction, Sister Rose White and two other Sisters left Emmitsburg for Philadelphia in September

1814. They traveled by land because the British fleet occupied the Chesapeake Bay; Father William DuBourg, PSS, their male superior, was with them for the first part of the journey. Upon reaching Philadelphia, the Sisters took control of an asylum established to care for the children of Catholic parents who had died in the 1797 yellow fever epidemic. They soon put things in order, retired the debt in three years, and increased the number of children. By 1832, the Sisters were in charge of not one but two Philadelphia orphanages—St. Joseph's with over forty children and St. John's with about twenty-five.[77]

The second-largest city in the United States after New York City, Philadelphia was the center of American medicine at the time of the cholera outbreak. Philadelphia housed the nation's first medical school and its first medical society, the College of Physicians of Philadelphia. Benjamin Rush, a signer of the Declaration of Independence and George Washington's surgeon general, was a founding member of the college. Students came from all over to attend Rush's lectures.[78] In the field of public health, Philadelphia was the country's leader. Its water system, known as the Fair Mount Water Works and designed by Benjamin Latrobe, supplied water of unusually good quality.[79] Philadelphia's board of health and its sanitary commission had good reputations.[80]

Opened in 1732, Philadelphia General Hospital was the city's almshouse.[81] Located just to the north of the African American and Irish neighborhoods, the almshouse contained a large number of foreign-born immigrants, almost one-half of the resident population. Many of the residents suffered from chronic disorders or disabilities, making them unfit for gainful employment. Discipline could be harsh. Those who failed to work or disobeyed the rules were confined to a cell or given smaller food rations.[82] Nurses were hard to find. The work was unpleasant and required little skill; the conditions were grim, and some of the inmates were violent. According to one assessment, "hundreds lived in overcrowded, ill-ventilated quarters, and shared contaminated latrines. . . . Unbelievable misery, reminiscent of 'the dark period of nursing,' existed in the Philadelphia almshouse and hospital."[83]

After the first cases of cholera appeared in early July, they rapidly increased in number. By August, more than one hundred cases were reported daily, the majority of them in the African American and Irish communities.[84] Philadelphia's doctors attributed the high rate of cholera cases on the south side to poverty and weak morals. In truth, the larger number of cases on the south side was because the residents got their water from wells, many of them contaminated from privies. Those living in more affluent districts on the north side of the city got their drinking water from the Fair Mount Water Works.[85]

Doctors and nurses at Philadelphia General Hospital were woefully unprepared for the cholera epidemic. Large numbers of poor people, with no one to care for them, inundated the facility. Frightened and overworked, the nurses demanded an increase in their wages to stay and attend to the patients. After the board of directors met their demands, many still left the hospital. "The few good nurses were broken down by loss of rest and by fatigue, and the remainder abandoned the sick from fear of disease or resorted to intoxication," the hospital's superintendent reported.[86]

Desperate, the hospital board asked Philadelphia's Bishop Francis Kenrick in early August to approach the Sisters. On August 9, Kenrick dispatched a letter to Emmitsburg.[87] Soon after receiving the letter, the motherhouse sent thirteen Sisters—eight from Emmitsburg and five from St. Joseph's orphanage. Most of them went to Philadelphia General Hospital, while others worked at nearby locations.[88] When the eight Sisters arrived from Emmitsburg, the disease was raging, the number of sick persons staggering. At St. Augustine's Catholic Church, which had opened its doors to accommodate the sick, two Sisters ministered to 370 patients.[89] Between August 18 and August 24, there were 358 new cases and 85 deaths from cholera in Philadelphia. By early September, the epidemic was almost over.[90] Remarkably, none of the Sisters died from the disease in Philadelphia, though two passed away while nursing cholera patients in Baltimore.[91]

The Sisters received much praise for their work during the cholera epidemic. A grateful board of directors at Philadelphia General Hospital lauded their efforts, their "courage" in the face of a deadly disease, their "mode of government," their refusal to accept compensation, and their ability to instill "morals and discipline."[92] The directors expressed "respect and admiration . . . for the conduct of the Sisters. . . . As nurses, their services [were] invaluable."[93] At a ceremony on November 15 to give thanks, city officials sought to present silver plates to each of the Sisters. But the Sisters declined and requested that any money go toward St. Joseph's orphanage.[94]

The Sisters continued to work at Philadelphia General Hospital until May 1833. The board of directors wanted them to stay permanently, but their male superior, Father John Hickey, PSS, refused the offer. In his letter to the board, Hickey alluded to the "rude assaults of such persons as are necessarily in your institution."[95] "I do not consider their longer stay in the Almshouse to be the department of charity in which they can be most usefully employed," he advised the directors.[96] Though the Sisters left the almshouse, they did not abandon Philadelphia. They remained at their orphanages, and in 1859, the Sisters (now Daughters) took charge of St. Joseph's Hospital, which was under the administration of another religious community, the Sisters of St. Joseph. The Daughters stayed at St. Joseph's Hospital for eighty-eight years under a lease agreement with the Philadelphia diocese.[97]

Buffalo, 1848 to 1861

Situated at the juncture of the Erie Canal and the Great Lakes, Buffalo commanded a strategic location for goods passing east and west in the mid-1800s. From a small frontier outpost with only 2,500 people in 1825, Buffalo's population expanded exponentially. In 1847, when many of the immigrants escaping famine in Ireland began to arrive, Buffalo's population was about thirty thousand. By 1860, it exceeded eighty thousand.[98] German and Irish immigrants dominated the new arrivals. The vast majority of the men were unskilled workers who labored in close proximity to the city's waterfront as longshoremen, dockworkers, grain scoopers, and canal diggers. Single Irish women often worked as domestic servants, while married women with children struggled to live on their husbands' meager wages. When men died or abandoned their families, the women and children often ended up in the Erie County Poorhouse. By the late 1840s, foreign-born Irish immigrants had surpassed native-born Americans as a percentage of the poorhouse population.[99] Conditions at the poorhouse were bleak, to say the least. According to one account, "the well, the sick, the mentally retarded, 'lunatics,' and newborn babies were crowded together in small wards."[100]

Austin Flint, a prominent Buffalo physician, tried to address the situation. Calling the death rate at the county poorhouse "without parallel in any similar institution in the country," Flint prevailed on civic leaders to build "a public hospital where the poor who were not yet reduced to indigence could receive timely care."[101] Civic leaders made the attempt, but the effort failed for lack of money. In desperation, Flint turned to Buffalo's presiding bishop, John Timon. Timon implored the Sisters to come to Buffalo and open a hospital.[102] Upon receiving Timon's request, the Emmittsburg motherhouse sent six Sisters. They arrived in Buffalo on June 3, 1848. There was no hospital when they reached Buffalo, but Timon was able to locate and purchase a three-story building near Main Street in the lower Fifth Ward three weeks later. Acting quickly to prepare the building, the Sisters "repair[ed] and convert[ed] the rooms . . . into hospital wards."[103] On October 1, 1848, Sisters of Charity Hospital opened for the admission of patients.

Soon after the hospital opened, another cholera epidemic struck America, killing about one out of every three who contracted it.[104] Many children were left without parents and many mothers without the means to care for their children. Lacking an alternative location for the orphaned children and the destitute mothers with children, the Sisters housed them in a separate unit at their hospital. When a wealthy benefactor donated land to the Catholic Church in 1853 for the construction of an asylum for "widows, . . . foundlings and lying-in women," the Sisters (now Daughters) moved "three frame cottages" from the hospital grounds to the new location, which they named St. Mary's Infant Asylum.[105]

"Poor women and needy children" flocked to St. Mary's, quickly exceeding the scant accommodations.[106] The situation was desperate when Sister Servant Rosaline Brown, DC, arrived from Detroit in 1854 to assume charge of the undertaking.[107] Written accounts reflect that there was much "poverty and hardship." Food and clothing were in short supply.[108] New to Buffalo and without connections, Brown appealed for help in the local newspapers.[109] "The [Daughters] have no revenue—no funds, their good efforts are impeded and contracted by the burden of debt," her notice in the *Buffalo Daily Republic* imparted.[110] Seeking "money, provisions, clothing or anything that would contribute to" the care of the residents, Brown and her companions "traverse[d] the city."[111] By the end of 1857, they had scraped together sufficient funds to begin construction on the donated property. During the new building's construction, Buffalo's business community joined the effort. Fourteen years later, in 1874, the asylum housed 223 "infant orphans and foundlings," 126 patients, and five widows.[112]

With St. Mary's on strong financial footing, Brown turned her attention to the plight of the mentally ill. On one of her "daily excursions" around Buffalo, she "called at" the Erie County Poor House, where she found the "condition in the insane department" to be "truly appalling." As one of the Daughters described it, the residents had been "strapped down to benches or chained to posts or anything to which they could be fastened, and most of them half naked, so that they appeared more like wild animals than anything human."[113] The experience "made a lasting impression" on Brown and her companions. Brown met no resistance from her superiors in Emmitsburg or Bishop John Timon when she proposed to open an institution for mentally ill persons. Timon was forthcoming, finding the money to purchase a twenty-three-acre tract of land on the city's outskirts. By this time, Brown's reputation as a frugal, efficient, and effective administrator and her openness to all denominations had been firmly established. Buffalo's mostly Protestant business community supported the project, lending much of the money and resources to begin construction.[114]

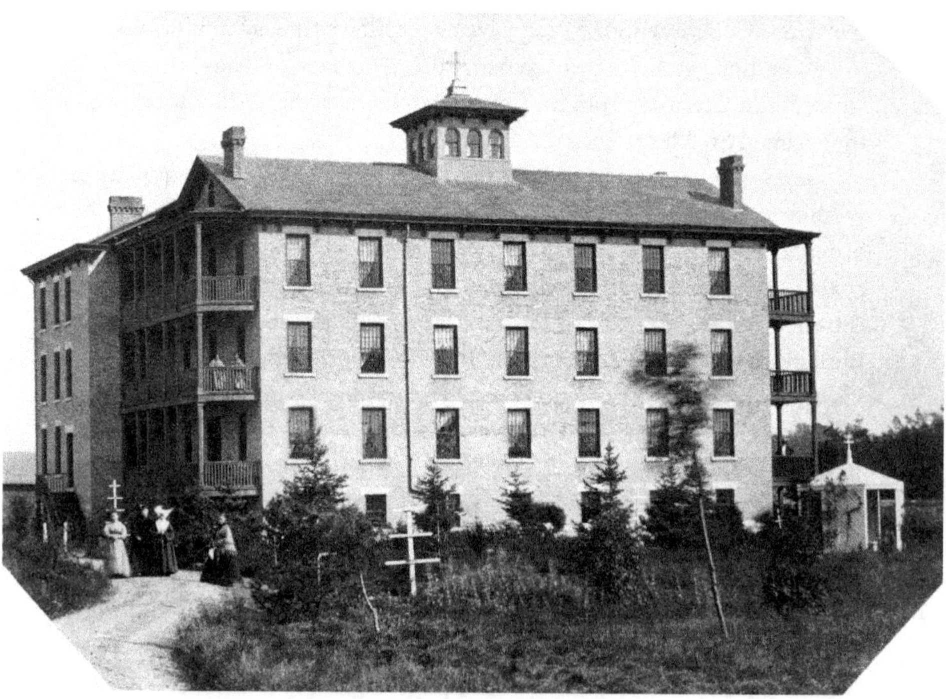

Figure 1.2. Providence Retreat asylum, Buffalo, NY, 1861.

Construction began in October 1860. Though the property was within the city limits, the work was difficult because of its location—"the roads were bad and water had to be carried in hogsheads by horse and wagons from springs almost a mile away to supply the masons who mixed the mortar for the buildings."[115] Yet only one year later, the first part of the asylum was completed, "70×40 feet in extent, and four stories high including the basement."[116] Brown was closely involved in overseeing the building's design and managing its construction. An article appearing in the *Buffalo Courier* noted that "the Institution is being erected under the charge of Sister Rosaline Brown, the present zealous and excellent Superintendent of the Widow and Foundling Asylum." Calling the building's design "ingenious," the *Courier* extolled the comfortable and secure environment that Brown had created.[117]

Providence Retreat, the name of the new facility, admitted its first patients on August 15, 1861. By all accounts, Providence was "well managed." An article in the *Buffalo Medical and Surgical Journal*, written by the attending physician at the asylum, Julius F. Miner, was quite glowing. Miner praised the Daughters' ability to "control . . . even the most violent" inmates. "Often times five or six strong men accompany a patient to the hospital," but when a Daughter is in charge, "kind words, and firm assurances" often suffice, he stated.[118]

The founding of St. Mary's and Providence Retreat were watershed events. Before the Sisters came to Buffalo, poor persons who were too sick to care for themselves, destitute mothers with small children, orphans, and mentally ill persons crowded together in the Erie County Poorhouse. Over the course of thirteen years, from the opening of Sisters of Charity Hospital in 1848 to the construction of Providence Retreat in 1861, the Sisters and then the Daughters established three facilities—a hospital, an infant asylum, and a mental health institution. Many of Buffalo's "unworthy" poor had alternatives. They did not have to languish in degradation and squalor in the Erie County Poorhouse.

TWO

IMMIGRATION, EPIDEMICS, ANTI-CATHOLICISM, AND SLAVERY

From 1820 until the outbreak of the Civil War in 1861, over five million immigrants came to the United States, the majority of them from Ireland and Germany.[1] Ireland accounted for about two million, Germany another 1.5 million. Religious persecution and the blight that destroyed the potato crop in 1846 and 1847 brought Irish immigrants to America's port cities.[2] Mostly poor and unskilled, Irish immigrants usually stayed near places they landed, taking almost any job available. German immigrants, on the other hand, often settled in Midwestern towns and cities such as Milwaukee, Saint Louis, and Cincinnati, where they pursued farming and urban craft trades, including baking and carpentry.[3] A majority of German immigrants were Protestant, but a substantial number, about one-third, were Catholic.[4] Many of the hospitals the Daughters established were in or near sizeable communities of mostly Irish immigrants.

The American Daughters employed traits and assets stemming from their dual heritage to address the needs of the new immigrants. Because there were few nurses who could match them for competent and reliable service before the arrival of other nursing sisterhoods, the Daughters were in high demand. Physicians, civic leaders, and Catholic bishops clamored for their assistance. Requests often came during epidemics, when the situation was most desperate. Epidemic diseases overwhelmed community almshouses, spurring the need for Daughter-owned facilities, particularly in port cities where poor Irish immigrants congregated.

Anti-Catholicism was an important factor prompting the Daughters to establish their own hospitals. Elected politicians threatened to oust the Daughters from public facilities, nativists opposed the use of public funds for Irish immigrants, and Protestants barred priests from community hospitals.[5] Before the 1850s, anti-Catholic bigotry stoked occasional violence. The first major attack against a group of Catholic nuns occurred in August 1834. Incited by rumors that young women were being held against their will, a mob burned a schoolhouse attached to the Ursuline convent in Charlestown, Massachusetts, outside Boston. Almost ten years later, in May 1844, a nativist mob set fire to twenty-nine houses, two churches, and a convent in Philadelphia, killing several people. As the number of Irish immigrants expanded, America's Protestant majority viewed the new arrivals with apprehension. Some members of the Protestant clergy stirred fear and prejudice, proclaiming that the newcomers represented the vanguard of a conquering "Romish" or "Popish" hoard that threatened to destroy American democracy and religious liberty. Secret nativist societies emerged to oppose them. Violent assaults on Catholic churches, schools, homes, and convents escalated.[6]

In addition to immigration, epidemics, and anti-Catholicism, the Daughters confronted local customs and practices concerning the care of Blacks, slave or free, in hospitals and other settings before and after the Civil War. The position of the Catholic Church was often mixed on the matter of slavery in antebellum America.[7] Bishops, priests, and sisterhoods largely adhered to "prevailing societal structures."[8] Some of them owned slaves in areas of the country where slavery was a common practice.[9]

EPIDEMIC DISEASES OF THE NINETEENTH CENTURY

The leading epidemics of the mid-nineteenth century, which many associated with the squalor and bad habits of Irish immigrants, were typhus, cholera, and yellow fever.[10] No one truly knew how epidemics started, if the disease was contagious, or what remedies afforded the best treatment. Large numbers of people became sick all at once, overwhelming family caregivers and physicians. Watching the advance of the disease in neighboring towns and cities, fathers and mothers who had the means to do so often gathered their children and fled the area. The Daughters cared for those left behind in their homes and in their hospitals. In the hardest hit locations, the motherhouse sent reinforcements if they were available. For many sick persons, this was their first encounter with the Daughters. In the course of their work, the Daughters helped to lay the foundation for nursing as an autonomous profession.

Typhus

Typhus or "ship fever," as it was commonly called, killed thousands of immigrants before, during, and after their difficult and lengthy ocean voyage to North America.[11] We know today that body lice carry the type of bacteria that causes typhus. Anywhere from five to fourteen days after being bitten, infected individuals experience severe headaches, muscle aches, high fevers, rashes, and general confusion. The typical treatment is a course of antibiotics. Untreated, the fever can last two weeks; death is a distinct possibility.[12]

Typhus outbreaks among mostly poor Irish immigrants escaping the potato famine in their home country recurred in US port cities from about 1847 to 1851. At the time of the outbreaks, many doctors suspected that typhus was contagious. In an essay on typhus fever, Nathan Smith, a professor at Yale's medical school, stated, "I consider typhus fever a disease *sui generis*, arising from a specific cause, and that cause contagion."[13] Another leading physician, W. W. Gerhard from Blockley Hospital in Philadelphia, refined Smith's observation. While "typhus is clearly a contagious disease," Gerhard asserted, it had strict limits. There has to be close contact with an infected person, he noted.[14] A committee of Maryland's state medical society confirmed Gerhard's observation. The medical society reported that "typhus is never active at [a] great distance from the person from whom it emanates; that it rarely extends its influence many yards or even many feet."[15]

Because typhus's incubation period was five to fourteen days, many passengers were unknowing carriers of the disease before they departed for North America.[16] Health authorities in England, Ireland, and Scotland were aware of the situation but did little to address it.[17] Some newspapers scolded the authorities for their inaction. Considering that "some of the Irish emigrants are in the incipient stage of fever before they embark," a British newspaper admonished, "it would certainly seem more consistent with common sense to ascertain, as far as possible, the state of health of the emigrants before the ship leaves."[18]

The holds of sailing ships making transatlantic voyages, often lasting eight to ten weeks, or longer in bad weather, were ideal locations for lice infestations. A ship's doctor gave a detailed account of the conditions. The typical immigrant vessel, he wrote, carried two to three hundred steerage passengers in "berths" below deck. On both sides of the boat, double rows of "bunks" about "six feet long, three feet wide, and three feet high" extended the entire length. A narrow passageway "about six to nine feet wide" separated the bunks. "Numerous boxes, bags, and mysterious-looking vessels" consisting of "chamber [pots], cooking, and parlor utensils" lined the passageway. The smell was intolerable. "Gases and filthy waters and odors collected in the bottom of the vessel."[19]

Newspapers on both sides of the Atlantic Ocean denounced the overcrowded and filthy passenger quarters. "Several British ships have recently arrived in the Mississippi River with hundreds of poor immigrants on board in a deplorable condition," the *New Orleans Crescent* reported.[20] "Any person who will step into the steerage of a ship with from one to three hundred emigrants huddled together, festering in the damp and fetid atmosphere of the place, will cease to wonder that sickness and death rage," a writer for the *Washington Union* related.[21] "The law says that vessels shall only carry a certain amount of passengers in proportion to their tonnage," but it seems clear that this "salutary provision is violated," an editorial in a Bristol, England, newspaper asserted.[22]

Public health officials in North American port cities often quarantined ships carrying passengers with typhus. After disembarking, health officers took the sick to temporary hospitals in isolated locations such as Quebec's Grosse Isle or New York's Staten Island, or to permanent hospitals with isolation wards, such as New Orleans' Charity Hospital. Such hospitals quickly became overcrowded with typhus patients.[23]

At Charity Hospital, the isolation wards filled beyond their capacity during an 1848 typhus outbreak. The New Orleans *Times-Picayune* reported that on Monday, February 21, "about one-half" of the hospital's 1,037 patients had ship fever. "These were taken from the ships lately arrived from Ireland," the newspaper indicated. Another ninety patients were admitted to the hospital on Tuesday. By Friday, the number of sick people exceeded three thousand. Patients "crowded together in such numbers [that] the beds touch[ed] each other. There [was] no room to pass between the invalids. Many [had] to lie upon the floors," the correspondent for the *Times-Picayune* stated. "The atmosphere in these crowded wards cannot be kept pure," he continued. "The sick of ordinary diseases are exposed to the infection of ship fever, which is confessedly contagious. Two of the Sisters of Charity have already fallen[,] sacrifices to their labors in the cause of humanity."[24]

Baltimore was another port city where the Daughters cared for sick travelers. Boats sailing to Baltimore in 1847 typically anchored at Fells Point, the city's natural deep-water harbor. During the months of April and May 1847, three ships sailing from Liverpool, England—the *Hampden*, the *Richard Anderson*, and the *Rio Grande*—arrived at Fells Point, Maryland. Combined, there were 674 Irish immigrants on the three vessels.[25] "Feeble and weak from a want of food at home, their situation has been rendered worse by the confinement of their passage," the *Baltimore Sun* reported.[26] The third ship to reach the harbor, the *Rio Grande*, carried the sickest of the immigrants. "Deemed in too foul a condition to be allowed to come into the harbor," the health officer quarantined the *Rio Grande* opposite Fort McHenry near the Lazaretto Point Light House.[27] Father James Dolan, chaplain to the Hibernian Society, an organization founded in 1803 to provide charitable relief to poor Irish immigrants, boarded the ship to inspect the passengers' quarters and report on their situation. "Horrified," Dolan related that many of the passengers would die unless they were quickly removed from the *Rio Grande* and given food, water, and medical attention.

Unable to secure a suitable structure for the sick immigrants, the Hibernian Society "bought lumber, employed carpenters, [and] hired laborers" to build a temporary shelter.[28] The Daughters were at the shelter when the passengers disembarked from the vessel. Though precise numbers are lacking, multiple sources indicate that several immigrants died at the shelter before they could be sent to the Baltimore Infirmary or other nearby hospitals.[29] Those who made it to the Baltimore Infirmary had a good chance of surviving. Of the 170 cases treated at the infirmary, less than 10 percent perished.[30] One of the Daughters also passed away while attending the stricken immigrants, as did Major James O. Law, a member of the Hibernian Society.[31]

Absent detailed descriptions in the Daughters' archival records, accounts contained in newspapers and other sources provide the only information concerning the Daughters' work during typhus epidemics. Based on these accounts, their efforts were substantial. At St. Mary's Hospital in Milwaukee and at a temporary facility on Jones Point, for instance, the Daughters cared for typhus-stricken patients disembarking from the immigrant vessel *Allegheny*. Two hundred of the passengers perished.[32] At St. Mary's Hospital in Detroit, which the Daughters also owned and operated, they nursed eighty-eight immigrants with ship fever. While caring for the immigrants, two of the Daughters contracted typhus. Both survived, but their recovery was difficult. Praising the Daughters for their "unwearied attention," the correspondent for the *Detroit Free Press* was effusive. They "deserve not only the highest commendation, but the gratitude of the community," he stated.[33]

Cholera

Major cholera epidemics struck the United States on three occasions in the nineteenth century—in 1832, 1849, and 1866. On each of these occasions, the rate and spread of the disease reflected the route and means of transport, slow-moving boats that plied rivers and canals in 1832, faster-moving steamships and trains in 1849 and 1866. "Cholera was probably the worst possible potentially infectious disease any theorist could choose to study in the mid-19th century because evidence about its mode of spread was so maddeningly contradictory," wrote epidemiologist and infectious disease specialist David Morens.[34] Outbreaks occurred simultaneously at separate locations, often several miles apart. The disease made a brief appearance for a few weeks at a time, only to disappear and then recur many years and decades later, often in the same location.[35]

Public health officials, typically doctors, attempted to determine how cholera started. Lacking knowledge of the microorganisms that caused "fevers," a word used to describe a large number of illnesses, including cholera, health officials could only speculate about their origin.[36] The most common explanation was that "miasmas," poisonous odors and gases coming from the ground, triggered fevers.[37] During hot and humid weather, the sun's rays, they conjectured, released a miasma (stench or cloud) in damp places where garbage and other decomposing substances had accumulated.[38]

"The localities in which I found the cholera to prevail most frequently," a Philadelphia physician wrote in 1832, "were low and damp; the houses generally with wet cellars, very closely built, dark and badly ventilated, and the stench arising from some of them, and many streets, was intolerable."[39] For many observers, miasmas explained why poor people living in low-lying areas and under crowded conditions disproportionately fell sick during epidemics. For others, bad habits were the main reason why poor people more readily contracted cholera. Poor Irish immigrants became convenient targets of public scorn when cholera epidemics started.[40]

Though most physicians blamed miasmas, a few careful observers claimed that impure drinking water was responsible for spreading cholera. John Lea's mapping of the 1849 cholera outbreak in Cincinnati correctly linked the spread of the disease to contaminated water. So did John Snow's detective work in South London five years later.[41] As we know today, the cholera bacillus enters the water through human excrement contained in raw sewage. Warm temperatures and draught conditions during the summer enhance the conditions for the germ's incubation. At the height of an epidemic, flies and contaminated food, in addition to water, can spread cholera.[42]

Lacking any real understanding about the cause of the disease, doctors often aggravated the situation through purging and bleeding, the customary forms of treatment. For well over two thousand years, from Hippocrates to the discovery of microorganisms, humoral theory guided medical practice. Humoral theory held that individuals in good health exhibited a proper balance of the four humors or bodily secretions—blood, phlegm, yellow bile, and black bile. Sick persons, on the other hand, manifested an imbalance of one or more humors. Physicians' main task was to restore the balance, typically by eliminating excess secretions.[43] Though opinions and techniques differed concerning how to go about it, doctors frequently bled their patients to remove excess heat associated with fever, prescribed calomel or mercury chloride to purge phlegm, and administered laudanum to reduce pain and suffering.[44]

Physicians' harsh remedies and lack of results undermined the standing of the medical profession in the mid-1800s. When a second cholera epidemic struck the United States in 1849, criticism of purging and bleeding was pervasive.[45] Though the Daughters did not join the critics, they resisted overzealous treatments.[46] They also worked independently with patients, observing their symptoms, alleviating their pain and suffering, and providing care and attention. Absent a cure for cholera, they offered the best care available. They kept the patient clean, they provided timely food and drink, they administered medicine in the prescribed doses, and they gave spiritual comfort.[47]

Cholera struck New York City and New Orleans in early December 1848. As in 1832, the disease spread up and down the East Coast from its point of origin in New York. But the path to the country's interior was different and more rapid than earlier. Instead of sweeping down from Canada and waterways flowing west and south, the disease made its way by steamboat up the Mississippi and Ohio Rivers after surfacing in New Orleans.[48] Cases emerged in rapid succession in Louisville, Cincinnati, St. Louis, Nashville, and Chicago. Small Midwestern towns along the Ohio and Mississippi Rivers and their tributaries were affected, towns named Gallipolis, Aurora, Rising Sun, Hanover, New Albany, and Vincennes. The death toll was high—4,557 in St. Louis, 5,969 in Cincinnati.[49] At their hospital in St. Louis, the Daughters recorded 510 deaths out of 1,330 cholera cases. Two Daughters perished while treating sick patients.[50] At Charity Hospital in New Orleans, 964 out of 1,400 patients died.[51]

In summer 1849, the first cases appeared in Buffalo. Steamboats traveling east from Chicago and Sandusky carried sick passengers to Buffalo on June 1 and June 4, 1849, while boats traveling west through the Erie Canal carried victims to Buffalo a few days later. The number of cases peaked at 103 toward the end of July and then "gradually diminished."[52] Dr. Austin Flint meticulously recorded the events in the *Buffalo Medical Journal*, which he founded and edited.[53] "Nine tenths of the cases" were in the Irish First and German Fourth Wards, where most of the poor immigrants had settled, Flint indicated.[54] Though Flint believed that the immigrants' "ignorance, recklessness, intemperance, and other vices" had contributed to their predicament, he noted that several prominent citizens living in better neighborhoods also had contracted cholera. "A small proportion of the cases were among a different order of our population, to whom none of the foregoing considerations are applicable."[55]

At Sisters of Charity Hospital, where Flint was a member of the medical staff, 52 out of 134 patients with cholera perished.[56] Flint applauded the care that the cholera-stricken patients received. Most of those who died, he said, "were already in the stage of collapse" when admitted.[57] Those who survived owed their lives to the Daughters. "Whatever credit is due to the Institution for the large proportion of recoveries, belongs to those under whose immediate charge the Institution is placed. . . . The degree of patience and endurance exhibited by the Sisters of Charity . . . during the period of the Epidemic, was a matter of astonishment not less than admiration."[58] Stephen Smith, the hospital's first medical intern, echoed Flint's assessment. "When pestilence or disaster came," Smith stated, "the Sisters did more than merely mourn with Buffalo in her grief—to allay suffering, to assuage misery, to dispel desolation, they lent willing hearts and hands."[59]

Yellow Fever

Yellow fever is an acute viral hemorrhagic disease transmitted by the bite of the *Aedes aegypti* mosquito. Called "yellow jack" for the jaundiced appearance of its victims, yellow fever proceeds in three stages. At the onset of the disease (stage 1), patients exhibit fever, headache, and muscle aches that, after three or four days, usually disappear. Over the course of the next ten to fourteen days (stage 2 remission), persons with yellow fever either fully recover or experience more serious symptoms (stage 3). Individuals entering stage 3 become delirious, suffer seizures, and undergo major organ failure. *Vomito negro*, or black vomit, another name for yellow fever, indicates that death is likely.[60] Absent modern medical treatment, about 50 percent of those who enter stage 3 will die from the disease.[61] Doctors could do little to change the outcome once the disease advanced beyond remission. Use of castor oil and calomel to empty the kidneys and intestines, the customary approach based on the appearance of excess bile in the liver, often aggravated the patient's condition.[62] Newspapers broadcast physicians' failures. "It seems quite out of the question that the doctors will ever afford us the smallest relief," one such newspaper contended.[63]

Though the Daughters offered no antidote, they alleviated patients' pain and suffering and helped them to recover during remission. "Although there are a variety of fevers," Matilda Coskery noted in *Advices*, "they all have a general, as well as a particular plan of treatment." Yellow fever, she observed, called for "a specific management."[64] "Bedclothing should be regulated," "cool drinks are proper [except] when perspiring," and "fresh air" and "nourishments" should be adjusted depending on the patient's condition.[65] Nurses should resist the excessive use of purgatives, mustard plasters, blistering, and bleeding, Coskery instructed. "Bleeding must be used with great judgment as to time and quantity. Blood must not be taken when the fever has, or is about to subside, or [is] in a sweating stage—and there are very rare exceptions to this."[66]

In 1853, New Orleans sustained its worst outbreak of yellow fever. New Orleans historian Joseph Baudier compared it to "the Black Plague of London for the appalling number of deaths and persons stricken."[67] "Every person who could, fled from the city," he reported. "Deaths were so numerous that riots took place at the Mortuary chapel [when] families sought to [carry out] the last rites for loved ones."[68] According to historian John Kendall, the 1853 outbreak was the worst ever in America—"the most terrible catastrophe of the kind that city has been called on to endure." Sanitation was "very bad," Kendall noted. Garbage and raw sewage collected in the streets, forming "pools of stagnant water," prime conditions for breeding mosquitos.[69]

The epidemic lasted from mid-July to early November, claiming over eight thousand lives in New Orleans and surrounding areas.[70] Five of them were Daughters.[71] Charity Hospital filled to capacity. "It was not uncommon to see a line of cabs and dark-covered wagons . . . lined up at [the hospital's] gate," medical historians S. L. Kotar and J. E. Gessler indicated. Sick patients came to Charity because the hospital's "well-regulated system provided for prompt care and attention," they stated. Because of the large number of people afflicted, the city's board of health opened several infirmaries, as did the Howard Association, a philanthropic organization founded in New Orleans to aid the sick poor during epidemics.[72]

From New Orleans, the disease spread to Donaldsonville and Natchez, Mississippi, and then to Mobile, Alabama. By mid-December, the number of deaths in Mobile had reached twelve hundred.[73] Some of the Daughters sought permission to go to the hardest struck locations, but the fast pace of the disease made this difficult. "When the scourge raged . . . at New-Orleans, my sister Chrysostom of Natchez, always indefatigable in the service of the sick," requested permission to go to Charity Hospital, but "it was not possible to grant it," Mother Etienne Hall, DC, wrote to the superioress in Paris. We feared that yellow fever would soon "reach . . . Natchez [and spread] to Mobile and Donaldsonville," making it best for the Daughters to stay in those areas. When the disease made its appearance at Donaldsonville, two of the Daughters fell sick with the fever, "but they escaped," Hall related. Unfortunately, two Daughters died at Mobile, where they "had the care of a temporary hospital."[74]

In 1855, yellow fever struck Norfolk and Portsmouth, Virginia. The source of the epidemic, which ultimately claimed about 3,200 lives, was the *Benjamin Franklin*, a cargo ship traveling from St. Thomas in the West Indies and bound for New York City. While in transit, the boat detoured to Portsmouth for repairs to its boiler. Suspecting that several of the sailors had yellow fever, based on a report that two crewmen had died after leaving St. Thomas, health officer R. H. Gordon ordered the *Benjamin Franklin* quarantined under a yellow flag near Craney Island in the Elizabeth River between Norfolk and Portsmouth.[75]

More deaths occurred while the ship was under quarantine, one from yellow fever and others from drowning when panicked crew members jumped overboard attempting to escape the fever. Rather than report the death of the sailor from yellow fever, the ship's captain secretly disposed of the body. When health officer Gordon returned eleven days later, the captain told him that there was no fever. Promising that he would not break open the ship's hold, the captain convinced Gordon to release the *Benjamin Franklin* for repairs at Portsmouth. After reaching Portsmouth, however, the captain discharged "the ballast . . . upon the wharf" and had "her bilge water . . . pumped out."[76] Health officer Robert Archer later determined that "the effluvia arising from the bilge-water was the immediate cause" of the epidemic. "Every individual . . . exposed to its influence, and almost every one [*sic*] who had come within its atmosphere was more or less affected by it," Archer recorded.[77]

The first cases appeared in early July among dockworkers, clerks, and other shipyard workers. From Portsmouth, the fever spread to Barry's Row, a squalid tenement district on the Norfolk side of the Elizabeth River where many poor Irish resided. Seeking to confine the disease to Barry's Row, Norfolk authorities erected "a 24-foot wooden wall . . . around" the district, "removed" the inhabitants when the epidemic persisted, and burned the houses while spectators and fire companies watched and gathered.[78] By early August, most people had fled Norfolk, a city of about sixteen thousand inhabitants. Though "probably not more than 1500 to 2000 whites remain[ed]" behind, a Portsmouth newspaper reported, the epidemic continued unabated.[79]

Doctors arrived in large numbers, as many as one hundred at the height of the epidemic, offering their help and assistance.[80] Nurses, however, were scarce. "There are a great many doctors here . . . and all doing what they can to alleviate the suffering of this dreadfully afflicted city," a correspondent covering the epidemic for the *Richmond Dispatch* indicated. But what we really need are "more nurses, and them quickly," he stated.[81]

The Central House at Emmitsburg responded. All told, "eight [Daughters] gave full time to the stricken," Sister Aloysia Dugan wrote in her compilation of the Daughters' work during the 1855 epidemic in Portsmouth and Norfolk.[82] Two Daughters treated sick orphans at St. Mary's Asylum, an orphanage near Portsmouth where "several" children contracted the fever. Most of them recovered.[83] Three Daughters worked at the US Naval Hospital in Portsmouth, which, under orders from President Franklin Pierce, opened its doors to civilians.[84] The remaining three Daughters went to a temporary hospital erected on the grounds of the Julappi racetrack near Norfolk. The death toll among the sick at Julappi was significantly less than in Norfolk. Seeking to explain the disparity, a reporter for the *Richmond Dispatch* credited the Daughters. Julappi hospital "is kept scrupulously clean and neat, and everything through the kind [Daughters] goes on with the regularity of clock work," he stated.[85]

By early October, the epidemic had subsided. Newspaper accounts indicated that returning residents were shocked at the number of fatalities. Among the dead were Norfolk's mayor, ten local physicians, seven ministers and several members of their families, the president of the Seaboard and Roanoke Railroad, members of the Select and Common Councils, Norfolk's postmaster, the senior editor of the local newspaper, and three Custom House officers.[86] Ann Plume Behan Herron, a wealthy Irish philanthropist whose uncle had donated the property for St. Mary's Asylum, also perished. Over the protests of her brother, Ann refused to leave Norfolk, electing to stay in the city and care for the suffering. She invited many into her home, called "Plumesville." Witnessing the work of the Daughters during the epidemic, the care and attention they gave to poor patients, Ann told her brother that she wanted to give Plumesville to them for use as a hospital. Though Ann died before she could make the necessary legal arrangements, her brother fulfilled her request. On June 11, 1857, Norfolk's first hospital (DePaul Hospital, as it later came to be known) opened on the site of Plumesville.[87]

ANTI-CATHOLICISM AND THE KNOW-NOTHING PARTY

In the early to mid-1850s, the rise and stunning electoral successes of the anti-Catholic Know-Nothing Party (officially the American Party) brought nativists out of the shadows and into the public arena. During its brief reign, the Know-Nothing Party gained nationwide standing. Members included former Whigs who felt that the Catholic vote in the 1852 presidential election had led to the defeat of Winfield Scott, their candidate. Know-Nothings were most active in and around East Coast cities and in the border states of Delaware, Maryland, and Kentucky.[88] In the statewide elections of 1854 and 1855, the party won governorships and carried state legislatures in Massachusetts, Rhode Island, New Hampshire, Connecticut, Maryland, and Kentucky. The movement also made solid gains in New York, Pennsylvania, California, Virginia, Georgia, Alabama, Mississippi, and Louisiana. But after 1855 support plummeted as differences arose over slavery. Know-Nothings in the North typically joined the Republican Party, while those in the South joined the Democrats. After 1856, the Know-Nothing Party largely ceased to exist as a viable political entity. Its last remaining stronghold was in Maryland, where Millard Fillmore, the party's nominee for president in the 1856 election, received his only electoral vote.[89]

The Removal or Threatened Removal of the Daughters from Community Hospitals

On their election to public office at certain locations, Know-Nothings assailed the Daughters, undermining their fundraising activities and, in some instances, leading to their ouster from community or government-owned facilities. In Mobile, Alabama, for instance, accusations of proselytizing and mismanagement were lodged against the Daughters after the Know-Nothings gained control of the local city government.[90] On May 15, 1854, James McGarahan, the vicar general or second in command of the Mobile diocese, wrote to Father Francis Burlando, CM, the Daughters' provincial director, informing him that "bigoted and malicious . . . assailants" had leveled "foolish, absurd, and unfounded charges."[91] The Daughters were alleged to have "mismanaged funds," removed Bibles, and prevented Protestant ministers from "convers[ing] or pray[ing] with the Sick."[92] When

McGarahan wrote Burlando on May 15, the Daughters were awaiting the results of a hearing that had taken place before the "Governors of the Hospital," a three-person body comprising the mayor, the head of the city council, and the representative of the board of aldermen. Apparently, the hearing had gone well from McGarahan's perspective. "The originators and advocates of this vile attack seem now heartily ashamed," he wrote Burlando.[93] Exuberant, McGarahan predicted that the Daughters "will not only be invited to stay, but amply protected from similar intrusions and impertinence in the future."[94]

McGarahan's optimism was unfounded. On June 30, the governors released their report, finding the Daughters "guilty of making the Hospital instrumental in the propagation of Sectarian principles."[95] Infuriated, McGarahan wrote Burlando on July 3, stating, "The Mayor, I am sorry to say, deceived us all." He "affected friendship to the last, but in his report the cloven foot appears."[96] The adverse ruling did not dampen the demand for the Daughters' services, however. With McGarahan's prompting and support, the Daughters remained in Mobile following their ouster from City Hospital. In May 1855, they opened their own hospital, a two-story structure, which they named the Providence Infirmary (the name was later changed to Providence Hospital).[97]

The Daughters' mission to New Orleans followed a similar pattern. Responding to an invitation from the State of Louisiana in 1833 to take charge of Charity Hospital, the motherhouse dispatched ten Sisters. They arrived at Charity in January 1834. Another group of ten Sisters soon followed.[98] For the next eighteen years, the Sisters worked at Charity Hospital free from controversy. That changed when the Know-Nothings gained control of the common council and various city offices in the mid-1850s.[99] Though no formal accusations of wrongdoing were lodged against the Sisters (now Daughters), as had occurred in Mobile, there was considerable apprehension.[100] In 1852, the Daughters agreed to manage an infirmary that Dr. Warren Stone, Charity's house surgeon, and his partner, Dr. William Kennedy, had started. Stone had been trying to attract the Daughters, but they rebuffed his efforts until the Know-Nothings assumed power. Fearful that they might have to leave Charity, five Daughters led by Sister Servant Theresa Francis (Ellen) Sheridan began working at the infirmary, which they called Maison de Sante.[101]

The Daughters' work at Maison de Sante was temporary; they wanted their own hospital. On July 20, 1855, they purchased "a square of ground" close by Charity, but it took several years for them to accumulate sufficient funds to start building.[102] Construction began in early 1858 and was complete by December. On January 2, 1859, the hospital opened, and the first patients, "four Negro slaves and one white man," were admitted.[103] The Daughters called their new hospital "Hôtel Dieu" after "the famous establishment of that name in Paris."[104]

Nativist Resistance to Public Funds for Irish Immigrants

As in other parts of the country, Buffalo experienced a rise in anti-Catholic activity in the mid-1800s. The Whig Party, which many nativists supported, controlled most of New York's elected offices. Though the Whigs were a mild lot compared to the Know-Nothings, Buffalo had its flamethrowers, led by the Reverend John Chase Lord, pastor of the Central Presbyterian Church. When the state appropriated nine thousand dollars in aid to Sisters of Charity Hospital in 1849, Lord assailed the legislature for its pro-Catholic position.[105]

Because it was the only hospital in Buffalo, Sisters of Charity was eligible for state funds subject to three conditions: The hospital had to serve the immigrant poor, be open to all religious denominations, and not engage in proselytizing. Lord and his followers claimed that the Daughters proselytized, that they sought to convert patients to the Catholic religion.[106] Bishop Timon was away from his diocese when Lord cast his aspersions, leaving Timon's second in command, Vicar General Bernard O'Reilly, to answer Lord's charges. A very public letter-writing campaign ensued on the pages of the *Buffalo Morning Express*, with O'Reilly responding to Lord and Lord responding to O'Reilly.[107]

Largely because of the negative publicity that the public confrontation between Lord and O'Reilly generated, the state legislature denied funds in 1850 and again in 1851 for Sisters of Charity Hospital. In 1852, the State of New York restored much of the funding. The main reason was the charitable service that the Daughters performed during the 1849 cholera epidemic. The epidemic had run its course before the funding was suspended, but the Daughters' role in the epidemic was not widely known in the state legislature. Eager to restore funding, Austin Flint penned an article in the

November 1851 edition of the *Buffalo Medical Journal* extolling the Daughters' efforts. Flint wrote that the "degree of patience and endurance" the Daughters "exhibited . . . was a matter of astonishment." He attributed "the large portion of recoveries" of hospitalized patients to the [Daughters'] skills in nursing and administration.[108]

A similar situation transpired in Rochester. Irish immigrants began arriving in Rochester in the 1820s to work on the Erie Canal. Many of them lived on the east side of the city in an area known as "Dublin." By 1845, Rochester's foreign-born population was overwhelmingly Irish, and by 1860, the Irish were the largest ethnic group in the city.[109] Sensing the need for a hospital, Bishop Timon approached Rochester's leading citizens in 1856 and asked them to form a committee. They were not interested.[110] The Know-Nothings had taken control of most city offices in the 1855 election, winning races for mayor, city treasurer, city assessor, justice of the peace, and sealer of weights and measures. Corruption and mob violence accompanied the Know-Nothings' brief tenure. Only one year after the 1855 election, the Know-Nothings were removed from office in the wake of a grand jury investigation into their methods and practices. Anti-Catholic bigotry nonetheless persisted. Those in charge of the Home for the Friendless, a Protestant-run facility for "poor and friendless females," continued to exclude Catholic priests from ministering to the Catholic women in residence. Rochester's reform schools and almshouses also restricted access to Catholic clergy.[111]

Despite nativist resistance, Timon moved forward. After surveying the area around Rochester, he purchased a parcel of land known as the Sibley estate. The estate contained "two small one-story stone stables connected by a dilapidated woodshed." At Timon's request, the Central House in Emmitsburg transferred three Daughters from Buffalo to Rochester. On September 8, 1857, the Daughters founded St. Mary's Hospital on the Sibley estate and began to admit the first patients. Led by Sister Hieronymo O'Brien, DC, the Daughters persevered over the course of the next six years, slowly transforming the "small, single-story, dilapidated" structures that Timon had acquired into a properly equipped, three-story building with sufficient space for three hundred patients.[112] Money was scarce in the beginning; even the basic necessities, food and beds, were lacking. According to one account, "The sisters slept [in the loft of a stable] on . . . pallets of straw with little more than their habits for covering. . . . [R]ats scamper[ed] across their beds at night."[113]

During the first year of its existence, St. Mary's Hospital served 250 patients, a remarkable achievement considering the harsh conditions. The Daughters' determination and unwavering devotion to poor patients gained notice. Several local physicians provided free medical care and donated money for operating expenses. O'Brien was gracious in the face of local hostility. She announced that St. Mary's would welcome the "sick of all denominations."[114] When a "Protestant visitor" toured St. Mary's in March 1858, he extolled the Daughters' liberality, stating, "The sisters have in no instance, refused an application for admission to the hospital."[115]

By fall 1858, O'Brien was sufficiently confident to approach Rochester's Board of Supervisors for money. She was not disappointed. On November 15, 1858, the board reached a "favorable decision." Though the amount was small, it indicated that the Daughters were achieving notice, that civic leaders, though mostly Protestant, realized that the Daughters were a valuable and needed asset.[116]

The Exclusion of Catholic Priests from Protestant-Run Hospitals

Anti-Catholicism also expressed itself in the exclusion of Catholic priests from Protestant-run facilities. Exclusion of Catholic priests was a prominent reason why Bishops John Hughes and John Timon wanted church-owned hospitals.[117] The circumstances surrounding the founding of Daughter-owned St. Agnes Hospital in Baltimore in 1862 are a good example.

On October 31, 1839, Sister Mary Ann McAleer departed Emmitsburg for Baltimore, where she would stay for the next forty years. Her first assignment was the Baltimore Infirmary, which Mother Rose White and Mistress of Novices Mary Xavier Clark considered a good place to send young sisters for their initial training.[118] Though McAleer craved nursing, her superiors initially sent her to housekeeping. But after only two months in housekeeping, she took charge of "St. John's Ward," which housed sick sailors.[119] St. John's Ward received funding under the Seaman's Sickness and Disability Act of 1789, which paid for the healthcare of sick or injured sailors. Despite the guaranteed income, many hospitals were reluctant to admit sailors because they often were drunk and disorderly.[120] St. John's Ward was an exception. "The dear good souls loved and respected the Sisters," McAleer wrote in one of her letters. "You would never hear them saying a bad word if they knew a Sister would hear them."[121] McAleer "regarded each [of the sailors] as her own brother and they, one and all, had an inexpressible veneration for her," another Sister wrote in her journal. "When vessels hailed each other at sea," the Sister related, "the first salute was 'Hallo there; are you from Baltimore? . . . How is Sister Mary Ann?'"[122]

McAleer spent eighteen years on St. John's Ward before becoming sister servant of the Baltimore Infirmary in 1860. As sister servant, McAleer showed great compassion for chronically ill and elderly patients, those with long-standing afflictions affecting the heart, lungs, or kidneys, or simply those who were too old to care for themselves. "I must not forget old persons who have no means," McAleer confided in one of her letters. "The poor old souls have raised large families." They are "now old & have no home." The children cannot or do not want to care for them. "We see plenty of this in hospitals," she lamented.[123]

Chronically ill and elderly patients had few options in the nineteenth century. Hospitals typically limited admissions to "curable" and "morally worthy" patients, using doctors and wealthy donors as gatekeepers.[124] Persons with means stayed home and paid for visiting nurses where they existed. In some cities, such as Charleston, Ladies Benevolent Societies aided the poor in their homes, but these societies excluded the "unworthy."[125] As the nineteenth century progressed and increasing numbers of mentally ill poor persons were sent to insane asylums, the percentage of elderly patients residing in almshouses rose substantially. By 1880, the elderly comprised one-third of the total US almshouse population.[126]

McAleer attempted to improve the plight of the chronically ill and aged. This was an area in which one's religion mattered. Because such people remained in one place for long periods, comfort and security often were more important than medical treatment. Access to a Catholic priest or a Protestant minister was an important consideration. So were the customs, habits, dietary choices, and attire of caregivers and neighboring patients.[127] McAleer's letters contained poignant stories of chronically sick and elderly patients struggling to survive under difficult and challenging situations. One of her accounts portrayed the predicament of an Irish seamstress known as "Hannah" who resided for over a year against her wishes in Baltimore's Union Protestant Infirmary, today's Union Memorial Hospital.

In 1857, Hannah found work in the home of a wealthy woman after traveling to the United States from Ireland. Three years later, Hannah suffered "a severe Hemerage [*sic*] from the lungs" and was taken to the Protestant Infirmary. Hannah protested, but her employer, who was one of the "Lady Managers of the Infirmary," told her that it was only temporary. "I will come for you myself," she promised, "as soon as" the doctor "thinks you are able."[128] Unknown to Hannah, her employer became sick and died, and no one returned for Hannah. When she arrived at the Protestant Infirmary, Hannah was "placed . . . in a large ward" where "all the suffering sick" around her were "strangers." She cried "all night, had [another] Hemerage [*sic*] . . . [and] a Fever." Feeling "very ill," she asked for a Catholic priest, but the matron refused, saying, "No Catholic Priest is allowed to administer any of the rights of the Roman Catholic Church here."[129]

Ridiculed by other patients for wearing Catholic religious objects, scapular and rosary around her neck, Hannah hid "them from their sight & made a small bag & placed them in it & carried it under her arm all day." McAleer's letters do not make it clear why Hannah did not walk out of the infirmary. Perhaps she was not able. Hannah had no friends or relatives living nearby who could help her. When she was working as a seamstress, Hannah sent her "hard earnings . . . every three months" to her "poor dear Father & Mother" living in Ireland. But after entering the Protestant Infirmary, she did not write them. "I could not find [it] in my heart to write, & tell them I was sick & in a Protestant Institution, as this would surely brake [*sic*] my poor dear parents [*sic*] heart."[130]

Hannah prayed for the "strength [to] walk over to the church," but her health continued to diminish. She asked the matron "to have her carried down to the sidewalk," but again, the matron refused Hannah's entreaties. Finally, after "remaining in [the] Infirmary one year to the day," Hannah's prayers were answered. A "gentleman" visiting a patient in the bed next to Hannah discovered her predicament. After leaving the infirmary, he alerted prominent members of Baltimore's Catholic community. Learning of Hannah's situation, McAleer sent for a priest who gained entry and took Hannah to the Baltimore Infirmary. Hannah was near death when she arrived at the infirmary. "To look at her, one could but think every breath must be the last," McAleer related. She "lived through the night, but next morning left us for her Home in Heaven."[131]

Hannah's symptoms—coughing up blood from her lungs, her confinement in bed for a year, and her slow but steady decline—indicate that she suffered from "consumption," the word used at the time for tuberculosis. Very little was known about tuberculosis. Because the disease took months and even years to develop and did not suddenly strike whole towns or cities like cholera or yellow fever, doctors and public health officials did not isolate tuberculosis patients. It was not until after German physician Robert Koch discovered the tubercle bacillus in 1882 that health officials realized that the disease was contagious and segregated people to prevent the spread of the illness.[132]

Less than a year after Hannah's death, the Daughters founded St. Agnes Hospital "to serve the Catholic poor" of Baltimore.[133] Five Daughters, with McAleer in charge, left the Baltimore Infirmary in April 1863 to staff St. Agnes.[134] McAleer worked quickly to enhance the hospital's reputation. By July 1863, St. Agnes was crowded with patients. Forced to "refuse admission" to sick patients because of "limited capacity," McAleer and others sought larger accommodations.[135] In 1875, Lady Elizabeth Caton Stafford, the granddaughter of Charles Carroll, who was the only Catholic to sign the Declaration of Independence, donated a thirty-acre parcel of land for a new building. Construction soon began, and by October 1876, the new facility was complete and ready for patients. McAleer remained at St. Agnes Hospital until September 1879. She spent her final days at Emmitsburg.[136]

THE SCOURGE OF SLAVERY

When the Know-Nothing Party split over slavery, Northern nativists joined the newly formed Republicans, while Know-Nothings in the South changed their allegiance to the Democrats. In the North, the political alliance between abolitionists and nativists drove most Irish toward the Democrats.[137] Seeking to court the Irish vote, Northern Democrats "purged" their party of the "Know-Nothing element," becoming outwardly "hostile" to most anything that the Know-Nothings represented.[138] For most Southerners, however, preserving slavery was more important than resisting Irish immigrants.[139] After the Know-Nothings lost in Mobile, the environment changed considerably.[140] Seeking to entice the Daughters back to City Hospital, the newly elected officials praised the Daughters' efforts at the Providence Infirmary. "We were gratified in observing the cheerfulness, neatness and comfort" at the infirmary, they stated.[141]

Local customs and traditions influenced hospital administration.[142] Treating slaves in Southern hospitals before the Civil War was not uncommon. While large plantations often had their own facilities, smaller ones contracted with physicians or hospitals.[143] In 1859, Hôtel Dieu's first year of operation, "a total of 523 patients" were admitted, New Orleans historian Joseph Baudier reported. "Of these, 285 were slaves, or more than half of the total intake," he indicated. During the hospital's second year, there were "536 patients . . . an increase of only 13." A substantial portion were "slaves sent by brokers as well as some masters."[144]

Free Blacks, on the other hand, rarely gained entry to Southern hospitals.[145] "To care for African Americans [in Southern hospitals], even in segregated wards, was a drastic departure from custom," wrote church historian Christopher Kauffman.[146] Northern hospitals were not much different. They typically confined Blacks to segregated wards "in undesirable locations such as unheated attics or damp basements."[147] Though they segregated the races, the Daughters often admitted free Blacks to their hospitals, even in Southern localities.[148] Not only slaves, but "free men of color and free women of color" received treatment at Hôtel Dieu in New Orleans.[149] Mullanphy Hospital in St. Louis cared for Blacks, "slave" or "indigent free."[150] Norfolk's Saint Vincent De Paul Hospital had separate wards for Black and White patients.[151]

While there is no discernable evidence that the Daughters owned slaves in the early 1800s, they benefited from their labors at several locations. Approximately ten to fifteen slaves worked in the fields, farms, kitchens, and washhouses at Mount St. Mary's College (the Sulpician priests owned them). Slaves also assisted the Daughters at Charity Hospital in New Orleans and at Mullanphy Hospital in St. Louis.[152] When the Daughters took charge of Charity Hospital in 1834 under a contract with the State of Louisiana, there were sixteen slaves at the institution. Sister Regina Smith, Charity's sister servant, could not replace them with paid workers; they were the hospital's property.[153]

After the Civil War, segregation of the races became formal church policy. Fearing Protestant incursions on the Catholic faith when large numbers of immigrants came to the United States beginning in the late 1800s, the Third Plenary Council of American Bishops, meeting in Baltimore in 1884, declared that Blacks and Whites should have their own schools and churches.[154] There was some resistance, particularly in New Orleans, where Whites, Mulattos, and Blacks traditionally had worshipped together. But any opposition to the separation of the races crumbled following Reconstruction, the enactment of Jim Crow laws, and the US Supreme Court's 1896 *Plessy* decision upholding racial segregation.[155]

The scourge of slavery and racism reverberated well into the twentieth century. The Daughters did not admit Blacks into their community until the second half of the twentieth century, nor did they mix Black and White children in the schools and orphanages they founded, except on a couple occasions—St. Joseph School in Baltimore and St. Euphemia's School in Emmitsburg.[156] Some sisterhoods attempted to integrate the races in the nineteenth century, but the clergy refused to allow it, citing state segregation laws in several instances.[157] The Oblate Sisters of Providence, a religious community for "Coloured Women" formed in Baltimore in 1828, was one of the few concessions that Blacks won from church prelates in antebellum America. Comprising free Blacks, many from Baltimore's "middle class," the Oblates were teachers. Though not trained nurses, they readily volunteered their services at Baltimore's makeshift hospitals during the 1832 cholera epidemic. The Oblates received limited financial support, frequently were omitted from church directories and press clippings, and were otherwise "marginalized . . . within the religious community."[158]

Black physicians founded hospitals for the training of Black doctors because internship programs for them were limited. White-run hospitals typically excluded them, including those that civic leaders and philanthropists established for Blacks in their cities.[159] The situation was the same for Black nurses. "It is not at all likely that any general hospital in a White community would dare to employ Negro women in its nursing service, no matter how competent they might be," a short note in the February 1926 issue of *The Modern Hospital* stated.[160] Black-run hospitals included Provident Hospital and Nurse Training School in Chicago; Tuskegee Institute and Nurse Training School in Tuskegee, Alabama; Frederick Douglass Memorial Hospital and Training School in Philadelphia; and Home Infirmary in Clarksville, Tennessee.[161] In 1912, there were 63 Black hospitals in the United States (Black-owned and White-run for Black patients only); by 1919, there were 118; and by 1944, there were 124.[162]

THREE

WARTIME SERVICE

Approximately seven hundred Catholic sisters from at least twenty different religious communities served in the US Civil War. Three hundred of them, the largest group by far, were Daughters.[1] The Daughters were also the largest contingent of Catholic nurses in the Spanish-American War and World War I. Almost four hundred Daughters served at nine different army encampments and two battlefield locations during the Spanish-American War. Ninety-three sisters from seven other Catholic communities also worked as nurses.[2] Only ten Catholic sisters participated in World War I as part of a base hospital unit.[3] All of them were Daughters.

The Daughters' wartime service thrust them into the national spotlight. They received recognition from military leaders, federal officials, and surgeons for their organizational capabilities, for their professional nursing, and for their administrative skills. Just as their proficient nursing distinguished them from caregivers and relief workers, so their compassionate treatment of wounded soldiers from different parts of the country and classes of society helped to diminish prejudice against them. Taken together, these various factors placed the Daughters in a favorable position to assume a leading role in the formation and development of America's healthcare industry after these wars were over. Their work in the 1918 flu pandemic at the end of World War I added to their growing list of achievements.

THE CIVIL WAR

There were approximately 620,000 casualties in the Civil War, two-thirds from disease and one-third from combat.[4] The number of deaths exceeded those in World Wars I and II, Vietnam, and the Korean War combined.[5] Among the survivors, one in thirteen lost one or more limbs.[6] Military leaders in the North and the South could not find equivalent substitutes for the Daughters, particularly at the war's beginning.[7] New York physician Elizabeth Blackwell sought to establish a program for training skilled nurses, but she had to step aside when President Lincoln's secretary of war, Simon Cameron, chose Dorothea Dix instead.[8] Known for her pioneering work in mental health, Dix was not a trained nurse, nor did she fully appreciate the rigors that nurses faced during wars and epidemics. Her criteria for selection emphasized age and social standing over youth and experience. From the beginning, the Daughters refused to serve under Dix, and much to Dix's dismay, US Surgeon General William Hammond granted their request.[9]

Ultimately, Dix recruited and assigned over three thousand nurses to hospital positions, more than four times the total number of all Catholic sisters.[10] But her emphasis on age and social standing over youth and experience soon became a problem. The lack of preparation surfaced in the summer of 1862 when the Union army bogged down in the woods and swamps east of Richmond during the North's aborted attempt to end the war quickly by seizing the South's capital city. Several of Dix's nurses served on transport boats or hospital ships outfitted to carry wounded soldiers and take them to military hospitals in Washington and elsewhere. The conditions on the transport boats were harsh, the soldiers' wounds often severe and festering. Though a few of the nurses persevered, "many . . . returned home as quickly as they had left," wrote historian Judith Giesberg.[11]

Women's role in the Civil War evolved as problems with male nurses surfaced (almost all army nurses were male) and as the Union and Confederate armies developed and instituted systematic approaches and standard procedures for the recovery, transport, and care of the wounded. The prevailing belief throughout the war was that women, particularly White women from the middle and upper classes, should refrain from nursing strange men in public places. This attitude was more pervasive in the South than in the North.[12] "There is a good deal of trouble about the ladies in some of the hospitals of this department. Our friends here have advised us to go home," Kate Cumming, a Southern lady from Mobile, wrote in her journal on September 8, 1862, while tending sick soldiers at Buckner Hospital in Chattanooga. "I must confess, from all I had heard and seen," Cumming confided, that "I wavered about the propriety of it; but when I remembered the suffering I had witnessed, and the relief I had given, my mind was made up to go into [a hospital] if allowed to do so."[13]

Prejudice against female nurses diminished on both sides as the war continued, at least in hospitals if not on battlefields. Sick soldiers generally preferred caring women to gruff men whom one Southern officer called "rough country crackers who have not enough sense to be kind."[14] In July 1862, Surgeon General Hammond ordered that female nurses receive roughly one-third of all hospital appointments, while in September of the same year, the Confederate Congress passed a law requiring that hospitals engage "matrons" to oversee hospital operations, stating that "preference [should be given] in all cases to females."[15] Still, there were certain restrictions. Matron duties were to be administrative, not clinical; there was no provision in the law for women to pursue nursing.[16]

The distinction between skilled nursing and battlefield aid or relief work is important to understanding the Daughters' involvement in the war effort. In the mid-1800s, most people associated the word "nurse" with women's domestic skills—cooking, cleaning, and running a household.[17] But to Elizabeth Blackwell and the Daughters, nurses were trained medical professionals, comparable in many respects to physicians. The men in charge of the United States Sanitary Commission (USSC), a private relief agency formed at the beginning of the war and authorized by President Abraham Lincoln, refused to acknowledge the distinction, claiming that, if "women would learn their true place," then their "work . . . would be more useful than even the work of the Sisters."[18] Educated Southern women of the middle and upper classes, such as Kate Cumming, also did not perceive a difference. Cumming was perplexed that Catholic sisters could enter hospitals while she and her companions often were prohibited. "It seems strange," Cumming wrote, "that they [referring to Catholic sisters] can do with honor what is wrong for other Christian women to do."[19]

Seeking to explain why most doctors preferred Catholic sisters, contemporary observers and several historians frequently stressed their discipline and obedience. Charles Tripler, US surgeon general when the war began, remarked that Catholic sisters were "far preferable" to other nurses because they were "better disciplined, more discrete and judicious, and more reliable."[20] "Doctors requested permission to appoint Sisters of Charity" because of "their efficiency, calm demeanor, lack of prejudice, and probably most important, their obedience to authority," wrote historian Mary Elizabeth Massey.[21] "Obedience" notwithstanding, doctors wanted experienced nurses to assist them, and in most instances, they favored Catholic sisters because their nursing skills were superior.[22]

A common misperception is that aid or relief workers, such as Clara Barton, were nurses just like the Daughters.[23] They were not. They carried wagonloads of supplies that they distributed at field hospitals and army depots, and they helped to bandage, shelter, and provide food for sick and wounded soldiers. Most other female volunteers, many of them with the USSC or other relief agencies and societies, were also not trained nurses; only 20 percent of them may have worked in field hospitals.[24] The Daughters, on the other hand, were experienced hospital nurses. While they served in several different locations (in army encampments, on transport ships, and in field hospitals) in the first two years of the war, during the last two years they principally worked in military or general hospitals.[25] Military hospitals were the end points in a chain of care or "tiered hospital structure."[26]

Though there were no major medical breakthroughs during the Civil War on the scale of germ theory, American medicine made some important strides, particularly in surgical and postoperative procedures. Before the war began, few physicians had performed surgery of any consequence. By war's end, most of them had. The traumatic wounds that soldiers suffered in battle, often related to advancements in weaponry—the Minié ball, a half-inch hollow bullet that expanded on impact, and the "Napoleon," a portable cannon that fired exploding canisters—placed a premium on certain surgical techniques, such as amputation and resection (removing a portion of a bone). Surgeons had to discern if and when to operate, and what approach to use. Fatality rates following amputation were high, over 40 percent. Once gangrene or erysipelas, a bacterial skin infection, set in, the chances of recovery were slim.[27] In the third year of the war, Union army doctors were experimenting with various antiseptics in military hospitals. One promising antiseptic, bromine, significantly reduced the incidence of gangrene and erysipelas. The growing realization that a clean environment and proper hygiene helped to reduce the spread of disease focused attention on nursing and hospital administration.[28]

Though high-ranking officers and doctors on both sides revered the Daughters, many of those wounded on the battlefield were not familiar with them, particularly Confederates from Virginia and other states where there were few Catholics. "Several of these poor soldiers had never seen a cornette" and believed that Catholics were "taught to hate the very name of Protestants," Sister Euphemia Blenkinsop, DC, remarked during a visit to a Southern hospital. "One of the [soldiers] could not control his emotions on learning that the Sister who served him was a Catholic; he wept aloud; but his prejudices soon vanished on witnessing the care that was taken of him," Blenkinsop related.[29] "They dress in a different way from any other women. I wish you could see their bonnets," a soldier wrote home from a hospital in Lynchburg, Virginia, where the Daughters were in attendance. "I think you would laugh till you could not stand. . . . They remind me of some great foul [*sic*] with its wings spread," he stated.[30]

Early in the war, prejudice against Catholics almost prevented the Daughters from serving in Confederate military hospitals. "It remains with the Confederate authorities to overrule the deplorable prejudice which would exclude from the military hospitals this most precious and spontaneous order of the Volunteer Sisters of Charity," an October 4, 1861, article in the *Richmond Enquirer* commented.[31] Fortunately for the sick and wounded soldiers, the Daughters' reputation for extraordinary care and service overcame the opposition against them.[32] Indeed, Richmond became a hub for the Daughters' outreach to cities such as Lynchburg, where in November 1862 they occupied two hospitals and the city's "infamous Pest House."[33]

The Daughters operated out of seven hubs or regional centers during the Civil War. Three were in the North, and four were in the South. The three in the North were St. Joseph's Central House, Providence Hospital in Washington, and St. Philomena's Asylum in St. Louis. The four in the South were Charity Hospital in New Orleans; St. Mary's Asylum and School in Natchez, Mississippi; St. Vincent de Paul Hospital in Norfolk; and St. Joseph's Asylum and School in Richmond.[34] Some of these hubs, such as St. Joseph's Central House and St. Mary's Asylum and School in Natchez, were near key battlegrounds. Others, including St. Philomena's Asylum, Charity Hospital, and St. Vincent's Hospital, were in strategic port cities. Still others, such as Providence Hospital and St. Joseph's Asylum and School, were in the capitals of the North and the South, respectively.

As events unfolded from 1861 to 1865, as cities came under siege and shifted from Southern to Northern control, the Daughters adjusted when communications were cut and supplies were low, when military leaders left and new ones emerged, and when the numbers of sick and wounded soldiers fluctuated from high to low and high again. In addition to their skilled nursing, what made the Daughters so effective during the war was their community identity, their governing structure, and their spirituality. They worked together as a unit whether large or small; they adhered to community rules and standards; they followed orders, not so much from army officers, but from female and male superiors at Emmitsburg and regional centers; they were highly mobile and could travel on short notice; and they persevered under difficult circumstances. Mother Ann Simeon Norris, DC, was their visitatrix throughout war; Father Francis Burlando, CM, was their provincial director. The following events, in chronological order, capture key features of the Daughters' evolving role in the war effort.

Harpers Ferry and Winchester, Virginia, June to August 1861

One of the first requests for the Daughters' aid came on June 7, 1861, from Confederate soldiers stationed at Harpers Ferry, Virginia (today's West Virginia). Seeking rifles and ammunition, and the machinery needed to manufacture them, Colonel Thomas J. (later General "Stonewall") Jackson's forces seized the federal armory. Surrounded by steep hills, ledges, and heights on all sides, Harpers Ferry was difficult to defend, and Jackson planned to leave as soon as the armory's tools and machinery could be dismantled and shipped south to Richmond and Fayetteville, North Carolina. As the work progressed, however, a significant number of soldiers among Jackson's forces, many of them from isolated rural towns and villages, fell sick from mumps, measles, and other communicable diseases.[35]

The Central House responded quickly, sending Matilda Coskery and two other Daughters. "[We] left [Emmitsburg] by stage . . . with a good outfit of prudence and caution," Coskery wrote in her account of the events at Harpers Ferry and later Winchester, Virginia. Traveling south through Maryland, "Southern pickets" appeared, seeking the Daughters' "intention," Coskery related. They were allowed to proceed, though the "passports" announcing their arrival had not yet reached these distant "outposts." Traversing the bridge at the Potomac River into Virginia, they noticed that "kegs of powder were placed here and there so that in case the Northern Army approached, [the bridge] could be instantly" destroyed, Coskery continued.

After reaching Harpers Ferry, Confederate officers took the Daughters to a makeshift hospital where they immediately set to work, tending to soldiers with "measles, sore throat, fever, and pneumonia."[36]

The three Daughters were not in Harpers Ferry very long "when suddenly [a] telegraph dispatch ordered everyone to leave." A Union force was advancing, and the retreating Confederate forces burned everything "they could not take" and blew up the bridge. With great difficulty, the Daughters made their way to Winchester, "about 30 or 40 miles distant," Coskery stated. Three days passed before they took charge of a hospital. Supplies of food and medicine were "of the roughest kind. The whole Town seemed to be but one family of men and as silent as death. Scarcely a female was to be seen," Coskery noted. The "lack of nourishment" and the relentless work took a toll on the Daughters, she asserted. They needed reinforcements, but they could not get word to Emmitsburg.

Desperate for help, Coskery returned to Emmitsburg with great difficulty, taking a cart, then a stage, and "crossing the Potomac in a kind of flat canoe."[37] Learning of the Daughters' plight in Winchester, the Central House dispatched three more sisters. The Winchester contingent, now "[six] in number[,] continued to labor . . . until the sick were either cured or dead." When there were only about a dozen soldiers left in the hospital, the Daughters told the doctors that they were needed in Richmond. At first the "Doctors said no," but they later "consented."[38]

New Orleans and Corinth, Mississippi, August 1861 to April 1862

Farther south in New Orleans, the Daughters struggled to maintain communication with the Central House in Emmitsburg. In April 1861, Union ships blockaded Confederate ports where the Daughters were working, including New Orleans, Mobile, Norfolk, and Portsmouth. The strategy, known as the Anaconda Plan, was to strangle the South into submission. But the blockade took several months after it began to substantially weaken Confederate commerce. The Union navy was not large enough and the South's coastline too vast and intricate (numerous barrier islands, shallow shoals, and narrow passages made navigation difficult) to prevent small ships from getting past the blockade.[39] Scoffing at the North's "feeble" attempt, an August 1861 editorial in the New Orleans' *Times-Picayune* stated,

"They have had it for three months, and they have got too much of it. By land and by water it is the worst of failures—a self-confessed blunder."[40]

Notwithstanding the newspaper's bluster, the blockade had a noticeable effect. From the month of June 1861, "we began to feel the results of the blockade," Sister Regina Smith, DC, wrote from Charity Hospital, where she was the administrator.[41] Communication between New Orleans and Emmitsburg had virtually stopped by midsummer. Because of the difficulties in communication, Mother Norris dispatched Sister Euphemia Blenkinsop, DC, her assistant, with instructions to report on the activities of the Southern missions. On November 3, 1861, Blenkinsop departed Emmitsburg for Richmond.[42] After a "short" stay in Richmond, she traveled to Pensacola, Mobile, and Natchez, arriving in New Orleans for Christmas.[43] Blenkinsop remained in New Orleans for the "Christmas holidays," leaving at the beginning of the New Year. "It was well" that she left when she did, one of the Daughters recounted, "for had she lingered in the far South until Spring, she would have found herself separated from her charge of the Southern missions."[44] On April 25, 1862, Union forces captured the "Cresent City."

The fall of New Orleans occurred three weeks after the Battle of Shiloh, an important Union victory. Located on the Tennessee side of the state line bordering Mississippi, Shiloh was among the war's bloodiest battles. Union casualties exceeded thirteen thousand, while Confederate losses surpassed ten thousand.[45] On April 9, 1862, soon after learning of the carnage, Smith sent five Daughters from New Orleans to Corinth, Mississippi, a strategic railroad crossing close to the battlefield. The Confederate army had established field hospitals in Corinth to care for the wounded soldiers. It took the Daughters seven days to reach their destination; under normal circumstances, it should have taken only two. The railroad "cars were densely crowded with passengers of all kinds, soldiers, doctors, nurses and ladies in pursuit of their wounded husbands," Sister Ann Patricia Morgan, DC, reflected.[46]

While the Daughters were in Corinth treating wounded soldiers, the Union navy advanced toward New Orleans. Facing little resistance (most of the soldiers from Louisiana were fighting in Tennessee and Virginia), the navy easily captured New Orleans, and by May 1 an occupying force of fifteen thousand Union soldiers was in the city.[47] The seizure of New Orleans significantly restricted the use of Charity Hospital as a hub for sending Daughters to missions in Confederate-held territory. "All communication was cut off with our Sisters [in] Mobile, Richmond and the temporary hospitals," Smith recounted. We could not contact the Daughters we had sent to Corinth. "At length, we heard indirectly that all had reached Mobile." Somehow, they made it back to New Orleans before early August. "They came just in time, for since" they arrived, Charity Hospital has been "full of wounded federals."[48]

White House Landing, Washington, and Richmond, June to September 1862

As Union forces advanced in the West, the Army of the Potomac under the command of General George McClellan moved on Richmond. Referred to as the Peninsula campaign, the operation began with McClellan massing troops in March 1862 at Fort Monroe, located on the Chesapeake Bay between the York and James Rivers. With one hundred thousand troops in place by May, McClellan began marching toward Richmond. Failing to discern that he had the numerical advantage, McClellan stalled the offensive. When McClellan began advancing again at the end of May, the Confederate army was much stronger.

From the end of May to early July 1862, the Union and Confederate armies fought a series of fierce engagements in the woods and swamps east of Richmond. Going by the names of Fair Oaks (the South referred to it as Seven Pines) and Seven Days, the battles produced huge casualties, about fifty thousand combined, but no clear victories.[49] Unable to advance any farther, McClellan withdrew his forces, establishing encampments or extraction points at Harrison's Landing and White House Landing on the James and Pamunkey Rivers.[50] Large numbers of sick and wounded soldiers gathered at the encampments, waiting for hospital ships or transports to take them to military hospitals.

After receiving an urgent plea on June 17 from Surgeon General Hammond asking for the Daughters' help in the evacuation, the Central House dispatched sixty sisters.[51] At White House Landing, one group of Daughters led by Matilda Coskery took charge of the *Vanderbilt*, a hospital transport, while another contingent boarded the *Commodore*.[52] Once on the transports, the "Sisters shared with their poor patients every horror [save] bodily pains," Coskery reflected. The sick and wounded were "on beds on the floor" of the lower cabins "with only space to stand or kneel between" them. One of the sisters "in charge of [a] lower Ward was so persevering," Coskery wrote, "that even the Dr. declared" that he did not "know how [she] could endure" it.[53]

Several of the transports went to Washington, while others traveled to East Coast cities, such as New York and Baltimore. Washington had no permanent hospitals, save the E Street Infirmary and Providence Hospital, the latter a small general hospital the Daughters owned and operated. Though the military did not take over Providence Hospital (it remained a civilian hospital throughout the course of the war), the hospital admitted as many wounded soldiers as possible. Because space was limited, the army set up tents on the hospital grounds that the Daughters attended.[54]

Needing more space for the wounded soldiers coming from White House Landing and other locations, the Union army opened twenty-two temporary hospitals in Washington and the surrounding area. Twelve of the temporary hospitals were in churches; several others were in hotels, schools, and private homes.[55] Fourteen Daughters tended to sick soldiers at Cliffburn, a converted army barracks. According to army surgeon John Shaw Billings, who worked at Cliffburn, the buildings and grounds were "in an extremely filthy and dilapidated condition."[56] "We have but a plank to shelter us," Sister Helen Ryan, DC, wrote in mid-September. There were "about twelve hundred sick and wounded, tents are [being] constructed to receive those who are continually coming; it is expected that we shall soon have sixteen hundred," she indicated.[57]

The South was in a similar situation when the Confederate wounded arrived from the battlefields east of Richmond. The Confederate army converted "abandoned buildings, warehouses, tobacco factories, and schools" into hospitals.[58] The Daughters worked in three Richmond hospitals—St. Ann's Military Hospital, the Louisiana Hospital, and St. Francis de Sales Infirmary.[59] The military possessed the first two, while the Daughters owned the third. Opened on May 3, 1861, St. Francis de Sales was a fifty-bed facility. One month after it opened, St. Francis de Sales exceeded capacity, housing three hundred soldiers on peak occasions.[60]

On September 27, 1862, almost three months after the Peninsula campaign was over, the Confederate army's medical department took total control of all hospitals housing wounded soldiers. Before that date, private and state-supported facilities provided most of the care in Richmond and elsewhere. The medical department proceeded to shut down several of the private hospitals on the grounds that they were too small and inefficient. Women in charge of private hospitals often became matrons at the military hospitals.[61] Hospital inspector William Carrington supervised the closures in Richmond. Though he closed most of the private Richmond hospitals or placed them under military control, Carrington did not shut down the facilities the Daughters owned or operated, observing that "they are most faithful, efficient and tender nurses."[62]

Fredericksburg, Philadelphia, and Washington, June to December 1862

When the Army of the Potomac marched again on Richmond in December 1862, stalling at Fredericksburg, Virginia, the Army Medical Corps' ability to transport medical supplies and wounded soldiers had improved considerably. USSC aid workers and others, such as Clara Barton, were still needed, but the corps now assumed most of the burden.[63] Several of the Daughters confirmed that the system was improving, that the corps was making better use of their expertise as skilled nurses and hospital administrators. Before the Battle of Fredericksburg, the Union army had called them to battlefields, camps, and military hospitals as needed, and rather haphazardly. But when the North evacuated its soldiers at Fredericksburg, the Daughters were caring for the wounded at military hospitals in Washington, Philadelphia, and elsewhere.[64] Writing on October 18, 1862, Sister Camilla Bowden, DC, conveyed an orderly scene at Eckington military hospital in Washington: "We have a great many servants and infirmarians; the Sisters have charge of distributing the medicines, of superintending the wards, and preserving the order and cleanliness, and in general of everything that concerns the welfare of the sick, their food, and the little delicacies for the patients."[65]

Improvements also occurred in the design and construction of military hospitals. Consistent with the growing stress on environment and hygiene, there was a distinct change in hospital architecture. Several of the military hospitals that the Union and Confederate armies constructed utilized a "pavilion style" design, devised to improve the flow of air and its circulation. Pavilion-style hospitals had become popular in Europe at the end of the Crimean War. Florence Nightingale's *Notes on Hospitals* touted the new design, featuring several pavilions or wards branching out from a central core in a hub-and-spoke pattern.[66] Surgeon General Hammond oversaw the planning and construction of the military's pavilion-style hospitals. The first one that Hammond established was Satterlee in West Philadelphia. When complete, Satterlee contained twenty-eight wards, two interconnecting corridors, and an administration building two stories high.[67] Satterlee was "so massive," medical historian Ira Rutkow observed, that its "various structures" covered "more than four acres."[68]

Hammond wanted the Daughters to come to Satterlee even before the hospital was finished. On May 28, 1862, he requested twenty-five Daughters. The initial group, numbering twenty-one, arrived on June 9, 1862. They traveled to Satterlee from all over the country, from Detroit, Buffalo, Rochester, Albany, Baltimore, Troy, and Washington.[69] Sister Gonzaga Grace, DC, was their sister servant. Born in 1812, Grace had served at Charity Hospital in New Orleans and at St Joseph's Orphan Asylum in Philadelphia.[70] Joining her was Chief Surgeon Isaac Israel Hayes. Only thirty years old at the time, Hayes had distinguished himself as an arctic explorer, naturalist, and surveyor.[71] When making hospital rounds, Grace and Hayes were "a strange contrast," remarked one of the Daughters—"the proud Military Officer in full uniform and the humble Daughter of St. Vincent to whom he shows every respect and attention."[72] Between June 9, 1862, and August 3, 1865, a total of ninety-one Daughters served at Satterlee at one time or another. While at Satterlee, they cared for more than eighty thousand sick and wounded soldiers.[73]

Another of the North's large pavilion-style hospitals where the Daughters worked was Point Lookout, Maryland. Constructed in June 1862 and located near the lighthouse at the end of the peninsula, the hospital complex at Point Lookout comprised twenty buildings housing 1,400 beds, "storehouses and stables," "laundry and dining facilities," and facilities for soldiers, doctors, and nurses.[74] Between August and December 1862, Hammond oversaw the construction of five more hospitals, all of them in the vicinity of Washington. The Daughters moved from Cliffburn to Lincoln General Hospital, the last of the five to open. Eventually comprising twenty wards and 2,575 beds, Lincoln was a major improvement over Cliffburn.[75] In addition to Cliffburn and Lincoln, the Daughters cared for Union and Confederate soldiers at two other military hospitals in Washington, Eckington and Stanton. At one time or another, fourteen Daughters were

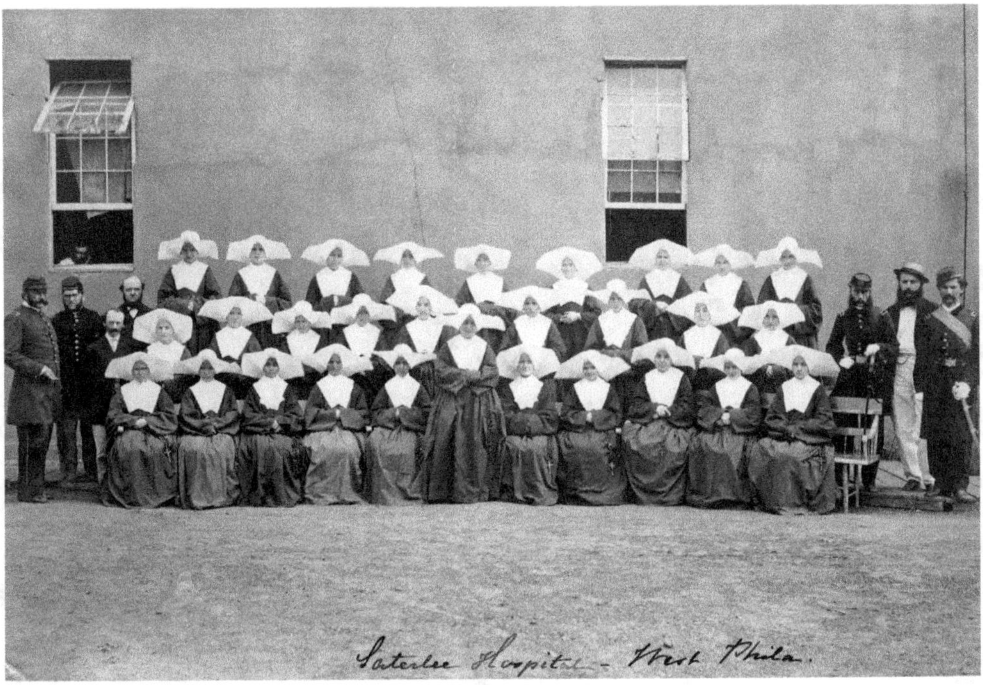

Figure 3.1. Daughters at Satterlee Hospital, West Philadelphia, PA, 1862.

at Cliffburn, eight were at Eckington, ten were at Stanton, and thirty were at Lincoln.[76]

Gettysburg, June 27 to July 5, 1863

Except for Confederate General Robert E. Lee's brief foray into Maryland, culminating in the Battle of Antietam, most of the battles during the war's first two years were fought on Virginia soil. Though outnumbered and outsupplied, Lee's army repeatedly repulsed Union advances. After the South's victory at Chancellorsville in early May 1863, Lee once again drove his forces across the Potomac. Virginians needed a respite from the interminable war, Lee determined, and Pennsylvania's resources and farmlands were inviting. Meanwhile, the dispirited Union army under the command of General Joseph Hooker moved in an "arc" northward from Washington. On June 27, Hooker resigned, and on June 28, General George G. Meade took charge of the Army of the Potomac.[77]

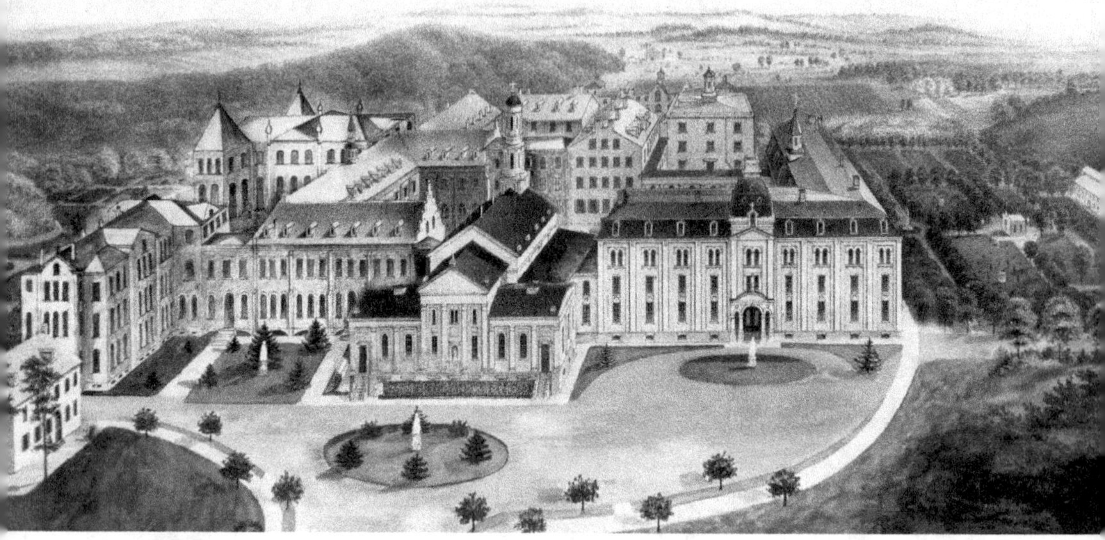

Figure 3.2. St. Joseph's Central House and St. Joseph's Academy, Emmitsburg, MD, ca. 1890s.

Lee's forces converged on Gettysburg from the north and west while Meade's forces came from the south and east. The Daughters' motherhouse in Emmitsburg was in Meade's path. Soldiers began to arrive at Emmitsburg on Saturday night, June 27. Aroused from her bedchamber, Mother Norris dressed quickly and climbed the stairs to the observatory, where other Daughters had already assembled. From the top of the observatory, they had a commanding view of St. Joseph's Valley. Though the night was dark, Norris could see the lights and make out the sounds of horses, wagons, and artillery. By the next morning, the immense size of the undertaking had become clearer. Over the course of the next three days, additional divisions and regiments encamped in the surrounding fields, exacting a significant toll on the Daughters' property. "The field opposite [St. Lazare's] was in fine clover at sunset Saturday, but when the sun rose on Sunday was barren and bare as a board," Sister Marie Louise Caulfield, DC, recounted.[78]

After the Union soldiers decamped and marched northward on July 1, the Daughters spent the next three days at St. Joseph's listening to the sounds of the cannons. Sister Camilla O'Keefe, DC, reflected on the course of events: "About noon on the first of July we heard very distinctly, the cannonading, *Boom! Boom!* So terrific, this kept on until the afternoon of the 4th, when the Confederates were defeated and retreated away as fast as they could that night. On Sunday morning the 5th July, some poor struggling Confederates came down [to St. Joseph's]. They told us that the battle ended late the evening before."

The Daughters moved as quickly as possible toward Gettysburg to aid the stricken soldiers. Maimed and injured soldiers filled Gettysburg's homes and buildings, requisitioned as makeshift field hospitals. At Penn Hall, the main building on the local college campus (today's Gettysburg College), four Daughters tended to six hundred wounded. We "could only take time to dress their wounds for surgeons were too scarce every place," wrote one of the four Daughters. Upon returning to the college each morning, there were "eight or ten bodies . . . at the entrance for interment."[79] At St. Francis Xavier Church, two Daughters assisted army surgeon William F. Norris. There was barely space to walk, one of them recounted. The wounded "lay in the sanctuary, in the gallery, on the pew seats, under the seats, [and] in the aisles." The floor was "constantly wet under our feet [with the] blood and bathing of their wounds." The smells were horrible. "Previous hardships had left [the soldiers] ragged and dirty and, added to these, were vermin and corruption, maggots, and stanch." On top of this, "gangrenous wounds had [begun] to infect all the air. . . . [B]loody water . . . ooze[d] up" from the chests of those shot through the lungs, "the foul atmosphere thickening by every respiration."[80]

At Gettysburg Courthouse, where more wounded men lay, a Daughter attempted to treat a soldier who had been diagnosed with "lock-jaw." Though the attending physician said he would surely die, the Daughter continued to nurse him. She administered "a mild opiate," which she "repeated at certain intervals." She also "plac[ed] a kind, trusty man by" the wounded soldier's side, and told him that he was "to keep his face, especially his jaws, cheeks, neck and face constantly warmed by applying hot sponges." To the doctor's "great surprise," the soldier recovered. Another wounded soldier, having witnessed the event, called for the Daughter's assistance. The doctors had informed him that in order to survive he needed an amputation. She told "the man he had better take courage," baptized him, and placed "a medal . . . on his breast."[81] He too survived.

Over 150,000 soldiers fought at Gettysburg—about 82,000 wore the blue uniform, another 75,000 wore the grey. Battlefield casualties exceeded 50,000 (approximately 7,000 dead, 33,000 wounded, and 11,000 missing), about one-third of those involved. Almost one hundred Daughters came to Gettysburg in the days and months following the battle. Some stayed for a few days or weeks, while others remained for several months or until the last of the wounded recovered.[82]

Vicksburg to Appomattox, April 1863 to April 1865

At Vicksburg, Mississippi, another important battle was unfolding. Taking Vicksburg was "key" to Union victory, President Lincoln and his generals determined. Dislodging Confederate forces from Vicksburg would be very difficult, however. From Vicksburg's heights atop a two-hundred-foot bluff at a hairpin turn on the Mississippi River, Confederate cannons repulsed Union gunboats. In order to take Vicksburg, Northern commanders devised a joint water and land strategy. In November 1862, General Ulysses S. Grant, commander of the Union army in the West, began marching toward Vicksburg, eventually taking positions to the west and south of the city. Concurrently, Union gunboats concentrated their weapons on less fortified towns south of Vicksburg on the Mississippi River, including Donaldsonville, Louisiana, and Natchez, Mississippi.[83]

The Daughters had missions in both Donaldsonville and Natchez (the Sisters of Mercy were at Vicksburg). Gunboats spared the Daughters' orphanage at Natchez but not at Donaldsonville. "Miraculous[ly]," the orphanage at Donaldsonville remained standing after the first attack. "We have been told that not a house remains except the church and the dwelling of the Sisters and the [Vincentian] Missionaries," wrote Sister Regina Smith, DC. Threatened with a second bombardment, the Daughters left Donaldsonville, seeking refuge several miles away with another community of Catholic sisters. Thinking that they would be safer "in the city than in the countryside," Smith implored them to come to New Orleans. But the Daughters stayed. "It is so hard to travel during these times," Smith acknowledged, "that if they do make up their mind to come, I hardly know how they will manage it."[84]

Following a forty-seven-day siege, Vicksburg fell on July 4, 1863. Several months later, on March 12, 1864, President Lincoln gave Grant command of the entire Union army. Grant moved on Richmond in summer

1864, determined to avoid the mistakes of his predecessors. After several pitched battles north of Richmond produced no clear victories and large numbers of casualties, Grant turned his forces east and south of the Confederate capital and advanced toward Petersburg, a strategic railroad junction. The siege of Petersburg lasted ten months, from June 1864 to April 1865.[85] Though Lee escaped following his eventual defeat, he could not evade the Union army. Surrounded, Lee surrendered at Appomattox Court House on April 9, 1865.

The Daughters were not with Grant or other Union generals during the final stages of the war. Instead, they nursed wounded soldiers at well-equipped military hospitals miles away from the conflict.[86] After the war ended, the Daughters resumed their daily activities. Despite the war's costs (sixty-two Daughters died during the struggle), the community expanded. The Daughters opened two new hospitals while the war was ongoing, Providence in Washington and Carney in Boston. Though the future looked promising, the healthcare environment would soon change considerably. Medical discoveries in the succeeding decades would enable doctors to perform surgery more safely and effectively and control the spread of diseases.

THE SPANISH-AMERICAN WAR

Unlike the Civil War, the Spanish-American War was relatively short-lived, lasting only four months. Despite advances in medical science, most of them occurring in Europe in the final decades of the nineteenth century, many of the problems experienced in the Civil War persisted. Historical accounts of the Spanish-American War and other conflicts typically highlight battlefield casualties. Yet battlefield casualties were often small compared to germ-related deaths and diseases. Many of those in charge of the war knew before it started that the main threat to American lives was not the Spanish forces but instead the dreaded yellow fever and other diseases such as malaria, dysentery, and typhoid.[87]

It was not on Cuban soil that most soldiers fell sick and perished; rather, it was in US army camps and field hospitals where large numbers of volunteer soldiers had congregated for deployment. Of the two hundred thousand volunteers, about thirty-five thousand, or less than 18 percent, went to Cuba or Puerto Rico. The rest remained in the army camps until the war was over, marching, drilling, and training. During the month of May, about 7 percent of those in the camps were reported sick, but by early August, the number had reached 53,705, or well over 25 percent.[88]

When the United States declared war against Spain on April 20, 1898, the army employed only 520 hospital corpsmen and 103 stewards. As occurred at the beginning of the Civil War, men and women rushed to volunteer their services. But once again, there was no established organization or means in place for selecting and screening nurses.[89] Learning of the need for qualified nurses, Dr. Anita Newcomb McGee, a graduate of Columbian University Medical School (later George Washington University), formed a special committee of the Daughters of the American Revolution (DAR), of which she was a member, and prevailed on the army's surgeon general, George M. Sternberg, to have her committee conduct the screening.[90] Sternberg agreed and assigned McGee to head the effort. On August 29, McGee became acting assistant surgeon general of the US Army.[91] Members of the American Red Cross, which had been involved in various relief efforts since the association's founding, including the 1889 Johnstown, Pennsylvania, flood disaster, chaffed at the surgeon general's selection.[92]

While Red Cross members and Sternberg's office were attempting to resolve their differences, McGee and her staff proceeded to screen applicants. "As many as sixty women at [the DAR's] office in Washington" were involved in the effort, the *Brooklyn Daily Eagle* reported.[93] Seeking to recruit the Daughters, McGee assigned Eleanor Dorsey, a writer for *Vanity Fair* and the *Chicago Tribune*, to head the effort.[94] Working closely with Sternberg's office, Dorsey secured the Daughters' services and arranged for their deployment to army camps and field hospitals. In early August, at the outset of the Daughters' deployment, Dorsey and Mother Marianna Flynn, DC, met with President McKinley at the White House. According to a newspaper account of the meeting, McKinley told Flynn "that he remembered the services the [Daughters] had rendered during the civil war, and was glad to welcome them back to the army."[95] By August 24, 1898, ninety-four Daughters were at army camps and field hospitals caring for sick and wounded soldiers.[96]

Camp Wickoff, Montauk Point, Long Island

Among the Daughters' initial assignments was the evacuation of sick and wounded soldiers at Santiago, Cuba. Five Daughters sailed from New York

City on August 11; another seven left from Tampa a few days later. All twelve were "immunes," which meant that they were resistant to yellow fever. Soon after the twelve Daughters arrived in Santiago, General Leonard Wood, later installed as Cuba's military governor, ordered them back to the United States on the hospital ship *Yale* with 1,300 sick soldiers. Their destination was a facility in the early stages of construction, known as Camp Wickoff, situated on Montauk Point, Long Island.[97] Located 125 miles from New York City, Montauk Point was isolated yet accessible to transports returning from Cuba. Over the course of three months, almost twenty-two thousand soldiers, most of them involved in the Santiago campaign, passed through Camp Wickoff.[98]

Despite the favorable terrain—"the place is healthful and during the summer cool and comfortable," a government report indicated—there were scant facilities to house, feed, and care for the sick and wounded when the first of the transports arrived from Santiago on August 7.[99] The situation was not much better on August 25 when the twelve Daughters aboard the *Yale* disembarked at Montauk. Because of the lack of cots, many soldiers slept on the floor weeks after the camp opened.[100]

Sister Adelaide D'Aunoy, DC, was the sister servant at Camp Wickoff. Described as a "most experienced nurse" in the newspapers, D'Aunoy had served at Hôtel Dieu and St. Simeon's School in New Orleans, the latter for fourteen years as its superior.[101] D'Aunoy and the other Daughters assisted in the hasty preparations, "putting up" tents and cots for the sick soldiers.[102] The situation was chaotic. "Our camp is being enlarged every day," D'Aunoy reported at the end of August.[103] The Daughters oversaw the "annex hospital," a misleading designation since it quickly exceeded the size of the main hospital. They also managed wards A and B of the main hospital, each ward containing "about forty-eight [soldiers]."[104]

Many of the soldiers were in poor physical condition when they emerged from the transports. "Some of [the men] are actually dying of starvation," Sister Blanche Hooper, DC, wrote to the Central House in Emmitsburg.[105] I could "scarcely . . . recognize" some of my parishioners, their "features distorted with pain . . . half naked and half famished," a priest from Boston told a correspondent from a local newspaper.[106] Chief surgeon Nicholas Senn forecast an outbreak of typhoid fever should the troops remain at Montauk much longer.[107] "Unless this camp is broken up within six weeks," Senn told reporters on August 31, "I predict that it will . . . rank with the infamous pest holes of the civil war."[108]

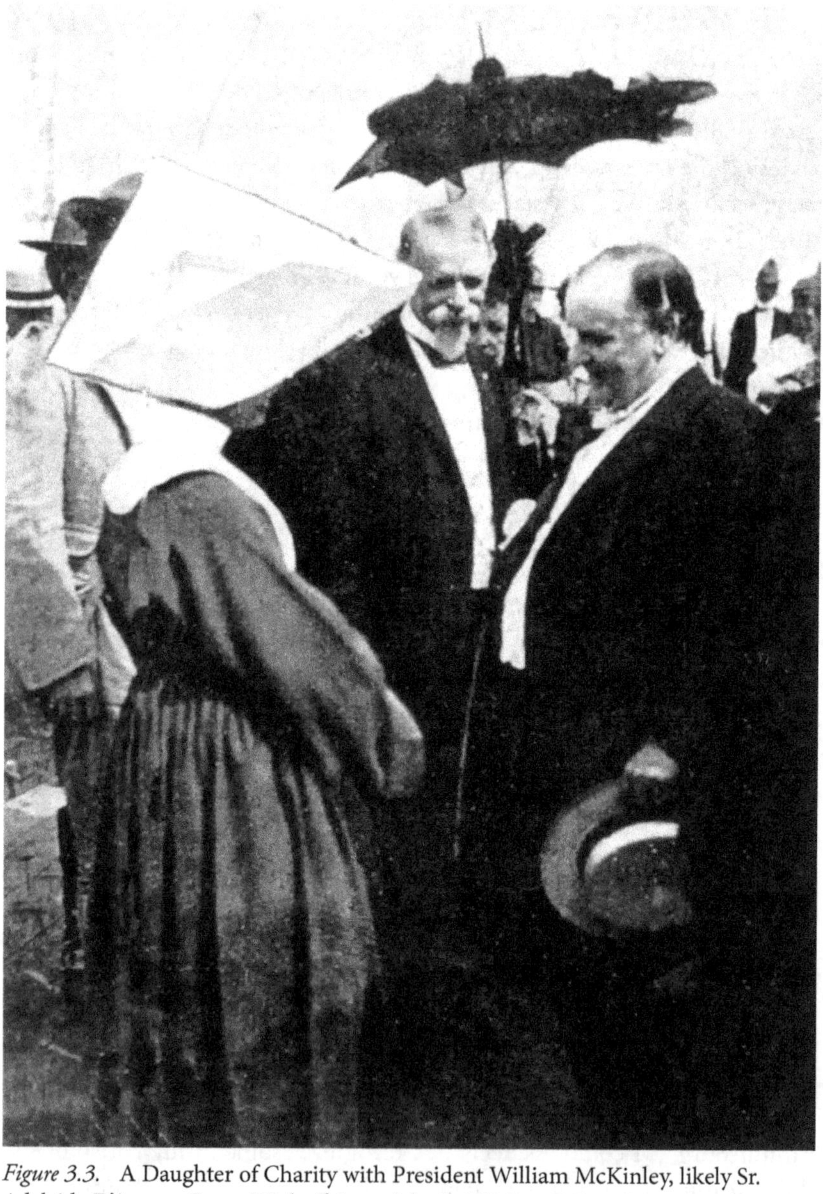

Figure 3.3. A Daughter of Charity with President William McKinley, likely Sr. Adelaide D'Aunoy, Camp Wickoff, Long Island, NY, September 10, 1898.

On September 2, President McKinley visited Camp Wickoff. The inspection tour was not on his original itinerary, but he wanted to "inform himself [if] the [adverse] reports . . . were accurate."[109] Accompanied by Secretary Alger and other dignitaries, McKinley visited several wards, met with D'Aunoy, and queried the officer in charge about the camp's "water supply" and sanitation.[110] Following his inspection, McKinley announced that he was "satisfied" with the conditions. But his actions belied his verbal assessment. He issued orders that the regular troops return to their posts "with the least possible delay" and that the volunteers be furloughed "as soon as possible."[111]

Camp Thomas, Chickamauga Park, Georgia

When President McKinley was at Camp Wickoff, typhoid was already raging in many of the camps where most of the volunteer soldiers had mustered while awaiting orders to go to Cuba, Puerto Rico, or the Philippines. Before the war ended, over twenty thousand troops or one-fifth of those at army camps contracted typhoid, and more than 1,500 perished, making typhoid the principal cause of wartime losses.[112] Created by the War Department on August 18, 1898, the Typhoid Board, consisting of three army surgeons with Dr. Walter Reed in charge, investigated the matter. Reed and his colleagues traveled to several army camps, gathering evidence.[113]

The board's preliminary findings, announced in May 1899 (the full report was not published until five years later), disclosed "myriad" sources of infection—"sub-surface privy pits that frequently flooded," "latrine-visiting flies" that "alight[ed] on people, their food, and their possessions," asymptomatic soldiers who carried the pathogen from one location to another, and sick persons in surrounding towns and villages.[114] The worst of the camps was Camp George H. Thomas, located at Chickamauga Park, Georgia, the site of the famous Civil War battle. Regular soldiers began arriving at Camp Thomas in mid-April, volunteers a month later. Most of the regulars left for Cuba in early May, but the volunteers kept coming. At the end of June, the camp housed 58,548 soldiers from several states and the District of Columbia.[115]

Early indications were that everything was fine at Chickamauga. Newspapers reported that the volunteers were acclimating to the hot environment, that they were pursuing their drills with "great energy, accuracy, and remarkable precision."[116] But in early July, the weather changed abruptly. "Heavy rains" turned the hot, dry ground into mud, causing the nearby "sinks . . . carrying . . . fecal matter" to overflow.[117] By mid-July, there were reports of a typhoid fever outbreak. Writing from Camp Thomas on August 5, Father Chrysostom Schreiner, a Catholic priest, told the *Brooklyn Daily Eagle* that "there is a great deal of malaria and typhoid" and that most hospitals lacked basic supplies and were "overcrowded."[118] On August 6 and 7, Red Cross officials visited Chickamauga. They noted that there were over 1,200 sick soldiers, 300 with typhoid, far more than the general and division hospitals could handle.[119]

Upon their arrival in late August, the Daughters seemed optimistic. There were "about five hundred cases of typhoid," but things "were improving," one of the Daughters indicated.[120] Yet only a few days later, their assessment was completely different. "The surroundings at the Hospital are simply horrible," Sister Stella Boyle, DC, informed Mother Flynn in her September 3 letter. Several Daughters were "not well," she stated.[121] Though Boyle indicated that the Daughters suffered from "sick stomachs and dysentery," many of them had typhoid.[122] All told, four Daughters perished from typhoid at the various army encampments.[123]

Not long after the Daughters arrived, the army took steps to close Camp Thomas, starting with the furlough of volunteers, as President McKinley had instructed. Issued in late August, the orders called for their immediate departure. But the deployment of troops did not happen fast enough to staunch the public outcry once the newspapers revealed the poor conditions at Chickamauga.[124] Many of the sick soldiers who left Chickamauga went to army camps at Knoxville, Tennessee, and Lexington, Kentucky, to recover. Several Daughters followed weeks later. On September 21, twenty Daughters left Chickamauga for Knoxville (Camp Poland), and on September 26, another twenty-five departed Chickamauga for Lexington (Camp Hamilton).[125] The conditions at Knoxville and Lexington were much better than Chickamauga, the "result of dearly bought and consequently appreciated experience," an army investigation of the conditions in the camps later determined.[126] But what happened at Chickamauga was not easily forgotten—nor forgiven. "The boys here blame Chickamauga for everything," Sister Teresa Carlin, DC, reported from Camp Poland on October 11.[127]

On September 24, 1898, President McKinley formed a commission under the leadership of Grenville M. Dodge, a railroad engineer and former brigadier general in the Union army, to look into the matter.[128] From October to December 1898, the Dodge Commission took testimony from 495 witnesses at seventeen different locations and visited nine army camps and field hospitals.[129] The commission's report, issued on February 9, 1899, while exonerating several department officials, found a significant number of deficiencies. The deficiencies included inadequate numbers of skilled doctors and nurses, the lack of medical supplies, and poor sanitation connected to an "epidemic" of typhoid fever.[130] The commission offered several recommendations for future action. Among the recommendations was the need for more women nurses. It is with "much regret," the commission stated, that army officers failed to "fully realize . . . when the war commenced" the value of "well-trained women nurses." Congress, the commission advised, should establish "a reserve corps of selected trained women nurses, ready to serve when necessity [requires]."[131]

WORLD WAR I

World War I marked a turning point in the Daughters' wartime service. Only twenty years earlier, in the Spanish-American War, the Daughters worked as head nurses, administrators, and organizers of numerous field and emergency hospitals. But by World War I, the American Red Cross (ARC) had emerged as the principal entity responsible for organizing humanitarian relief at the national level, subsuming the relief efforts of other charitable groups and organizations such as the Daughters. Still, the Red Cross had to rely chiefly on voluntary facilities for the delivery of healthcare services. ARC did not own any hospitals.

The transformation of the hospital in the early twentieth century from a chronic- to an acute-care facility replete with surgical suites, X-ray machines, laboratory equipment, and a professionally trained staff of doctors, nurses, and technicians was a remarkable feat of organization and scientific ingenuity. In less than twenty years, US healthcare progressed from a marginally skilled and disjointed enterprise into a generally well-planned, specialized, and integrated operation. Despite these advances, the US military lacked the means on its own to transfer these innovations to the combat setting. Some mechanism was needed to bring emergency medicine and surgical techniques performed in the best hospitals to the front lines of the war in Europe. The principal mechanism that policy planners developed was the base hospital unit, a joint public-private undertaking.

Army specifications for establishing a base hospital unit called for a sponsoring entity (typically an academic medical center comprising a medical school and an associated teaching hospital) to enter into a contract with the Red Cross for the formation of a five-hundred-bed (later one-thousand-bed) facility.[132] The number of nurses in a base hospital unit, according to the specifications, was one hundred, while the number of doctors was fifty.[133] The director of a base hospital unit, typically a leading physician, appointed a chief nurse, who then chose the other ninety-nine nurses. While the chief nurse could use her discretion, the nurses she selected had to meet certain criteria, including graduation from a recognized school of nursing. Experience and specialized skills were also important. Each base hospital unit needed assistant chief nurses, charge nurses, operating-room nurses, dietitians, and contagious disease specialists. Those chosen became members of the Army Nurse Corps and donned a Red Cross uniform.[134]

Though ARC provided much of the equipment and supplies for base hospitals—beds, linens, drugs, uniforms, sterilizers, ambulances, kitchen facilities, and more—the investment in personnel and resources that sponsors had to make was substantial. Not surprisingly, the largest and most prestigious medical schools and their associated teaching hospitals were best suited for establishing a base hospital unit. Sponsoring hospitals included Bellevue, Presbyterian, and Mount Sinai in New York City, Massachusetts General and Boston City Hospital, Lakeside Hospital in Cleveland, Pennsylvania Hospital in Philadelphia, and Johns Hopkins Hospital in Baltimore.

Few, if any, of the smaller hospitals, such as the ones the Daughters owned and administered, could muster sufficient resources to form a base hospital unit. Seeking to encourage medium-sized and smaller hospitals to join the effort, the Army Medical Department eventually allowed for "smaller units about one-half the size of a base hospital." Still, the resources required were too much for most of the smaller hospitals. Only nineteen hospitals sponsored smaller units, many of them also the products of large university systems.[135]

The Daughters, as it turned out, were the only Catholic sisters to participate in World War I as part of a base hospital unit.[136] Because large numbers of Catholic sisters previously had functioned as wartime nurses, many people questioned why so few were selected. Catholic newspapers fueled rumors that the Red Cross was discriminating against them.[137] But this was not why so few went to Europe. Rather, the principal barrier to greater involvement was the criteria for forming a base hospital unit and the process for selecting nurses. Assembling a base hospital unit of one thousand beds or even five hundred for oversees deployment required more resources than most Catholic hospitals could muster.

The reason the Daughters went to Europe was because New Orleans surgeon Joseph A. Danna organized a base hospital unit and asked them to join it. Having worked beside several of the Daughters at Charity Hospital, Danna eagerly sought their services. Danna initially requested six Daughters, eventually securing ten.[138] The ten Daughters selected were seasoned veterans, "the best the Community had to offer," wrote Sister Catherine O'Rourke, DC, in her account of the Daughters' experiences in Northern Italy.[139] On January 8, 1918, the army and the Red Cross accepted Danna's offer to form a base hospital unit and appointed him director. The official army designation was Base Hospital Unit No. 102, often referred to as the "Loyola Unit" after the name of its sponsor, Loyola University.

The Loyola Unit was assigned to the 332nd Infantry Regiment of the American Expeditionary Forces located in Northern Italy. Danna chose Sister Chrysostom Moynahan, DC, an 1894 graduate of Carney Hospital's nursing school, to oversee the nurses. The other nine Daughters served in various management positions—as assistant chief nurse or head nurse of a particular ward or department. Most of the ninety lay nurses who accompanied the Daughters were graduates of nursing schools at the Daughters' hospitals.[140]

The Daughters' fourteen-day ocean voyage from Baltimore to Italy by way of Gibraltar on the Italian steamer *Umbria* was eventful. Fearing an attack from a German U-boat, the Daughters had to wear life preservers and, if needed, put on an "all-rubber suit" over their habit "within the time limit of one minute." The "all-rubber suit" proved to be quite difficult. During training exercises on the *Umbria*, "the cornette had to be removed, and the habit skirt slid [with great difficulty] into the rubber garment," O'Rourke recounted.[141]

After arriving in Gibraltar, the Daughters sailed to Genoa, disembarking on August 27 and staying several days before departing for their base hospital unit in Vicenza, almost forty miles west of Venice. Once in Vicenza, they took over an industrial school the Italians had converted into a military hospital. They were close to the field of battle. "As I am sitting here," Sister Angela Drendle, DC, wrote in her diary, "I can hear the roaring of the large guns at the Front. The nearest point of the Austrian line is only 12 miles from here."[142] "If the Austrians had crossed the Piave [River]," Sister Mary Catherine Coleman, DC, reflected, "they could have reached us in less than an hour."[143]

The fighting in Northern Italy began more than three years before the Americans arrived, ever since the Italians had declared war on Austria-Hungary on May 23, 1915. Neither the Italians nor the Austrians won a significant battle until six German divisions joined the Austrians in October 1917 and launched a major offensive. By mid-November, the Austrians and Germans were on the Piave River, about twenty miles north of Venice, having pushed the Italians back over 150 kilometers. Unable to advance any farther after British and French soldiers came to the aid of the Italians, the German divisions returned to the Western Front, leaving the Austrians to defend the newly seized territory.[144]

Before the 332nd Infantry Regiment went to Italy, American troops had been fighting German forces in France and Belgium. Notwithstanding its small size, less than four thousand soldiers, the 332nd played an important role in the allied counteroffensive, known as the Battle of Vittorio Veneto.[145] The regiment's principal contribution was to trick the Austrians into believing that the American force was much larger. Instigating the deception, Colonel William Wallace split the regiment into several groups wearing dissimilar headgear and had them march "in double file, not in squad formation," along several roads in different directions. Convinced that the Americans had as many as six divisions or almost three hundred thousand soldiers, the Austrians "hastily retreated" soon after the battle started, stopping to blow up bridges rather than mount a stiff resistance. On November 4, 1918, one month after the counteroffensive began, the Italians and the Austrians signed an armistice.[146]

During the seven months that the Daughters were in Vicenza, from September 1918 to March 1919, they cared for about three thousand sick and wounded soldiers—Americans, Italians, and British.[147] On the eve of the Battle of Vittorio Veneto, the Daughters were busy treating about four hundred patients with flu-like symptoms.[148] The addition of large numbers of wounded soldiers proved almost too much for the base hospital to handle.

There was "great excitement" when the battle began, Sister Florence Means, DC, stated—"Three operations in one night. Ninety-six cases admitted."[149] Only a few days later, however, the excitement had diminished, and the search for new quarters to house the sick and wounded had begun in earnest. "Everything is crowded," Means reported. We are having "great difficulty . . . moving between cots to do the dressings of the wounded."[150] Many of the flu-stricken soldiers were sent to a converted orphanage, but by the end of November, the orphanage also was overcrowded. When I "went on night duty" on December 1, Drendle wrote in her diary, "nearly every bed [was] filled." There were "220 patients in in the Hospital—About 210 suffering with Spanish Influenza."[151]

At the end of December, the flow of patients had greatly diminished. "We still have many [influenza] cases but [they aren't] increasing," Means indicated.[152] Wards closed and several nurses took furloughs.[153] The patient load increased again in mid-January when the Italians, French, and British closed their nearby hospitals and sent their surgical and convalescent patients to Vicenza. We "have reopened our Wards," Coleman related. The hospitals remained "very busy" through the month of February, but the "new patients coming in from the [other] hospitals . . . were not very sick," Coleman stated.[154] By early March, "the patients [were] leaving in large numbers," and plans were in place for the closure of the converted orphanage on March 9 and the main hospital a week later.[155]

The return trip to America was less eventful than the crossing to Italy. Upon the Daughters' arrival in New York City on April 15, 1919, Red Cross ambulances drove them to a clinic for their physical examinations. From New York, they traveled to Emmitsburg, where Mother Margaret O'Keefe, DC, was there to greet them. While in Emmitsburg, they learned of the devastating effects of the flu pandemic on the American population.[156]

THE 1918 FLU PANDEMIC

Far from obsolete at the end of World War I, the Daughters' nursing skills were greatly needed during the influenza pandemic that spread across America and Europe in 1918, killing by some estimates over thirty million people.[157] Because neither the knowledge nor the technology existed, doctors were unable to isolate the virus responsible for the 1918 outbreak. Many of the important discoveries and techniques related to the imaging of viruses and the determination of their essential characteristics did not begin to develop until the mid-1900s.[158] Public health workers could not mount an effective campaign to address the disease's spread and the social dislocations occurring from it. As the death toll mounted along with the number of orphaned children, the Daughters labored in hospitals, orphanages, schools, and the homes of sick families. Many Daughters fell ill and died from the influenza, just as they did while treating people with cholera, typhoid, and other infectious diseases.[159]

The disease passed through three stages as the virus mutated. It began with a mild outbreak at US army camps in spring 1918. As the infected soldiers traveled from one place to another, the disease spread throughout much of the country, crossed the Atlantic Ocean with American troops in April, and then struck British and German forces fighting on the Western Front two months later. The virus then became dormant before appearing again in more virulent form at the Commonwealth Pier in Boston on August 27. By mid-September, about 20 percent of the soldiers at Camp Devens near Boston were seriously ill and in the hospital. From Boston, sailors carried the disease to several US port cities, including New Orleans and Philadelphia. The greatest number of cases appeared in October, but by mid-November, the second phase was over. Once again, the virus mutated, emerging for the third and last time during the months of December and January.[160]

Throughout the flu pandemic, the Daughters struggled to care for fever-stricken persons in their hospitals, schools, and orphanages. Conditions at Carney Hospital were "appalling," Sister Raphael Jones, DC, reported in early October. "U.S. Navy Patients, U.S. Army Patients and civic patients have been coming in day and night," she stated.[161] Carney was without Dr. Thomas F. Leen, its chief physician. Leen had died on September 16 after contracting the virus while treating the first patients.[162] Many of the children were also sick in Boston's schools and orphanages. At St. Vincent's Orphan Asylum on Camden Street in South Boston, thirty children contracted the illness. Two of them died, the head sister reported on October 11.[163] "We never had such a siege of sickness before," wrote one of the Daughters from Boston's Home for Destitute Children. "The Sisters [have] been so sick and miserable [that] nearly every one [has] had a turn in bed," she stated.[164]

The situation was even worse in Philadelphia. By mid-October, the death toll in Philadelphia exceeded that of any other city.[165] The mayor's office failed to respond quickly and effectively, Howard Anders, a prominent Philadelphia physician, claimed in a letter to the *Philadelphia Public Ledger*. "We knew . . . that . . . influenza was prevalent among the boys of the army and navy, in cantonments and in barracks," Anders stated, "but the authorities pooh-poohed the idea that the civilian population would be attacked, and virtually no preventive steps were taken."[166] Approximately two thousand Catholic sisters from the Philadelphia area, many of them teachers and day-care workers, volunteered their services.[167] Emergency hospitals opened throughout the city, but there were not enough trained nurses to staff them. Several of the city's hospitals, including St. Joseph's, where the Daughters were working, were short-handed.[168] "The sick are pouring in all day and all night," the head sister wrote from St. Joseph's Hospital. "We have lost three nurses, one of them was sick only 48 hours. . . . I feel like I have lived in a daze or dream for hundreds of days," she stated.[169]

The virus was so deadly and infectious that there really was no way to stop it, no matter the extent of the efforts made to prevent it from killing and spreading. "Our mortality rate has been high. . . . [S]o far we have registered 100 deaths [out of] 605 cases of Influenza," Sister Clarisse Bresnan, DC, reported from Baltimore's St. Agnes Hospital.[170] "The dead are piled one upon another waiting for burial; it is the most frightful thing that has ever been witnessed," Sister Lizzie Patterson, DC, wrote from Cathedral Day Nursery in Philadelphia.[171] The "death rate is climbing," Sister Blanche Summers, DC, related from Troy Hospital.[172] "Big strong men are dying off like flies. We can do nothing to relieve them," Sister Camilla Campbell, DC, corresponded from Detroit's St. Mary's Hospital.[173] The deaths of so many young parents greatly increased the number of orphans. Boston's Home for Destitute Children had "a full house" by mid-October with the addition of one hundred newly orphaned children. "There are so many children left without parents," the sister superior wrote from Detroit's St. Vincent's Asylum. In "one family," the mother and father "left ten children," she lamented.[174]

Stretched thin because so many nurses were serving in Europe, the Red Cross turned to the Daughters for assistance on several occasions. In Boston, local ARC officials contacted Sister Raphael Jones, DC, the sister servant at Carney Hospital, on September 27. They wanted her to assume control of district nursing in South Boston. Ready and willing to help, Jones engaged twelve Daughters and two lay nurses and soon had them visiting the homes of sick persons and their families. "What awful conditions they are meeting in the tenements," Jones wrote in her journal. There are "two [or] three families in the same house, all ill, death visiting many."[175] At Jackson Barracks in New Orleans, there were too many sick soldiers for the attending Red Cross nurses to handle—approximately eight hundred patients, many at an advanced stage with pneumonia. On October 9, the head nurse at Jackson Barracks reached out to the Daughters. As soon as arrangements could be made, twelve Daughters left Charity Hospital for Jackson Barracks, where they stayed until November 7.[176] Local Red Cross chapters also called on the Daughters for assistance at other army encampments, including Camp Dick near Dallas, Camp McArthur close by Waco, Camp Grant near Detroit, Fort Niagara outside Buffalo, and Camp Meade south of Baltimore.[177]

By late October, the worst of the epidemic was over in many of the East Coast cities.[178] Things were "beginning to look a little bit brighter," Sister Lizzie Patterson, DC, wrote in one of her letters.[179] On October 21, public health officials in Wilmington, Delaware, expressed the belief that "it will only be a short time until conditions get back to normal."[180] But in later-struck cities in the Midwest and on the West Coast, the virus raged until mid-November and then reappeared in December and January. Fortunately, the death toll was lower at most of these locations.[181]

The 1918 flu pandemic exposed the shortcomings of scientific medicine and America's public health system. Medical science and public health officials were largely impotent against a fast-spreading, unknown, and deadly virus. The focus on acute surgical care, while suitable for base hospital units in Europe, did not prepare the country's hospitals for an influx of influenza patients. Absent an effective antidote to the virus, the Daughters often provided the best care and treatment available. This is why many soldiers and civilians alike turned to the Daughters for bodily assistance and spiritual guidance.

FOUR

DAUGHTERS, DOCTORS, AND OUTPATIENT CLINICS

Between 1865 (the end of the Civil War) and 1919 (the end of World War I), just about anything having to do with healthcare changed significantly, a remarkable occurrence considering that advances in the previous two thousand years were relatively minor by comparison.[1] The catalyst was germ theory, the notion that germs from outside the body were responsible for certain diseases and that living organisms did not spontaneously generate from nonliving matter. Germ theory replaced humoral theory, the claim that disease resulted from an imbalance of the four humors (blood, phlegm, yellow bile, and black bile) and that restoring the balance through purging, bleeding, or other means was the proper course of treatment. Breakthroughs based on germ theory occurred in rapid succession following Louis Pasteur's discoveries on fermentation and putrefaction in the early 1860s. In 1867, Joseph Lister pioneered antiseptic surgery; in 1882 and 1883, Robert Koch identified the organisms causing tuberculosis and cholera, respectively; in 1885, Pasteur developed the first vaccine for rabies; in 1900, Walter Reed proved that mosquitoes spread yellow fever; in 1910, Paul Ehrlich formulated a treatment for syphilis; and in 1928, Alexander Fleming isolated the mold for penicillin.[2]

Not only did germ theory alter doctors' approach to diagnosis and treatment, it became a force for reorganizing healthcare delivery. Hospitals evolved to provide the institutional setting for the application and teaching of germ theory. Surgeons could perform operations safely and more effectively in hospital operating rooms with sterilized surfaces and advanced medical equipment than in homes or in their offices. Coupled with other contemporaneous discoveries and inventions, such as indoor lighting, plumbing, heating, mechanical ventilation systems, and fire-retardant materials, germ theory and its many applications allowed architects and builders to construct multistory hospitals in cities where land was scarce and increasing numbers of people resided. Sprawling pavilion-style hospitals with wards radiating out from a central core were no longer needed in order to contain the spread of infections in most instances. As Lister, Koch, Ehrlich, and other scientists demonstrated, antiseptic (germ-killing) and aseptic (germ-preventing) techniques could control or eliminate pyemia, gangrene, and erysipelas, even in confined spaces. Rather than long-term care centers for chronically ill poor people, most hospitals, including Daughter-owned hospitals, converted to short-term, acute-care facilities for all individuals.[3]

As hospitals shifted from long-term to acute-care institutions, doctors gained greater influence over hospital administration. So long as there was a surplus of physicians seeking medical staff positions, hospital governing boards comprising lay trustees could control the agenda. But when the number of doctors sharply declined following the closure of several poorly performing medical schools in the early 1900s and physician referrals of paying patients became the major source of hospital income, doctors demanded a greater role in hospital administration, including patient admissions, billing and compensation, staff appointments, and specialty department formation. Governing boards of small community hospitals were the first to relinquish operational authority to staff physicians. Lacking expertise in hospital administration, those who sat on governing boards, mostly businessmen, politicians, and community leaders, delegated important decisions to them.[4]

Most hospitals developed two distinct lines of authority—one of them clinical and the other administrative. Hospital medical staffs controlled the former, while superintendents or administrators oversaw the latter.[5] But this "dual pyramid," as some observers called it, did not emerge at the Daughters' hospitals or at other Catholic-owned facilities.[6] Sister superiors remained in charge of all areas except medical decisions concerning individual patients. They acted as board presidents, hospital superintendents, and chief fundraisers. They established hospital policy, handled the finances, oversaw the wards, and made all the important decisions concerning hospital operations, including appointments to medical staff positions. Decision-making at sister-owned hospitals remained hierarchical and unitary.[7] This extended to the training and supervision of student nurses.

Germ theory augured a significant rise in the political power of the medical profession. After the American Medical Association (AMA) reorganized in 1901, solo practitioners joined the AMA in record numbers. Membership soared from 11,211 or 10 percent of all doctors in 1900 to slightly over 145,000 or 77 percent by 1950. Advertising revenues, the principal source of AMA income, grew from less than $10,000 in the late 1890s to $1,750,000 in the late 1940s.[8] Fearing federal government intervention in healthcare delivery, the AMA and its constituent state and local medical societies became reactive, opposing most anything that smacked of "socialized medicine."

The Daughters faced a predicament. Reliance on income from paying patients in order to maintain their facilities reduced the number of charitable admissions, thereby jeopardizing their mission. Seeking to address the healthcare needs of the medically indigent, the Daughters and other Catholic sisterhoods extended hospital services into surrounding communities through outpatient clinics. There was initial support for these endeavors, but physicians' emerging professional interests worked against them. Doctors with office-based practices protested that clinics competed with them for paying patients. Funds for clinics, already precarious, decreased when economic conditions worsened during the Great Depression. Hospitals moved to contain costs as charitable donations diminished. Facing stiff opposition from organized medicine, federal lawmakers failed to support a government-financed healthcare system.

"ONENESS OF AUTHORITY"

Relationships with doctors could be difficult and challenging given the Daughters' various roles as nurses, owners, and hospital managers. From the beginning, the Daughters aligned themselves with regular or allopathic physicians, not irregular or unorthodox providers. Most doctors praised the Daughters for their compassionate care, endurance, and discretion. Differences of opinion sometimes led to significant rifts, as in the case of the Baltimore Infirmary, which the Daughters left in 1879 after managing it for fifty-six years.[9] Such incidents were rare before the advent of medical science, however. Members of hospital medical staffs in the 1800s were mostly elite physicians with established practices who often provided free care to poor patients in the hospital setting while simultaneously teaching medical students and residents about various diseases and medical conditions.[10] These elite physicians typically supported the Daughters' mission.

More often than not, relationships between Daughters and physicians were harmonious in the decades following the introduction of germ theory. Sister servants looked to hospital advisory boards comprising doctors to aid their decisions. Yet disputes over medical staff appointments and hospital privileges became more frequent. Differences emerged over the creation of specialty departments,[11] the generation of patient revenues,[12] and the right of "outside" physicians (doctors with "courtesy," not permanent staff appointments) to admit ward patients.[13] The Daughters were stern administrators. They overrode staff physicians on several occasions. In 1899, for example, the Central House in Emmitsburg dispatched Sister Blanche Hooper, DC, to investigate doctors' performance at Sisters of Charity Hospital in Buffalo. After discovering that certain physicians were not meeting expectations, she admonished them and secured their resignations.[14]

Confrontations between Daughters and doctors also occurred over the training and supervision of nurses. Germ theory called for "a different kind of hospital workforce," one that was educated and skilled in the new technology.[15] The first nurse training schools in the United States opened in 1873 at Bellevue Hospital in New York City, Massachusetts General in Boston, and New Haven Hospital in New Haven, Connecticut. These were secular institutions, patterned on the Florence Nightingale Model of nursing, which stressed discipline, good moral character, and practical nursing. Under the Nightingale Model, nurses were responsible for providing a healthy atmosphere that enabled patients to recover, for promoting a nutritious diet, good personal hygiene, and a sanitary environment.[16]

By 1900, there were over four hundred hospital-based nursing schools in the country, twenty-eight of them at the Daughters' facilities.[17] These early nurse training schools emphasized on-the-job training. Physicians and experienced nurses gave weekly lectures, though most instruction occurred on hospital wards, not in classrooms. Student nurses became an important part of the hospital's political economy, an inexpensive form of labor. They received a meager stipend or allowance, lived and ate their meals in hospital quarters, wore the same caps, and donned the same uniforms. Discipline was strict. The period of training lasted about two or three years, but there were few overlapping standards from one school to another. Training schools developed separate identities and allegiances. A small number of graduates received appointments as head nurses or superintendents; many others worked in homes as private-duty nurses.[18]

When nursing schools first opened in the 1870s, the Daughters could perform most of the tasks that schools imparted. By the 1890s, however, the need for technical training had increased largely because of advances in surgery and the formation of specialty departments.[19] Physicians clamored for better-trained nurses at the Daughters' hospitals. At Sisters of Charity Hospital in Buffalo, for instance, Drs. Herman Mynter and William Heath pressed the administration. "The system of nursing of twenty years ago" does not meet current needs, they wrote in November 1890. "Surgical cases of today require trained nurses who [know] how to act in an emergency."[20] At Charity Hospital in New Orleans, the Louisiana State Medical Society issued a terse warning. "How many lives are annually sacrificed upon the alter [*sic*] of careless nursing?" an editorial in the 1892 edition of the *New Orleans Medical and Surgical Journal* queried. "This is an anomalous state of affairs; it has existed for a number of years, and every physician in the city knows of it and deplores it." The Daughters should be stripped of their "power to appoint the nurses," the editorial asserted.[21]

The editorial reflected the culmination of a series of events at publicly owned Charity Hospital. In December 1881, Dr. Daniel C. Holliday, a member of Charity's medical staff, sought to establish a nursing school under the auspices of an independent board of directors. Independent boards were commonplace at nursing schools affiliated with public hospitals in the late 1800s. The typical model contemplated physician supervision of student nurses who provided a large share of patient services.[22] Believing he had the support of Charity's board of directors, Holliday met with a group of leading women from the New Orleans community. The women agreed to back the venture. They formed a nursing society to oversee the school and the supervision of student nurses.[23] Learning of Holliday's efforts in late

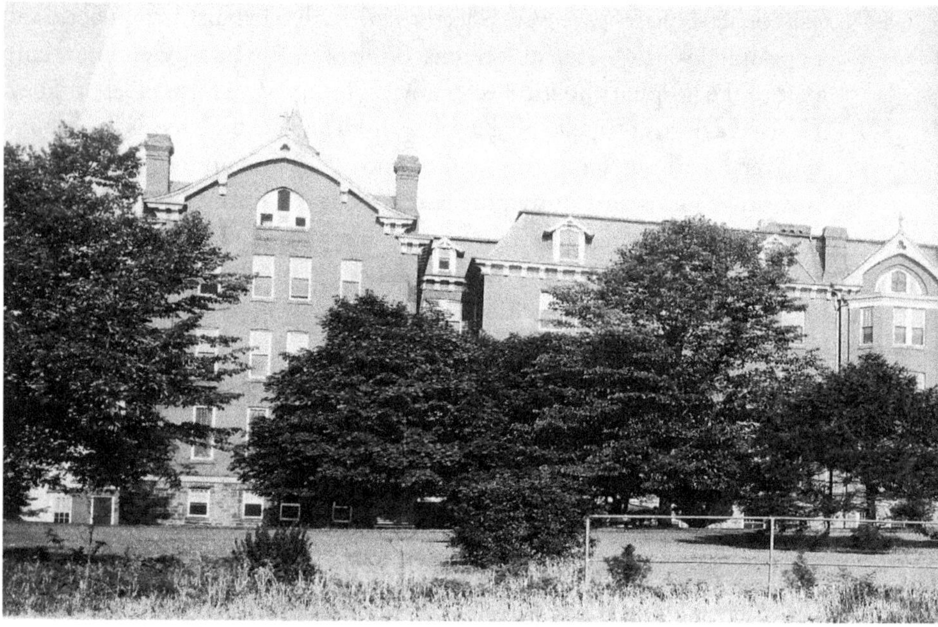

Figure 4.1. St. Agnes Hospital (Baltimore) Nursing School students, ca. 1890s.

January, the Daughters objected, claiming that the nursing society's involvement breached their contract with the hospital. On January 30, Holliday organized a public session in an attempt to placate the Daughters. Local newspapers covered the meeting. According to one of the reporters, Holliday "eulogi[zed] . . . the Sisters and their work, [stating] that there could be no interference with them." Maintaining that there was "nothing covert" about his proposal, Holliday contended that "every physician felt . . . the need for skillful nurses."[24]

When Holliday approached the hospital board in March with a formal proposal and a request for funds to get started, the board gave its preliminary approval "provided" the Daughters "consented." Attempting to frame his proposal to overcome the Daughters' objections, Holliday stated that "two wards in the hospital [would] be placed under the management of a matron and nurses subject to the orders of the Sister Superior."[25] Still, the Daughters objected. Because the school was an independent entity, Sister Agnes Slavin, DC, explained in her April 3, 1882, letter to board members, "the Sister Superior cannot exercise the same absolute authority over the

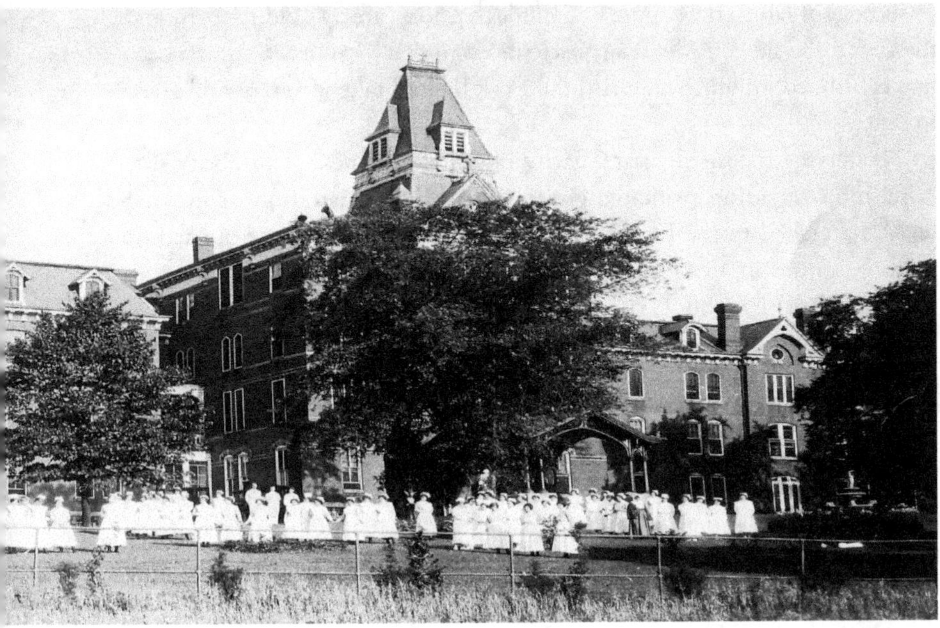

matron and the pupils which is now exercised over all other persons connected with the hospital." Such an arrangement, she claimed, violated the principle of "oneness of authority [which] in our opinion [is] essential to proper discipline."[26] After hearing Slavin's objections and perceiving an uphill battle, the hospital board abandoned the effort.[27]

At the end of the nineteenth century, the call to educate nurses in the new scientific paradigm gained momentum. Sister servants from several of the Daughters' hospitals gathered on April 19, 1892, at Mt. Hope Retreat in Baltimore to consider how best to move forward.[28] They realized that their nursing skills needed improvement, that the clinical instruction and hands-on experience they gained on hospital wards was no longer sufficient. During the next few years, several nursing schools opened at the Daughters' hospitals.[29] On August 9, 1897, almost fifty Daughters gathered in Emmitsburg to hear lectures on physiology and practical nursing. Their provincial director, Father Robert Lennon, CM, greeted them upon arrival, stating, "New methods of theory & practice in the hospitals requir[e] a course of study." While "older Sisters might find it hard [to make changes] after years of successful labor, they must not think that they are too old to learn and the young should consider it a conscientious matter." Failure to adjust, Lennon cautioned, might "result [in] the work [being] taken from us and given to others."[30]

Following the incident at Charity Hospital, "oneness of authority" became the overriding principle governing the administration of nursing schools attached to the Daughters' institutions. When Charity opened its nursing school in 1894, Slavin chose a Bellevue alumnus, Mary Agnes O'Donnell, as the school's superintendent. O'Donnell reported directly to Slavin, not to the hospital's governing board or the staff physicians.[31] Slavin's protégé, Sister Stanislaus Malone, DC, was among Charity's first graduates. With Slavin's urging, Malone went to Chicago, where she received advanced training under famed surgeon Nicholas Senn. Returning to Charity, Malone worked to upgrade the hospital's surgical facilities. In 1902, she became superintendent of the nursing school, and in 1914, Charity's chief administrator. For the next thirty years, Malone oversaw Charity Hospital.[32]

The Daughters typically selected one of their own for nursing school director if she had the required credentials and qualifications. In 1903, the surgical staff at Carney Hospital objected when Sister Gonzaga McCormick, DC, chose a Daughter for the position. They wanted a lay nurse for school superintendent. Unless McCormick changed her decision, several doctors on the medical staff said they would submit their resignations. Refusing to back down, McCormick accepted the surgeons' resignations at the hospital's annual meeting and announced their replacements.[33] The next day, the *Boston Globe* led with the following headline: "Entire Change: Carney Hospital Has a Big Shakeup; Surgical Staff Resigns, and New Man Is Placed in Charge."[34]

With resilience and determination, the Daughters survived some early conflicts with staff physicians. They maintained control over hospital finances and medical staff appointments, and they kept nursing within the confines of hospital administration. As the contest over nursing schools showed, they helped to advance the nursing profession during a period of significant upheaval and transition. By making the director of nursing responsible to the sister superior, they thwarted physician interference in nurse training and supervision. Though the Daughters did not engage in early efforts by nurses to organize for professional status—the formation in 1896 of the Nurses' Alumni Association (later, the American Nurses Association), for example—they advanced the struggle for nurse independence.[35]

CHANGING DYNAMICS, SHIFTING INTERESTS

The new scientific paradigm that took hold in the late 1800s gradually altered the physician workforce and the nature of medical practice. US medical schools tightened their standards for admission, increased the length of study, and added hospital internship training. Most of this occurred under the auspices of private professional organizations—the AMA, its component state and local medical societies, and the medical specialty boards that emerged in the early 1900s.[36] Though reforms to medical education and training enhanced physicians' qualifications, the higher costs and time involved discouraged (and largely excluded) students from the lower and working classes. "Under the emerging system," wrote medical sociologist Paul Starr, "young doctors could scarcely hope to be making a living before age thirty."[37] Catholic physicians were disproportionately few in number, largely because of the enhanced time and expense of medical school education. Discrimination against Catholics was also a factor, particularly at the elite medical colleges.[38] Responding to anti-Catholicism and seeking to advance Catholic values in medical education, nine Catholic universities started medical schools in the late 1800s and early 1900s. These included Marquette, St. Louis, Georgetown, Creighton, and Loyola Chicago.[39]

Technological innovation and increasing complexity fostered medical specialization. In the late 1800s and early 1900s, specialty societies appeared in several different areas, including pediatrics, urology, gynecology, psychiatry, neurology, pathology, dermatology, laryngology, and ophthalmology. Speaking before the Canadian Medical Association in 1900, F. C. Shattuck, a prominent Boston surgeon, warned about the ramifications. "Specialism divides up the organs and systems of the body," he noted. It "separates the sexes in a measure, and . . . steps in between children and parents." Still, Shattuck recognized that specialization was inevitable. "One fact stands out clearly—that specialism in medicine has come to stay. . . . Its advantages infinitely outweigh its disadvantages."[40]

By the second decade of the twentieth century, licensure or certification in a specialty area was a distinct possibility. The formation of the American College of Surgeons in 1913, the American College of Physicians in 1915, and the American Board for Ophthalmic Examinations (later the American Board of Ophthalmology) in 1916 moved the process forward. Several years passed, however, before specialty board certification became a reality. In 1934, the AMA and the specialty boards reached an agreement. Physicians seeking board certification in a specialty area had to graduate from an accredited medical school, complete three years of residency training at an approved hospital, and then pass an exam that a specialty board administered.[41]

Medical specialization reconfigured the nation's hospitals, creating internal divisions among departments and external boundaries between specialists and general practitioners. While specialists found a home in the hospital setting and used it to their advantage, general practitioners toiled in homes and private offices in small towns and rural areas, and they worked in dispensaries where the poor and working classes lived in the inner cities.[42] Though open staffing in hospitals remained the norm in America, closed staffing (the restriction of hospital privileges to a limited group of physicians) slowly gained a foothold. Whether a hospital's medical staff was open or closed did not really matter to general practitioners, however. They still needed to find a hospital department that was willing to accept them. "The uncoordinated drift toward specialism and medical complexity did not bode well for the future of the general practitioner," observed medical historian George Rosen. "The disappearance of the general physician of the nineteenth century was already accepted by the second decade of the twentieth," Rosen stated.[43]

The emerging configuration jeopardized the Daughters' mission. The Daughters were generalists, not specialists, and many of them were immigrants or children of immigrants with roots in working-class neighborhoods. The care they provided was holistic, spiritual as well as corporal, social as well as medical. As originally conceived, their hospitals were charitable institutions dedicated to the care of poor people.[44] The contrast with the "culture of medicine" that was taking shape in most hospitals could not have been more palpable. According to Charles Rosenberg, the new arrangement was "uncongenial to the holistic, individual, and moral understanding of health and illness" that for centuries had informed medical and nursing practice. "Personal interaction between doctor and patient . . . began to seem marginal, if not inconsequential." Charity care outside public hospitals and academic medical centers diminished in importance.[45]

Though the Daughters' approach differed from most doctors, they did not resist medical progress. Far from it, they championed reforms to medical education, clinical training, and specialization in order to enhance the quality of care in their hospitals. They sought ties with medical schools, they organized specialty departments, they recruited leading specialists, they acquired the latest medical equipment, and they built some of the most advanced laboratory and surgical facilities in America.[46] Providence Hospital in Washington, DC, provided clinical instruction for medical students at Columbian and Georgetown Universities beginning in 1882, while Sisters of Charity Hospital in Buffalo and Carney Hospital in Boston affiliated with Niagara Medical College and Tufts University in 1883 and 1920, respectively.[47] Carney had inpatient specialty departments for medicine, surgery, ophthalmology, obstetrics, gynecology, and pathology and outpatient specialty departments for aural care, laryngology, and dermatology by 1890.[48] Philadelphia's St. Joseph's Hospital had several specialists on its medical staff, including a laryngologist, an ophthalmologist, a neurologist, and a pediatrician in the 1890s.[49] And St. Vincent's Hospital in Norfolk had four surgeons, four physicians of "general medicine," three gynecologists, two pediatricians, four "eye, ear and throat" doctors, and one pathologist in 1901.[50]

Yet the Daughters did not embrace the culture of medicine. They maintained their Catholic identity and tailored the new configuration to fit their mission. "The notion of hospitals as inevitably and uniquely medical must be discarded," nurse historian Barbra Mann Wall has written. "In reality, Catholic sisters' hospitals were both medical and religious institutions," Wall asserted.[51] Writing about the Daughters' daily routine in the early 1900s at St. Mary's Hospital in Milwaukee, Monsignor Peter Leo Johnson observed that "spiritual training" was paramount. All other phases and things [are] really an effect of something inner and spiritual," Johnson indicated. "Virtue and industry are welded so finely that even the convalescent are kept occupied. . . . Because labor is deemed an excellent form of mortification, the Sisterhood is eager to cultivate it," he stated.[52]

THE DAUGHTERS' FINANCIAL QUANDARY

Between 1870 and 1910, the number of hospitals in the United States markedly increased from just under two hundred to over four thousand.[53] Before 1870, the Daughters founded a majority of US Catholic hospitals. But after 1870, several other sisterhoods joined them. Though the Daughters almost

Table 4.1. The Top Ten Sisterhoods by Number of Hospitals, 1869 to 1909.

Religious Community	*1869*	*1889*	*1909*
Sisters of Mercy (RSM) (2570, 2580)	6	17	68
Daughters of Charity (DC) (0760)	30	42	56
Sisters of St. Joseph (SSJ) (3830)	2	7	22
Sisters of Providence (SP) (3350)	1	11	20
Sisters of St. Francis of Perpetual Adoration (OSF) (1640)	0	10	17
Franciscan Sisters of the Poor (SFP) (1440)	9	13	14
Benedictine Sisters of Pontifical Jurisdiction (OSB) (0230)	0	3	13
Hospital Sisters of the Third Order of St. Francis (OSF) (1820)	1	11	13
Sisters of Charity of Leavenworth (SCL) (0480)	1	9	13
Sisters of St. Francis of Philadelphia (OSF) (1650)	2	6	11
Other	17	67	188
Total	69	196	435

Source: Stewart, *Marvels of Charity*.
Note: Order of ranking reflects the number of hospitals owned by a particular community in the United States in 1909. The *Official Catholic Directory* number following each order is the principal identifier for aggregating hospitals owned by a particular community, not the community's abbreviation.

doubled the number of their hospitals between 1870 and 1910 (from thirty to fifty-six), the combined output from other Catholic communities was much greater.[54] As shown in table 4.1, the Daughters accounted for 43 percent of all Catholic hospitals in 1869 but only 13 percent of all Catholic hospitals in 1909.

While demand for medical services was the main reason for hospital growth and development, urban migration and immigration were also important. In 1880, only 20 percent of the US population resided in urban centers; by 1900, 40 percent of the population did.[55] The newcomers came from rural areas of the United States and from foreign countries in search of jobs in steel, textiles, petroleum, automobiles, and other industries. Between 1881 and 1900, approximately nine million people immigrated to the United States; from 1901 to 1920, another fourteen and a half million arrived, the largest share originating in countries from eastern and southern Europe.[56]

The Daughters labored to find the money to build new hospitals or refurbish old ones. Though bishops and charitable donors often helped a group of sisters purchase property or obtain buildings to get started, their support was too meager to meet the costs of renovating, equipping, and maintaining modern scientific institutions.[57] The Daughters' situation differed from most other sisterhoods in certain important respects, however. Many of their hospitals as shown in table 4.1 predated 1870. The Daughters had to decide whether to upgrade these facilities or abandon them and start over. It was not uncommon for them to attempt renovation initially, only to discover that it was better to construct a new facility.[58] Because the Daughters oversaw an extensive network of hospitals from a central location, they could pool their resources, secure a loan from the Central House, or ask the Central House for assistance in obtaining credit from banks or other sources.[59] While most loans from the Central House came with interest (usually 6 percent), default did not incur foreclosure, and when hospitals defaulted on bank mortgages, the Central House typically assumed them.[60]

In 1910, the Daughters' US Province split in two, an Eastern Province headquartered in Emmitsburg and a Western Province located in Normandy, Missouri. Though the Eastern Province helped to finance construction projects as shown in some hospital records, the minutes from provincial meetings did not reflect them. The Western Province, on the other hand, kept detailed accounts of loans and other financial transactions in the corporate minutes. These minutes show that, between 1910 and 1920, the Central House in Normandy loaned money to St. Thomas Hospital in Nashville; to St. Joseph's Hospital in St. Joseph, Missouri; to St. Margaret's Hospital in Montgomery, Alabama; to Seton Infirmary in Austin, Texas; to Hôtel Dieu in New Orleans; and to St. Mary's Hospital in Evansville, Indiana.[61] The Central House in Normandy also helped to negotiate and secure loans and contracts with banks, contractors, and architects for St. Mary's Hospital in Milwaukee, St. Vincent's Hospital in Los Angeles, and Mullanphy Hospital in St. Louis.[62]

In addition to loans, the Daughters obtained money from patient revenues, government appropriations (federal, state, and local), and charitable donations (legacies, bequests, fundraisers, and subscriptions). Most of this money went to sustain daily operations—to purchase food, clothing, and medical supplies and to pay for salaries and general maintenance. Table 4.2 illustrates the breakdown between 1880 and 1929 of funds from patients, governments, and donors at Carney Hospital in Boston, Providence

Hospital in Washington, DC, Sisters of Charity Hospital in Buffalo (SOC), and St. Joseph's Hospital in Philadelphia.

As table 4.2 demonstrates, there was no shared pattern among the four hospitals from 1880 to 1904. Patient revenues far outpaced charitable and government funds at St. Joseph's, but that was not the case at the other three facilities. Among the four hospitals, Providence was in the best position to seek government assistance because of its location in the District of Columbia.[63] In order to obtain federal support for Providence, the Daughters had to lobby politicians,[64] work with heads of federal agencies,[65] and satisfy certain reporting requirements.[66] They also had to be on the winning side of an important US Supreme Court decision. In 1897, Joseph Bradfield, a citizen of the District of Columbia, filed a lawsuit claiming that the allocation of taxpayer funds to Providence violated the First Amendment's prohibition against a "law respecting the establishment of religion." After the case wound its way through the lower courts, the Supreme Court ruled against Bradfield on December 4, 1899, holding that the congressional appropriations did not violate the Establishment Clause of the First Amendment. Providence was a secular institution because it was incorporated under the laws of the United States for the "care of . . . sick and invalid persons" of any race or religion, the Supreme Court decided. It did not become a "religious or sectarian body" simply because the Daughters owned it.[67]

By 1915, the situation had changed considerably as the data from table 4.2 indicate. The Daughters could not rely on external grants or donations to meet daily expenses. Political considerations, budgetary constraints, and economic downturns caused fluctuations and created uncertainty. Hospital expenses had substantially increased as medical science advanced and flourished. Neither governments nor donors could timely respond to inflationary trends or changes in patient census.

A series of economic recessions from 1907 to 1921 partly explains the drop in government and charitable revenues. Another important factor was the consolidation of fundraising under the auspices of Catholic clergy. Founded in 1910, the National Conference of Catholic Charities (NCCC, today's Catholic Charities USA) advanced the formation of "diocesan bureaus." By 1918, seventeen dioceses had bureaus.[68] Catholic bishops used the bureaus to consolidate charitable giving for social services.[69] If the Daughters wanted some of the money a particular diocese collected, they had to meet certain requirements. Such requirements included the auditing of

Table 4.2. Profile of Funding Sources for Selected Hospitals in Five-Year Increments, 1880 to 1929.

Year	*Carney % PR*	*Carney % GR*	*Carney % CR*	*Providence % PR*	*Providence % GR*	*Providence % CR*	*SOC % PR*	*SOC % GR*	*SOC % CR*	*St. Joseph's % PR*	*St. Joseph's % GR*	*St. Joseph's % CR*
1880–1884	49	9	38	51	48	-	28	44	19	91	-	9
1885–1889	37	24	34	59	40	1	26	59	12	95	-	4
1890–1894	37	9	44	65	34	1	27	58	10	73	1	21
1895–1899	39	9	34	64	36	-	35	50	15	73	3	8
1900–1904	38	6	46	55	36	5	46	40	11	73	7	4
1915–1919	73	2	15	-	-	-	62	24	1	-	-	-
1920–1924	75	0	13	-	-	-	73	12	1	-	-	-
1925–1929	80	0	14	-	-	-	73	10	0	-	-	-

Source: Selected hospital collections, RG 11-2-1, APSL.

Note: PR = patient revenues; GR = government revenues; CR = charitable revenues (includes donations, legacies, subscriptions, and sundries). Percentages are based on five-year averages for corresponding periods. Data are insufficient for all four hospitals from 1905 to 1915. Data are also insufficient for Providence and St. Joseph's after 1904.

hospital finances, the provision of financial reports, and the inclusion of bishops' representatives at board meetings. Seeking to maintain their independence, many of the sisterhoods resisted. They refused to take "diocesan funds as long as possible," economist Mary Oates has written.[70]

Changing conditions affecting hospital finances created reliance on income from paying patients to cover expenses. While paying patients increased, charitable patients correspondingly decreased. Raising concerns about the shift toward paying patients, Father John Cronin, CM, Western Province director, admonished the Daughters: "The records show an unbelievably small number of charity patients [at your hospitals]. I would be derelict in my duty, if I were to fail in pointing out to you the situation. THE DOORS OF THE HOSPITAL SHOULD BE OPEN TO THE POOR. It would be a calamity if the poor were to be taken from you" (emphasis in original).[71] Notwithstanding Cronin's objections, the Daughters could not cover mounting expenses if they admitted large numbers of charity patients. Funds from governments and donors were insufficient. The situation called for a new approach or strategy if their hospitals were to remain the central focus of their mission.

THE RISE AND FALL OF OUTPATIENT CLINICS

Hospital inpatient care was not the only means for measuring the success of the Daughters' mission. Outpatient clinics attached to hospitals could be equally if not more effective in treating poor persons' afflictions, afflictions that, in the words of medical historian Rosemary Stevens, "were as much social as medical in their origin."[72] The Daughters had tended to the sick poor in the outpatient setting for epidemic diseases and debilitating conditions since coming to America. They now redoubled their efforts.

Beginning in 1880, the Daughters' hospitals reported the "No. of Extern Poor visited and relieved" (changed in 1901 to "Poor relieved at the House") to the Central House in Emmitsburg.[73] The figures the Daughters reported fluctuated, sometimes substantially, from hospital to hospital and even from year to year within hospitals, suggesting inconsistent recordkeeping and possible guesswork. Those visited and relieved at St. Joseph's Hospital in Philadelphia ranged from three thousand to six thousand poor people and their families in each of the years between 1880 and 1893, while those at Carney Hospital ranged from ten thousand to thirty thousand each year from 1887 to 1899.[74] An 1881 annual report from Mullanphy Hospital indicated that the Daughters visited 870 "poor families . . . in their homes and assisted or received [them] at the Hospital."[75]

Much of the work the Daughters performed under the category "visited and relieved" did not involve the treatment of diseases and ailments. It often took the form of food, clothing, and other material assistance. A 1911 report from the medical staff of Washington's Providence Hospital noted, for instance, that the Daughters offered "domestic" instruction to reduce "unhygienic surroundings," helped "families . . . move into healthful places," furnished milk for babies, delivered "hot lunch in the hospital building" for schoolchildren, and taught "class[es] at the hospital" in cooking and sewing. In addition, they established a "soup kitchen" in the hospital's "basement," took poor persons "to the markets" where they "instructed [them] in buying and preserving foodstuffs," and "distributed . . . baskets of food . . . each evening [from] the surplus of the hospital." In the case of pregnant women, the Daughters arranged "for the care of the mother through the obstetrical department of [the hospital's] dispensary" or outpatient clinic.[76]

Outpatient departments or clinics, such as the one at Providence, evolved from freestanding dispensaries.[77] As the word "dispensary" indicates, physicians who ran them dispensed prescriptions while occasionally performing minor operations, including suturing lacerations and mending fractures. Freestanding dispensaries were mostly for poor people; affluent patients went to private physicians. Dispensaries often appeared in locations where new immigrants congregated. Public health commissioner Michael Davis calculated that in 1862 "patients of foreign birth" accounted for "81,000 of the 145,000 visits" to New York City dispensaries.[78] After the Civil War, dispensaries frequently affiliated with urban charities, religious hospitals, and settlement houses.[79]

Just as the transformation from chronic to acute care in the hospital setting reflected the introduction and growth of medical science and technology, so did the shift from freestanding dispensaries to hospital outpatient departments. Many poor immigrants who previously went to dispensaries sought treatment from doctors and medical residents in hospital-based clinics (the Daughters used the terms "outpatient department," "outpatient clinic," and "dispensary" interchangeably in their reports and letters).[80] St. Joseph's in Philadelphia was the first of the Daughters' hospitals to add an outpatient clinic in 1867.[81] Several other hospitals the Daughters owned or managed soon followed St. Joseph's. St. Mary's Hospital in Rochester opened an outpatient department in 1870;[82] Carney started one in 1877;[83] Charity Hospital in New Orleans constructed "outdoor clinics" in 1891;[84] St. Vincent's Hospital in Norfolk organized an "out-door dispensary" in 1892;[85] and St. Agnes Hospital in Baltimore founded a "dispensary" in 1894.[86] Carney kept detailed records that closely tracked the amount of work performed in its outpatient clinics. By 1880, outpatients exceeded inpatients at Carney, and by 1899, there were five times more outpatients than inpatients.[87]

Between 1910 and the early 1920s, dispensaries and hospital-based clinics surged in popularity. According to the US Census Bureau, the number of "dispensaries," which the bureau defined as both freestanding and attached to hospitals, increased from 574 in 1910 to 2,526 in 1922.[88] Roughly 40 percent of dispensaries in 1922 were attached to hospitals, while the other 60 percent were freestanding.[89] Dispensaries and outpatient clinics received strong support from public health advocates, including many physicians. Articles appearing in *The Modern Hospital*, the American Hospital Association's lead journal, often praised clinics for the care they provided. "No form of service in medical institutions is capable . . . of rendering larger benefit to public health" than the dispensary, Michael Davis contended.[90] "The dispensary, or outpatient department, is a very vital part of the hospital, for it is here that patients come seeking advice, either in the early stages of acute disease . . . or for minor ailments," the assistant superintendent of Johns Hopkins Hospital stated.[91] "The dispensary acts . . . as a personal physician" for the "sick poor," wrote Samuel Lambert, the chief physician at New York's St. Luke's Hospital.[92] They are a "connecting link between the community and the hospital," a spokesperson for the Associated Out-Patient Clinics of New York City asserted.[93] Dispensaries offer an "effective channel" for the delivery of social services, maintained Alice Walker, the director of the Social Service Department for Detroit's Harper Hospital.[94]

The Daughters recognized the value of outpatient clinics and heavily invested in them.[95] When social service departments appeared in hospitals in the early 1900s, the Daughters placed them in their outpatient clinics. St. Louis's Mullanphy Hospital added a social service department to its clinic in 1918 after receiving a onetime cash outlay from the National Catholic

War Council for the care of discharged soldiers and their families. A Daughter and two laywomen trained as social workers ran the social service department at Mullanphy.[96] Washington's Providence Hospital also started a social service department in its clinic after receiving a grant from the National Catholic War Council. From 1919 to 1942, three people under the direction of Sister Berchmans Beltzhoover, DC, oversaw the work of purportedly "the busiest [social service department] in the city."[97]

Just as dispensaries and outpatient clinics seemed destined to become the principal means for delivering healthcare to large portions of the population, their appeal suddenly diminished. Articles appearing in *The Modern Hospital* in the mid- to late 1920s began to focus on their deficits rather than their benefits. "Experienced physicians" are lacking in outpatient clinics, New York physician John Osborn Polak indicated. "Recent graduates . . . fresh from [their] college or hospital training" are treating patients without "proper supervision," he stated.[98] Clinics are not the best places for treating chronic diseases, Ernst P. Boas, the medical director for New York's Montefiore Hospital, contended. "The perpetual clinic patient who wanders from one department to another and from one dispensary to another seeking, but not obtaining, relief" is a common and unfortunate occurrence.[99] "There are signs of unrest" in the outpatient clinic, E. M. Bluestone, the assistant director of New York's Mount Sinai Hospital, noted. "The greatest single cause of unhappiness in the life of the young clinician is [the lack of] economic [benefit]."[100] US Surgeon General H. S. Cumming did not even mention outpatient clinics when promoting the development of community health programs in a 1926 article. To Surgeon General Cumming, the most important link was the physician in "private practice."[101]

Changing attitudes concerning charitable obligation and service were among the reasons support for outpatient clinics faded. Professional achievement and economic gain had become more important. It was in the hospital, not outside it, where doctors garnered status and reputation.[102] "The criteria of sweet charity are being superseded by the criteria of scientific medical service," wrote the authors of a 1926 study of outpatient clinics at four of the nation's leading academic medical centers.[103] Opposition from private practitioners was also a significant factor. So long as outpatient clinics remained strictly charitable operations, independent physicians raised few objections. But when clinics began to charge patients a modest fee and pay doctors a fixed amount or salary for the services they provided, private practitioners protested. Many who went to outpatient clinics could afford a private physician, they asserted.[104]

Claims of so-called charity abuse first appeared in the late 1800s. At the International Congress of Charities, Correction and Philanthropy in 1883, John Shaw Billings, the founder of the National Library of Medicine, denounced "the increase in free dispensary work, or outpatient relief." This was "one of the signs," he said, "of the socialistic tendency of the age, of the increasing tendency to subordinate the individual to the community in attempting to equalize the burdens and pleasures of mankind."[105] Billings's remarks conflated physicians' growing discontent with the move toward government-financed healthcare in Europe. By World War I, ten European countries had some form of national health insurance.[106]

Led by Morris Fishbein, the editor of *JAMA* (the AMA's principal journal), the AMA joined forces with the nation's hospital associations to stop the trend toward "socialized medicine," a term Fishbein and others doctors pejoratively applied to any form of collective activity averse to their interests, whether government or corporate sponsored.[107] In 1934, the AMA codified Fishbein's prohibitions when it amended its Code of Medical Ethics to say that patients should have "free choice of physician." All patients, the free-choice principle held, should be able to select their own doctor, and no person or entity—hospital, government, or private insurance company—should come between them.[108]

Over the course of the next several decades (until the mid-1970s, when federal antitrust authorities intervened), medical societies invoked the free-choice principle against clinics and group payment plans in several locations throughout the country. Doctors connected to group plans and clinics faced expulsion from their local medical societies and termination of their hospital privileges.[109] The crackdown on clinics these actions generated undercut the Daughters' strategy to provide healthcare services for the indigent.

HEALTHCARE REFORM AND THE CATHOLIC HOSPITAL ASSOCIATION

Prompted by Pope Leo XIII's 1891 encyclical, *Revum Novarum*, US bishops in 1919 adopted a program of "Social Reconstruction," which embraced unemployment, health, and old-age insurance as well as minimum-wage laws and labor unions. Under the auspices of the National Catholic Welfare

Conference (NCWC), the bishops promoted government intervention to accomplish their objectives.[110] Father John A. Ryan, a leading reformer, headed the NCWC's Social Action Department. Though World War I and the fear of communism stalled Ryan's efforts, the Great Depression and the Roosevelt administration revived them. Another papal encyclical on social reconstruction, *Quadragesimo Anno*, issued in 1931, encouraged Ryan and the Social Action Department to help craft and support New Deal legislation.[111] Yet the Catholic Hospital Association (CHA), which spoke for the Daughters' hospitals, did not support legislative efforts to make healthcare more accessible. The primary reason was because the CHA's president, Father Alphonse M. Schwitalla, SJ, decried physician group practice and government-financed health insurance.

Schwitalla's resistance was deeply embedded. When the Committee on the Costs of Medical Care (CCMC) (Schwitalla was among the CCMC's forty-eight members), a private undertaking, formed in 1927 to address the rising costs of healthcare, most businesses were prospering. But there were warning signs on the horizon. Access to healthcare was decreasing, and there were huge health disparities depending on location.[112] When the CCMC issued its final report in 1932, the country was in the midst of the Great Depression. Persons of moderate means were unable to pay for medical services, not just low-wage workers.[113] "[Thirty-eight] per cent of the people in this country receive no medical, dental, or eye care. . . . The rest are served very unevenly, with uneven costs, and with some doctors receiving too little money for doing the same work that pays others well," the committee discovered.[114]

Though committee members believed that the situation called for action, they could not reach consensus on a set of recommendations. The members divided over two principal issues: (1) the organization of healthcare delivery—group versus solo practice; and (2) the manner of finance—group payment versus individual fee-for-service. A substantial majority of the members (thirty-nine out of forty-eight) determined that "comprehensive group practice" coupled with "comprehensive prepayment" was the best way forward. "Comprehensive group practice," that is, "organized groups of practitioners, organized regionally and preferably around hospitals," would make healthcare more accessible, the majority determined, while "comprehensive prepayment" through "group payment plans" would make it more affordable.[115]

Opposition from the nine-member minority, "eight physicians and one layman," was intense. The minority contended that group practice and group payment constituted an assault on the private practice of medicine.[116] Of the nine-member minority, eight were physicians. Given the connections of the eight physicians to organized medicine, their rejection of the majority's proposal was unsurprising.[117] But the inclusion of Schwitalla, the "layman" on the minority report, seemed striking considering the Catholic Church's support for social legislation.

Schwitalla labored to explain his position.[118] "Some Catholics," he acknowledged, "welcomed" the CCMC's proposals, "in which the duty of government is emphasized, to protect and care for the needy, the infirm, and, especially, the indigent." But this did not mean, he asserted, that "differences of opinion" should not emerge among Catholics concerning "the elements [of] legislative enactments."[119] Schwitalla railed against physician group practice, drawing from Catholic doctrine to do it.[120] "The personal relationship between patient and physician," Schwitalla wrote, is "the only concept that can justify the Church's traditional attitude toward the work of the physician." "Catholic ethics," he said, "can never justify a physician in shifting responsibility from himself to his employer in the care of the sick, even if the employer is the government and even if he himself is acting as a governmental agent."[121] Schwitalla equated the doctor-patient relationship to that of priest and penitent. "A friendship and intimacy develop[s]," he maintained, between "patient and physician" which "assumes priestly characteristics on the part of the physician." Group practice, he wrote, eroded the "individual relationship" between doctors and patients.[122]

Schwitalla's speeches, writings, and rhetoric closely tracked the AMA's position on free choice of physician. When Fishbein appeared before several local medical societies to criticize the CCMC's recommendations, Schwitalla frequently joined him.[123] Though Schwitalla typically showed more restraint than the flamboyant Fishbein, who in a hyperbolic and oft-quoted editorial accused the CCMC of representing "the forces of socialism and communism," he could be equally fervent when addressing a group of physicians. Speaking at a meeting of the Chicago Medical Society on January 4, 1933, Schwitalla called the CCMC's proposals "subversive to the development of medical science and a blow to [the medical profession]." The CCMC, he professed, asks us "to socialize our medical endeavors."[124]

Schwitalla remained wedded to the AMA's hard-line position long after the conflict with the CCMC had diminished. Organized medicine did not have a better friend and supporter, particularly in its quest to achieve a united front against national health insurance. During congressional hearings on a series of legislative initiatives in the late 1930s and early 1940s, Schwitalla conflated "the interests of the hospitals" with "the interests of medical practice." Testifying before a US Senate subcommittee on June 1, 1939, he maintained that hospitals and physicians were "united against any plans by which socialization of medicine or socialization of hospital service, *no matter how defined*, might be contemplated" (emphasis in original).[125] The AMA rewarded Schwitalla for his efforts. In 1948, it presented its prestigious Certificate of Merit and Gold Medal to him (the first nonphysician) for "outstanding effort for the public welfare on a national level and for his service to American medicine."[126]

THE DAUGHTERS' EARLY SKEPTICISM OF THE CATHOLIC HOSPITAL ASSOCIATION

Though there is scant documentation to show the Daughters' position on physician group practice and national health insurance, the lack of clear evidence should not be mistaken for acquiescence.[127] While they favored certain policies that the CHA promoted, such as the move toward hospital standardization in the 1910s and 1920s, Schwitalla's vigorous support for the AMA's program undercut their mission. Yet the Daughters could do little about it. The 1917 Code of Canon Law, religious studies professor Carol Coburn has written, "diminished . . . the sisters . . . decision-making abilities . . . in favor of rigidity, uniformity, [and] regulation."[128] Under the 1917 code and the CHA's founding documents, only priests and bishops could occupy the leading positions in the national association.[129] Schwitalla possessed sufficient organizational authority to pursue his agenda, and he used the political platform the CHA provided to do it.

Ostensibly a "sisters' organization," the CHA was not much different from a bishop's diocese or "demesne," as Monsignor John O'Grady, executive secretary of the National Conference of Catholic Charities, called it.[130] From 1915 to 1947, only two people served as CHA president, Father

Charles Moulinier, SJ (1915–28), and Schwitalla (1928–47). When Moulinier brought thirty-five sisters together in Milwaukee on April 8, 1915, to begin the planning process, two Daughters from nearby St. Mary's Hospital attended.[131] They did not have a good experience and did not want to go to any more meetings. On April 10, Sister Mary Dolores Gillespie, DC, St. Mary's sister servant, wrote Visitatrix Eugenia Fealy complaining that some of the speakers were demeaning. A surgeon "with the Mayo Bros. in Rochester, Minnesota . . . made a bold statement that the Sisters were far inferior to the nurses in the course of training," Gillespie stated. As for one of the priests, "I will not comment on [his] remarks. I might lose my temper."[132]

The CHA's inaugural convention in Milwaukee from June 24 to 26, 1915, attracted two hundred sisters, lay nurses, and physicians. No Daughters attended, though St. Mary's sent a chaplain and four lay nurses.[133] In response to the invitation from the archbishop of Milwaukee, Sebastian G. Messmer, Fealy stated, "We would not feel justified in permitting our Sisters, in a general gathering, to read papers, discuss questions, [and] take part in debates." By way of explanation, Fealy added, "We've been [meeting among ourselves] to achieve greater uniformity and efficiency. But all this, Your Grace, is within the family, and we cannot see that we can conscientiously approve of our Sisters doing the work otherwise."[134]

Notwithstanding the Daughters' absence, Messmer heralded the gathering at the Milwaukee convention, stating that the "intermingling of Sisters of different orders [was a] most excellent stimulant in all works of charity and religion."[135] The sisters established a constitution and bylaws and selected Moulinier as CHA president.[136] When the CHA held its second annual convention in 1916, also in Milwaukee, the number of people attending almost doubled to about four hundred. This time, Fealy sent Gillespie. The Daughters' Eastern Province also sent a representative, J. T. Bottomley, a physician from Carney.[137]

During the early years when Moulinier was its president, the CHA sought to increase its constituency, to extend beyond its roots in the upper Midwest. At the CHA's 1919 convention, the delegates passed a resolution expanding the association to include state or regional "conferences." The development of subsidiary organizations made good sense, particularly at a time when travel was difficult, money was scarce, and state laws governed most hospital operations.[138]

By all accounts, the conferences flourished in several states and regions, such as Indiana, Illinois, Missouri, Kansas, New England, Pennsylvania, and Maryland.[139] At the first annual meeting of the Maryland Conference held on April 25, 1925, "every Catholic hospital and high school in the archdiocese" sent representatives, including St. Agnes Hospital in Baltimore and Providence Hospital in Washington.[140] Even at these regional gatherings, however, the Daughters remained aloof and cautious. They were under strict orders from Father John Cribbins, CM, Eastern Province director, to refrain from "any agreement or promise that might bind you in any way to the Catholic Hospital Association."[141] Cribbins's instruction, coupled with their actions and Fealy's earlier letter to Archbishop Messmer, suggests that the Daughters did not want CHA leadership to speak for them, that they sought to retain their independence. Before Schwitalla had become CHA president, the Daughters were wary of political entanglements.

Despite canon law restrictions, several sisters served as CHA officers and board members almost from the beginning, though male clergy occupied the most important positions.[142] The Daughters were not among them. Those who sat on the board often served for lengthy periods and supported Schwitalla on most occasions. According to Father Robert Shanahan, the CHA's biographer, grassroots opposition did not really matter so long as Schwitalla had the support of the board and the sisters on it. "Always assured of complete backing from the sisters," wrote Shanahan, "Father Schwitalla was able at times to have policies adopted which reflected his own convictions rather than those of the majority of the membership."[143] Some of the sisters were ardent followers. Mother M. Concordia Puppendahl, SSM, for example, publicly criticized the CCMC majority recommendations at the CHA's 1933 annual convention. Puppendahl's principal complaint was that private health insurance would lead to the "commercialization of the medical profession."[144]

Given the AMA's reaction to the CCMC's recommendations, President Roosevelt decided not to pursue healthcare reform during his first term in office. But with economic conditions worsening and public support for a federal program increasing after his 1936 reelection, Roosevelt advanced several proposals, including aid to the indigent and federal dollars for the expansion of hospital facilities.[145] Senator Robert F. Wagner of New York introduced legislation in February 1939 based on the president's recommendations, but the AMA and Schwitalla, speaking on behalf of the CHA, opposed the legislation.[146] Before testifying in Congress on June 1, 1939, Schwitalla polled the CHA's membership.[147] Ostensibly seeking their endorsement, he sent a letter to the sisterhoods telling them "how to act in this matter."[148] While there are no documents to show how the Daughters voted, their history suggests that they would have been reluctant to support Schwitalla's position.

The outcome of the political conflict among reformers and interest groups in the 1930s and 1940s was a disjointed healthcare system at the local, regional, and national levels. There was no comprehensive strategy, no centralization or rationalization of healthcare finance and delivery. Not only poor patients but also patients who could pay for healthcare found their choices limited. Addressing Harvard's School of Public Health in 1963, preeminent hospital administrator Ray E. Brown asserted, "The failure to develop a comprehensive system of care forces the patient to go to bed in the acute facilities. In general, there are no organized outpatient services for the private ambulatory patient, no organized home-care program as an integral part of the hospital's operations for the pay patient and not very many long-term facilities integrated with the services of the general hospital for either the free or the pay patient."[149]

The situation was untenable. Pressure for change began to build following World War II as the costs of inpatient care, fueled by private health insurance, rose precipitously, and the disparity between those with insurance and those without it, the poor and the elderly, undermined the quality of the nation's healthcare delivery.

FIVE

"MORE ACTIVE, VOCAL, AND VISIBLE"

The Daughters did not remain on the sidelines much beyond the 1940s. The Sister Formation movement that took shape in the 1950s and the pronouncements of the Second Vatican Council (Vatican II), meeting from 1962 to 1965, spurred Catholic sisterhoods to social and political action. Sister Formation furthered postgraduate education in areas such as health-care administration, while Vatican II called for sisters, brothers, priests, and prelates to be more approachable and interactive, to assimilate societal changes. The resulting mix of the sacred and the secular transformed religious lifestyles and traditional institutions.[1] Though the Daughters altered their attire and some of their rules or regulations, these modifications were not as noteworthy as their enhanced engagement in political, social, and economic matters. A provincial document from 1984 acknowledged the shift, observing that "the Daughters [became] more active, vocal and visible."[2] Remarkably, several Daughters attained leading positions in the Catholic Hospital Association starting in the late 1960s. Using their platform as CHA presidents and heads of important committees, these Daughters lobbied for federal legislation that increased access to care for poor people.

This chapter examines how this transpired, how the Daughters moved from avoidance to active participation in the policymaking process. The Vatican II pronouncements were pivotal, as was the civil rights movement and the federal government's entry into the healthcare arena. Vatican II lifted the ecclesiastical restrictions on sisters' political activities, and the US civil rights movement strengthened their resolve. For the Daughters, these were important prerequisites to future health policy initiatives, but what ultimately made the difference, what spurred them into leadership positions within the CHA and other national associations, was the transformation of the healthcare industry following the enactment of the Medicare and Medicaid programs in 1965. During the 1970s and 1980s, government regulators and private insurers undercut the power of the AMA. The new regime that formed in the wake of the AMA's demise advanced market competition to control rapidly escalating healthcare costs and expenses.[3] The Daughters had to engage. They had to participate in order to sustain their hospitals and their mission to the sick poor. But to be effective, they needed qualified leaders who had the requisite education and experience in the workings of complex healthcare organizations. The Sister Formation movement laid the groundwork for their endeavors.

SISTER FORMATION

In the early 1940s, Sister Bertrande Meyers, DC, a forward-thinking educator, fostered a change in direction. Her doctoral dissertation on "Sister Formation" became the blueprint for sisters seeking a more integrated and heterogeneous education. In the mid- to late 1950s, several sisterhoods adopted the recommendations Meyers set forth in her dissertation, prompting the establishment of sister-run colleges that taught courses in the humanities and social sciences.

Born in Chicago on December 1, 1898, Meyers entered the Daughters of Charity in 1915.[4] Missioned to the Daughters' school and orphanage in Donaldsonville, Louisiana, Meyers forged a close and long-lasting friendship with Sister Catherine Sullivan, DC, who was working as a nurse at the National Leprosarium, which the Daughters administered in Carville, Louisiana.[5] Attracted to Meyers' keen intellect, Sullivan, who would later serve as visitatrix for the Western Province from 1952 to 1962, helped to further Meyers' education. When Meyers completed her doctoral dissertation at St. Louis University in 1940, Sullivan extolled its significance. In a letter to a fellow sister, Sullivan related, "When things settle down I shall send you a copy of her dissertation. We are negotiating now to have it published as the University thinks it will be of untold help to all teaching religious Communities."[6]

Meyers traveled all over the country in connection with her doctoral research, surveying provincial superiors and those responsible for the education of novices at over sixty different communities.[7] Her findings demonstrated pervasive "dissatisfaction . . . with prevailing educational practices." The sisterhoods were "totally unaware—even misinformed—[concerning] the educational policies and practices of [each] other," Meyers discovered.[8] According to Meyers, the widespread discontent stemmed from two factors: (1) educational requirements (typically a baccalaureate degree) for state teacher certification, and (2) pressure from bishops and priests for more teaching sisters. Seeking to address both concerns simultaneously, superiors often required young sisters to teach while obtaining their credentials.[9] The conditions were onerous. Many young and unprepared sisters labored long hours in overcrowded schools and then attended college in the evenings and during the summers. There was little time for community engagement, for religious training and social assimilation. "Getting the degree became the dominant motive," Meyers stated. "But the knowledge gained was far removed from the philosophy of true education. . . . [I]n the majority of cases, the experience seemed to have destroyed rather than nurtured any love of learning."[10]

Meyers did not simply present her findings and assess the consequences in her doctoral dissertation. She also offered a detailed solution, "a plan for a pre-service education" that called for at least two years of integrated study postnovitiate at a sister-run "community junior college."[11] Meyers believed that religious and professional training as currently provided were too segmented, that the latter (professional training at a secular university or college) was divorced from the former. By combining the curriculum at a "community junior college," the sister would obtain "the religious, social, cultural and professional development" she needed. Such combined or integrated training would "distinguish" the sister "from the lay teacher," while satisfying the requirements for state teacher certification, Meyers contended.[12]

But the type of "community junior college" Meyers envisioned did not exist in 1941, when her dissertation was published. If Meyers's plan was to succeed, several sisterhoods, including the Daughters, would have to embrace and implement its features. Because of the turmoil surrounding World War II and opposition from male clergy, it took several years before Meyers's proposal gained traction. In 1949, at the National Catholic Education Association (NCEA) annual conference, Sister Madeleva Wolff, CSC, the president of St. Mary's College in South Bend, Indiana, began to move things forward. Wolff announced in her well-publicized speech, "The Education of Sister Lucy," that the time had come to address the situation. The following year, in December 1950, Pope Pius XII echoed the concerns that Sisters Wolff and Meyers had been raising.[13]

At the NCEA's annual conference in 1953, the sisterhoods founded their own organization, which in 1954 became the Sister Formation Conference (SFC). The SFC became the forum for launching Meyers's initiative.[14] SFC leaders proceeded to survey the various communities, hold workshops, and with financial assistance from the Ford Foundation organize "demonstration" projects. By 1957, the SFC had determined that Meyers's original plan for combined study postnovitiate was warranted, that communities should establish "juniorates," sister-run colleges for sisters only, which would offer baccalaureate degrees in teaching, social work, and nursing.[15] Among the first of its kind, Marillac College in Normandy, Missouri, just outside St. Louis, was the Daughters' juniorate. Meyers served as its dean and then its president. The college attracted students and faculty "from over seventeen different communities." It "was the epitome of Sister Formation ideology, educating and housing American and international sisters," wrote historian Carol Coburn.[16]

Meyers's work on Sister Formation spurred the Daughters' involvement in professional and policymaking endeavors. In 1957, she wrote "The Place of Religious in Social Work," which encouraged more sisters to obtain an advanced degree so they could claim their position in the new professional discipline. "Works of mercy—now organized as a profession—are more than eighty percent in the hands of lay persons," she noted. "Even in the Catholic sector," Meyers asserted, "the Sisters do not have the influence they should have by reason of ownership and administration, nor by reason of their complete dedication to this apostolate."[17] Though the nursing profession was not Meyers's main interest, her "Aggiornamento of the Sister-Nurse," published in 1965, provided an outline for future action. Observing that sister-nurses were "the best educationally qualified of any group" and held "high office" in professional associations, she nonetheless warned about

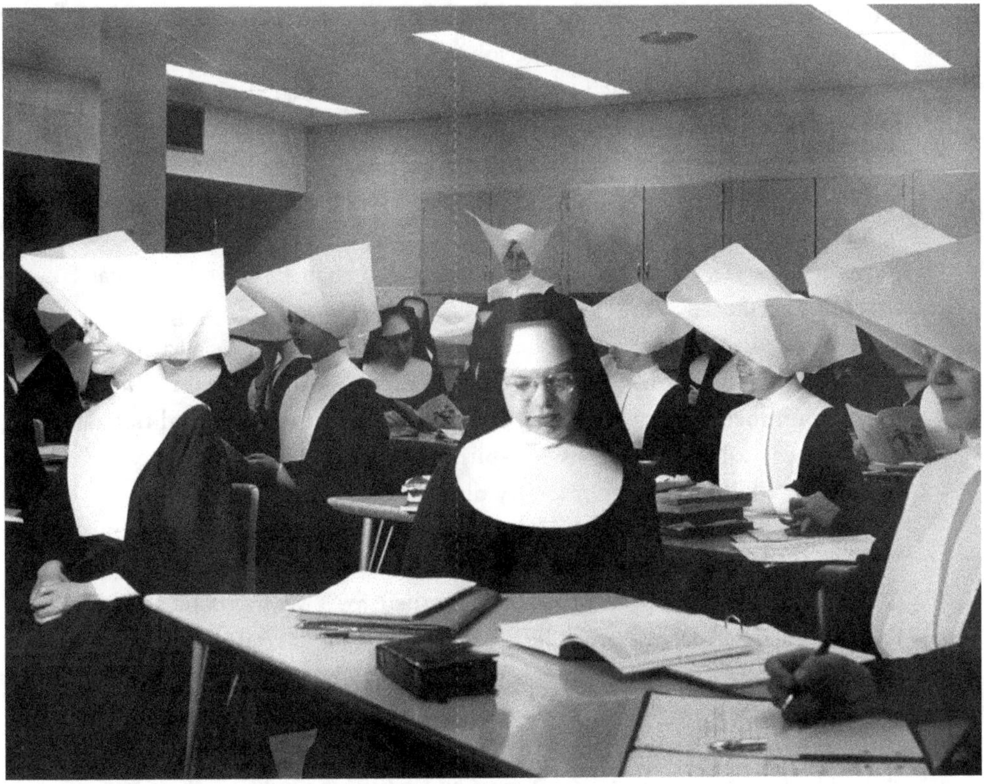

Figure 5.1. Marillac College students, St. Louis, MO, 1960.

the tendency toward "narrow specialization and self-containment." Nursing education should include the humanities and the social and behavioral sciences, "which give insight into the causes and effects of human conduct," Meyers argued. A broad-based education would advance "total patient care" and "teamwork," she stated.[18]

VATICAN II AND 1960S AMERICA

Between 1962 and 1965, thousands of bishops and "observers," including auditors, sisters, and laypersons, convened at the Vatican on four separate occasions to prepare for a spiritual renewal, a revitalization of the church's teachings and traditions under contemporary conditions.[19] Sister Suzanne

Guillemin, DC, the superioress general of the Daughters of Charity, was among the eight sisters whom Pope John XXIII invited to "audit" the proceedings.[20] After the council completed its work, it issued sixteen documents. The document affecting the sisterhoods most directly was *Perfectae Caritatis*. In calling on religious communities to reassess their rules and priorities in light of changing conditions, *Perfectae Caritatis* initiated a period of adjustment and discernment, a process that would lead to sweeping reforms in lifestyle, conduct, and community governance.[21] In her circular letter of February 2, 1968, Guillemin expounded on the meaning of *Perfectae Caritatis*. The Daughters, she wrote, are "invited to move away from a . . . position of authority to one of collaboration." "It must be said," Guillemin continued, "that this entails a true turnabout from our traditional position, and a long and persistent spiritual preparation. We must realize that we shall have to make some very difficult decisions."[22]

For the sisterhoods, the principal message of Vatican II was to strive to make the founders' teachings relevant, to work with laypersons and non-Catholics to achieve social justice. This called for a synthesis of church teachings and secular society, a difficult and sometimes controversial process. Church teachings, rules, and values flowed from the pope, the diocesan bishops, and the founders of religious communities and orders. Secular values, on the other hand, reflected societal norms and customs, some deeply entrenched in governmental structures and political systems, others constantly changing and evolving. Because America was a pluralist society with an uncharacteristic form of government, implementing the Vatican II pronouncements presented a unique challenge.

The social climate in 1960s America differed significantly from that in most other countries. Demographic changes occurring after World War II altered the racial composition of many US cities as Blacks migrated from rural to urban areas and Whites moved from the cities to the suburbs. Because those moving to the cities were often poorer than those leaving, "American society became more and more segmented by race and class," historian Jay P. Dolan noted.[23] The resulting segmentation in metropolitan regions of the country ignited the civil rights movement, a widespread undertaking involving courts, Congress, religious leaders, and others to end discrimination in schools, housing, and healthcare facilities. Coinciding with the message of Vatican II, these events stimulated the quest for social justice among priests and sisters. Some sisters emerged from the convent to participate in boycotts, marches, sit-ins, and other forms of civil disobedience, while others left teaching and hospital work to participate in new forms of engagement.[24]

In addition to racial and class tensions and divisions, the other prominent force in 1960s America concerned the rights of women. While the first wave of feminism, spanning from 1848 (the date of the first Women's Rights Convention in Seneca Falls, New York) to 1920, centered on women's suffrage, the second wave from the 1960s to the 1980s stressed educational and job opportunities. Betty Friedan's 1963 book, *The Feminine Mystique*, inaugurated the second movement. Friedan articulated many women's desire to work outside the home, to pursue a career apart from "domesticity." In 1966, Friedan's followers formed the National Organization for Women and pushed for an equal rights amendment to the US Constitution.[25]

The struggle for women's rights energized America's Catholic sisters. They too sought relief or "emancipation," though not from domesticity but from convent culture. In 1962, Leon Joseph Cardinal Suenens, Pope John's emissary to the United Nations and a key figure in the Vatican II proceedings, penned a treatise, *The Nun in the World*, criticizing rigid convent rules, traditions, and lifestyles. "It is well known," Suenens wrote, "that what one can only call the anti-feminist tradition has had a long inning."[26] Addressing four thousand "nuns" in New York City on May 18, 1963, Suenens stirred the sisters to action. I have "not come . . . to preach peace," he said, "but to call for a revolution, a revolution in the life of active nuns, the nuns in the world, so that they may be able to fulfil as perfectly as possible their mission of bringing Christ to the world of the twentieth century."[27]

Suenens's oratory colored Vatican II teachings. Most of the sisterhoods, including the Daughters, altered their dress and lifestyle to conform to the modern world. They abandoned the traditional habit and replaced it with more modern attire; they revised the horariums that dictated their daily schedules; they removed restrictions on family visits; and they gave sisters greater choice in the selection of their mission and ministry.[28] For the Daughters, the change of habit augured a new era. Since the late 1600s, they had worn the famous white cornette and blue-gray attire of French peasant women. But in 1964, they significantly altered their appearance. "Gone is the large, stiffly starched head covering [called] a cornette," the *New York Times* reported. "In its place the sisters will now wear a trim, white headdress covered by a shoulder-length blue coif."[29] Outwardly, these changes reflected "a new relationship with the larger society"; inwardly, they embodied a new form of governance that enhanced personal autonomy.[30]

THE PRECIPITOUS DECLINE IN THE NUMBER OF US SISTERS

An unintended consequence of the changes Vatican II and the civil rights and women's rights movements initiated was a sharp decrease in the number of US sisters. In 1966, there were 181,421 Catholic nuns and sisters in America. By 1980, there were 126,517, a decrease of just over 30 percent.[31] The US Daughters were no exception. Between 1969 and 1980, their numbers declined from 2,448 to 1,781, or about 27 percent.[32]

The precipitous drop among US sisters caused considerable alarm. "A rebellion—quiet but significant—is raging in America's convents. Nuns are leaving in record numbers," the author of a 1967 article in *Ladies Home Journal* reported.[33] "The falloff in sisters is a grave blow—to church-related institutions and programs, especially schools and hospitals," Russel Shaw wrote for *Catholic Answers Magazine*.[34] There was much speculation about the reasons, from the Vatican II reforms to America's feminist movement. Some observers blamed the church's "rigid and unreasonable restrictions."[35] Others pointed to women's increasing professional opportunities and the improving economic status of many Catholics.[36]

Just as their numbers had peaked and were about to plummet, the Daughters expanded the amount of provinces in 1969 from two to five, as shown in figure 5.2. The five new provinces were the Northeast Province, headquartered in Albany, New York; the Southeast Province, headquartered in Emmitsburg, Maryland; the East Central Province, headquartered in Evansville, Indiana; the West Central Province, headquartered in St. Louis; and the West Province, headquartered in Los Altos Hills, California. Adding new provinces seemed untimely given the reductions in sisters, yet it proved advantageous. By expanding the number of provinces, the Daughters created new hierarchies, new pockets of innovation, and new forms of collaboration that aided their ability to respond at the local, regional, and national levels to a rapidly changing healthcare environment.

The combination of fewer women entering the community and the advancing age of the sisters reduced the number of Daughters willing and able to work in hospitals. Effects varied from province to province depending on the quantity, size, and characteristics of their sponsored hospitals. In

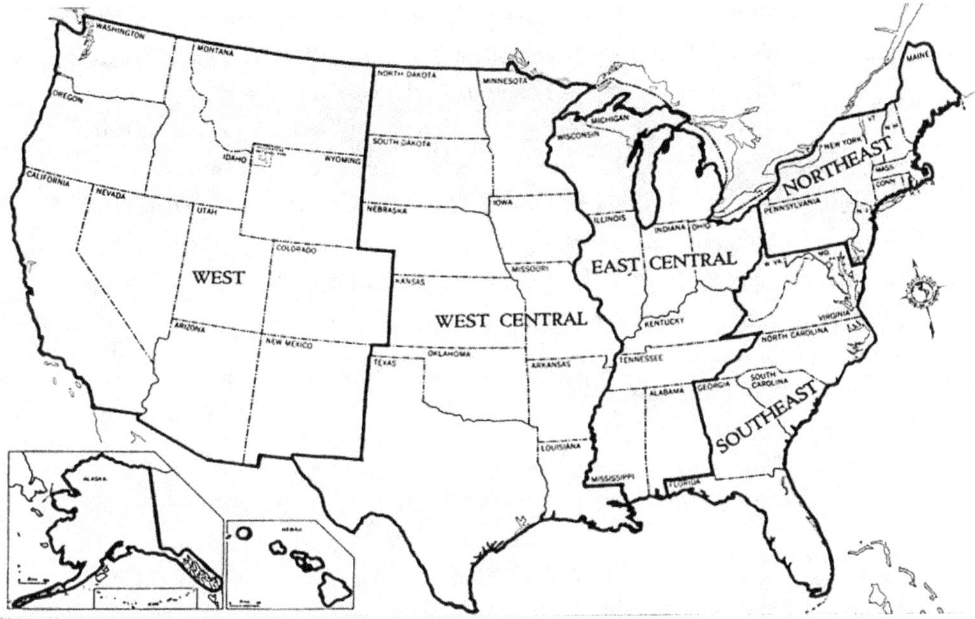

Figure 5.2. The Division of the Provinces, 1969.

1969, the Northeast Province had nine hospitals, the Southeast Province had nine, the East Central Province had ten, the West Central Province had thirteen, and the West Province had three.[37]

Acting independently but almost simultaneously, each of the five provinces initiated a review of its "works" or apostolates soon after the division. In 1970, the Northeast Province established an Apostolic Work Studies Commission under the direction of Sister Helen Kelley, DC.[38] One year later, in 1971, the West Central Province formed a similar committee for the purposes of determining which works "could be carried on [by laypersons] without the Sisters."[39] These efforts as well as others led to several withdrawals, sales, or closures. The West Central Province, for instance, withdrew "from about ten . . . works" including two hospitals—St. Joseph Hospital in St. Joseph, Missouri, and DePaul Hospital, a psychiatric facility in New Orleans—which the Daughters sold to non-Catholic entities.[40] Though provincial leaders resolved to stay at Charity Hospital in New Orleans and Lafayette Charity Hospital in Lafayette, Louisiana, both state-owned institutions, they opted to "gradual[ly] decrease" the number of sisters, noting "the pressing needs for sister personnel in other health areas."[41]

Instead of leveling off, the sharp decline continued, falling to 1,404 Daughters by 1990, a 43 percent reduction since 1969.[42] Data obtained from a 1983 assessment of their hospitals in the Northeast Province showed that the Daughters were overextended. Sisters of Charity Hospital in Buffalo, for instance, had 1,046 full-time employees but only eleven sisters.[43] Carney Hospital in Boston had more than two thousand part- and full-time employees but only ten sisters.[44] While provincial needs assessments continued, the piecemeal sale of hospitals to non-Catholic entities threatened the Daughters' healthcare ministry. Diminishing numbers of sisters, decreasing hospital revenues, and increasing competition in the 1980s called for new and bolder measures.

CIVIL RIGHTS AND ACCESS TO HEALTHCARE FOR RACIAL MINORITIES

In 1954, the US Supreme Court, in *Brown v. Board of Education*, held that the segregation of public schools by race was unconstitutional.[45] Subsequent Supreme Court decisions ruled that in addition to schools, public facilities such as buses, theaters, restrooms, libraries, cafeterias, parks, and hospitals could not exclude Blacks either.[46] The manner and course of desegregation differed by social sector.[47] Much depended on the ownership mix (public or private, sectarian or nonsectarian), the important stakeholders and organizations, the role of the federal government, and the means of financing the principal institutions in each sector.

In the field of education, most elementary and secondary schools were local and state institutions. Local school boards were engaged, as they are today, in policymaking and administration; they oversaw school budgets, allocated resources, and hired school superintendents. Resistance to public school desegregation was widespread in the South, yet state and local officials in Northern and border states, such as Maryland and Kentucky, often complied with the *Brown* decision. Catholic bishops followed the general pattern. Bishops integrated parochial schools in Washington, DC, Virginia, Texas, New Mexico, Kentucky, Tennessee, Oklahoma, and North Carolina.[48] But in the Deep South—in Alabama, Mississippi, Georgia, South Carolina, Louisiana, and Florida—the bishops vacillated.[49] They feared adverse reaction from the local populace, including the Catholic laity.[50]

Unlike education, the healthcare sector consisted of mostly privately owned, nonprofit hospitals and other facilities, such as nursing homes and doctors' offices. A 1950 survey of hospitals in major US cities showed that 66.9 percent of acute-care hospital beds were in nonprofit hospitals, 3.0 percent were in for-profit hospitals, and 32.5 percent were in public facilities. Twenty years later in 1970, the division was 76.5 percent nonprofit, 4.2 percent for-profit, and 19.3 percent public.[51] Hospital size over this twenty-year period increased substantially.[52] So did the percentage of nonprofit hospitals with medical school affiliations.[53] Many Southern hospitals refused to admit Blacks until the early 1960s, while others, Northern hospitals included, restricted Blacks to segregated wards, which often were overcrowded and housed in basements and attics.[54] One year after passage of the 1964 Civil Rights Act, the United States Commission on Civil Rights found that "nearly two-thirds" of the thirty-nine Southern hospitals it surveyed still maintained discriminatory practices. "No substantial change had occurred in patient admissions or assignment to rooms and wards," the commission discovered.[55]

Medical Staff Desegregation

The integration of Black patients was only the first step in the process. The second step, which proved to be more difficult, was the integration of Black doctors at White-run hospitals. Gaining admission to a medical school was challenging for most Blacks because few White schools would admit them. In 1955, only 216 Blacks attended a White medical college, but in 1962 there were even fewer.[56] Most Black physicians, roughly two-thirds in the 1950s and 1960s, received their medical degree from Howard University in Washington, DC, or Meharry Medical College in Nashville, both historically Black institutions.[57] The path toward success did not get any easier. Obtaining medical staff privileges and specialty training at an AMA-approved hospital was also problematic. Most doctors had to be members of their local medical society in order to secure hospital privileges and receive specialty training, yet many Southern medical societies denied membership to Black physicians until the mid-1960s.[58]

The Daughters were the first or among the first to integrate their hospitals' medical staffs depending on the particular location. They integrated the medical staff at St. Vincent's Hospital in Kansas City in 1952,[59] St. Paul's

Hospital in Dallas in 1954,[60] and Providence Hospital in the District of Columbia in 1955.[61] When researchers from Kansas University surveyed St. Vincent's Hospital in October 1952 in order to determine how things were proceeding, they were dumbfounded. "There were no demands for transfers to work situations involving less contact with Negroes," nor were there any apparent divisions among the Black and White physicians, the researchers discovered. In their final report, they concluded that "St. Vincent's is in so many ways a most peculiar institution." Believing that the situation was highly unusual, the researchers were "hesitant to generalize from St. Vincent's experience."[62]

The disposition of local physicians was an important factor in the Daughters' ability to desegregate their hospitals. If the medical staff was willing to accept Black physicians, then it was much easier for the Daughters to move forward. At St. Paul's Hospital in Dallas, for example, all three hundred staff physicians gave their approval.[63] And at St. Vincent's Hospital in Kansas City, the White medical staff welcomed their Black colleagues.[64] But at the Daughters' Alabama hospitals—St. Margaret's in Montgomery, St. Vincent's in Birmingham, and Providence in Mobile—the medical staff resisted.

In 1965, St. Margaret's administrator, Sister Catherine Fink, DC, accepted the applications of three Black doctors, "superseding" both the medical staff and the local medical society in the process.[65] Fink faced recrimination for her actions.[66] "In spite of the ignorance and hostility [surrounding you]," a physician from outside the South wrote in a letter, "I think you're doing a wonderful job at [St. Margaret's]. . . . We can certainly understand your feelings of frustration and hopelessness but thank God there are people like you."[67]

Not everyone felt that Fink was moving quickly enough to desegregate St. Margarets, however. John Leo, the associate editor at *Commonweal*, a progressive Catholic magazine from New York City, skewered the Daughters for providing only twenty-five beds for Black patients in a segregated wing at St. Margaret's.[68] Fink responded, writing Leo that she was doing everything she could under the circumstances. "A large segment of our employees are against integration to the point of being rude and not caring properly for the patients," Fink told Leo. If I "move too quickly," I will "jeopardize our apostolate to the Negro patients."[69] Montgomery's racial climate was particularly inhospitable. On March 7, 1965, known as "Bloody

Sunday," police assaulted demonstrators with nightsticks and tear gas as they marched from Selma to Montgomery, sending seventeen protestors to the hospital, many of them with serious injuries.[70]

Hostility toward racial integration was equally intense in Birmingham, where St. Vincent's Hospital was located. Attacks on homes and churches occurred with such frequency that some critics called the city "Bombingham."[71] On Sunday, September 15, 1963, the situation reached a climax when a bomb exploded at the 16th Street Baptist Church, killing four young girls and injuring fourteen other people. The publicity surrounding the bombing, coupled with the ensuing demonstrations and investigations, raised national awareness.[72] "Birmingham is probably the most thoroughly segregated city in the United States. Its ugly record of police brutality is widely known. . . . There have been more unsolved bombings of Negro homes and churches in Birmingham than in any other city in the nation," wrote Martin Luther King Jr. from his Birmingham jail cell.[73]

Black physicians could not obtain privileges in any of Birmingham's accredited hospitals, including St. Vincent's, before the mid-1960s.[74] Unable to gain appointments at the city's White-run hospitals, Black doctors left the area. In 1971, the US comptroller general reported that "only 15 black physicians were practicing at hospitals in Birmingham."[75] Despite the racially charged environment, the Daughters made some, if limited, headway. In 1963, St. Vincent's nursing school admitted four Black students. One of them, Quentine Johnson, worked in the operating room at St. Vincent's before beginning her education. Johnson noted that there were very few nursing schools that accepted Blacks when she first started. Upon her graduation in 1967, she expressed her appreciation for the instruction she received at St. Vincent's. "In my freshman year," she stated, "the faculty and students treated me so warmly, it was just like home."[76]

At Providence Hospital in Mobile, the Daughters were more successful. Despite intense opposition from White doctors, Providence was the first Mobile hospital to comply with the 1964 Civil Rights Act's antidiscrimination provisions and receive federal certification.[77] Protesting the Daughters' actions, several staff physicians sent their patients to the Mobile Infirmary, a White-only facility.[78] Providence's average daily occupancy plummeted from 99 percent in 1964 to 69 percent in 1967 following the staff physicians' actions, prompting a reevaluation of a planned expansion the hospital had submitted to Alabama's Department of Health for approval a couple years earlier. "While the 1967 occupancy . . . gives reason to doubt that the proposed addition [to Providence] is needed," an official from the health department stated, "the downward trend in utilization, if not immediately reversed, would appear to indicate that within a few years the hospital may be forced to close due to lack of patients."[79] Fearing further recrimination at Providence and other area hospitals, the federal government stopped the certification process until all healthcare facilities satisfied the act's conditions.[80] Providence eventually recovered.[81]

Hospital Relocations

The First Great Migration of Blacks from Southern to Northern states occurred from 1916 to 1940, while the Second Great Migration took place after World War II and lasted until about 1970. Chicago, Cleveland, Detroit, Buffalo, New York, and Philadelphia experienced large changes in racial composition, from predominately White to predominately Black in many neighborhoods. But this was not simply a matter of displacement and replacement, of Whites leaving as Blacks entered. The number of departures substantially exceeded new arrivals. More than half of large US cities (those with populations exceeding two hundred thousand in 1950) suffered population losses between 1950 and 1980.[82] Two of the cities in which the Daughters owned hospitals—Buffalo and St. Louis—lost more than 20 percent of their residents.[83]

A principal reason for the exodus was greater access between central cities and suburbs, the construction of roads and highways connecting the two locations.[84] Members of the growing middle class could now enjoy the benefits of suburban life—larger homes, better schools, lower crime rates, and lower taxes—and still work in the downtown area. For those Blacks and Whites remaining in city centers, residential segregation was the common pattern. "Regardless of their economic status, Negros rarely live in 'White' neighborhoods, while Whites, no matter how poor, rarely live in Negro residential areas," sociologists Karl and Alma Taeuber discovered while conducting research in the mid-1960s.[85] Government policies significantly contributed to the situation, including loan restrictions, racial covenants, redlining, racial zoning, and the construction of roads and highways dissecting Black and White communities.[86]

Many urban hospitals either shut down or relocated to the suburbs during the transition. One study showed that 210 hospitals closed or relocated in fifty-two cities between 1937 and 1980.[87] The largest number of closures occurred from 1972 to 1978.[88] For-profit hospitals were most likely to discontinue during this period, followed by voluntary, nonprofit hospitals, and lastly government, nonfederal facilities.[89] Among the reasons for hospital closures or relocations were financial difficulties, outdated facilities, low occupancy rates, and insufficient staffing.[90] But there was one overriding determinant, one dominant factor associated with hospital closure or relocation that stood out among the others—the racial composition of the surrounding neighborhood. Almost 50 percent of hospitals located in predominantly Black neighborhoods closed or relocated between 1937 and 1977, while just over 14 percent of hospitals in predominantly White neighborhoods closed or relocated.[91]

Yet few of the Daughters' urban hospitals shut down or moved from the cities to the suburbs during this period. Reasons included their medium to large size, their medical school affiliations, their good fiscal management, and their accessible locations, such as proximity to a major thoroughfare or highway.[92] Still, the Daughters had to rebuild or renovate several of their hospitals. Rebuilding often meant moving to a different site that allowed for future expansion and more room for parking. Sometimes the new location was in close proximity to the old one, across the street or on abutting property. On other occasions, it was a few miles away, in an area bordering a middle-class White neighborhood. In 1948, Buffalo's Sisters of Charity Hospital moved to a new facility several blocks northeast on Main Street, to the north of the Humboldt Parkway and Kensington Avenue;[93] in 1953, Boston's Carney Hospital relocated from South Boston to South Dorchester, about five miles from its original location;[94] in 1956, Washington's Providence Hospital opened a new hospital in the Michigan Park section of Northeast Washington, DC;[95] in 1964, Chicago's St. Joseph Hospital moved from 2100 N. Burling Street in the Lincoln Park neighborhood to 2900 N. Lake Shore Drive;[96] and in 1972, following years of "considerable interior renovation," New Orleans's Hôtel Dieu rebuilt across the street from the old one.[97]

At the end of the Second Great Migration in 1970, two of the Daughters' hospitals, St. Mary's in Rochester and DePaul in St. Louis, were in predominantly Black communities. While St. Mary's did not change location,

DePaul moved to the suburbs.[98] "In choosing [to stay]" in Rochester, Sister Daniel Hannefin, DC, wrote, "the [hospital] board gave witness to the commitment to care for the poor and underserved."[99] Community associations, Catholic churches in the area, and municipal leaders supported the Daughters. This "is certainly one of the most neglected areas of the city," a document contained in the parish records of Ss. Peter and Paul Roman Catholic Church stated. "We are trying to make ourselves known to the people. . . . We are trying to communicate [to] Black people that S[s.] Peter and Paul welcomes them."[100] In 1979, a regional health agency approved an eight-million-dollar renovation to St. Mary's Hospital.[101]

The Daughters also sought to remain in St. Louis, but the obstacles were more substantial than in Rochester. Over the course of fifty years, from 1950 and 2000, St. Louis lost more than 60 percent of its residents, dropping from number eight to number fifty in population among major US cities. "Not since the Romans leveled Carthage has a city lost so much of its population," an urban policy analyst hyperbolically stated.[102] East St. Louis, the location of DePaul Hospital, was the epicenter of the out-migration. From the mid-1950s to the mid-1960s, many middle-class Whites left East St. Louis, leaving behind poor and largely unskilled Black workers.[103] Unemployment reached 21 percent by 1967, the crime rate soared, and large numbers of retailers either closed or left the vicinity.[104]

On November 20, 1968, the Daughters commenced discussions about relocating to the town of Bridgeton in northwest St. Louis County. Three years earlier, the Daughters had purchased a tract of land in Bridgeton near the intersection of Interstates 70 and 270 with the intention of eventually expanding their operations. By 1968, pressure was mounting to move the hospital to the new location. Sixty staff physicians signed a petition advocating relocation, listing as reasons the losses of paying patients, nursing staff, and doctors; the "futility" of renovating the old facility; the inability to attract young physicians; and the "need for hospital beds in fast-growing [St. Louis County]."[105] Still, the Daughters refused to leave East St. Louis. Sister servant Josephine Aitchison, DC, and her fellow Daughters examined the options. At a meeting on September 19, 1969, they reached a conclusion. The proposed "medical complex" in Bridgeton should proceed, they determined, but the old hospital should convert to a "comprehensive community health care center" and remain at the old location.[106]

The conversion failed to materialize for lack of funding, however, as discontent increased among the staff physicians.[107] By 1971, DePaul's financial situation had become desperate. Citing "decreasing medical staff use," a 7.5 percent decline in patient census over the previous two years, and "inflationary construction costs," Anthony Bunker, the first lay administrator of a Daughter-owned hospital, announced that DePaul would move to Bridgeton.[108] Construction began in 1973, and the new hospital opened for patients five years later.[109]

The Renewed Emphasis on Outpatient Clinics

As the DePaul Hospital situation demonstrated, the Daughters struggled to reconcile the needs of the poor Black community with the hospital's future prosperity. When the Daughters raised concerns about those left behind, proponents of relocation argued that the sisters were not abandoning the Black residents, that government programs and public or teaching hospitals were available to them.[110] DePaul Hospital "is not making an impact on the health care needs of the poor," Dr. William Smiley, one of DePaul's staff physicians, maintained at a December 1968 meeting. What the Black community needed, Smiley claimed, was access to primary care services. Acute-care hospitals could not replace the "family doctor," he asserted. Federally funded "neighborhood clinics . . . tied to a hospital/medical complex may be the answer," he suggested.[111]

Smiley's observations and advice to the Daughters was timely. By the late 1960s, the dearth of physicians engaged in the general practice of medicine was a serious problem as chronic diseases including diabetes, asthma, hypertension, and various heart conditions escalated. In 1949, 50.1 percent of all US doctors were generalists, but by 1970, only 18.6 percent of US doctors practiced general or primary care medicine.[112] Public health advocates clamored for a new type of physician who could replace the aging and obsolete general practitioner. The search officially began in 1963 when the AMA formed a commission under the leadership of John Millis, the president of Western Reserve University (the predecessor to Case Western Reserve University). Three years later, the Millis Commission issued its report, declaring that "primary physicians" (general internists, pediatricians, and family practitioners) could fill the void if they provided "comprehensive and continuing health care."[113] Rather than focus on a specific body part or disease, primary physicians should care for the whole person, the Millis Commission determined. The AMA endorsed the commission's report and, in 1969, approved a specialization in family medicine.[114]

But even if the number of primary physicians increased, few poor persons would have sufficient access to them. This was because family doctors were often among the first to leave the inner cities when their patients migrated to the suburbs. Rather than reverse the trend, the Medicaid program, which provided health insurance for the indigent, aggravated the situation.[115] Medicaid reimbursed doctors at lower rates than private health insurers, typically below the cost of services rendered. Doctors who took on large numbers of Medicaid patients frequently made up the difference by multiplying, sometimes excessively, the volume of services to Medicaid patients.[116] Given the economic constraints and the deteriorating condition of the surrounding community, many family practitioners, including those at DePaul Hospital, followed their middle-class patients. When the Daughters criticized DePaul's physicians for moving, one doctor retorted, "The Sisters . . . cannot accept [the] fact that it is the patients, not the Doctors, who do not want to go to DePaul Hospital."[117]

The Daughters faced a growing reality—their acute-care hospitals were not the best means for handling the healthcare needs of poor people. Decades earlier, they had tried to care for the poor through their hospital outpatient clinics, but opposition from organized medicine, increasing specialization, and changes in medical education and training had undermined their good intentions. By 1970, less than 30 percent of voluntary, nonprofit hospitals operated outpatient clinics.[118] DePaul Hospital in St. Louis closed its clinic and terminated its internship and residency programs in medicine, OB/GYN, and surgery in the early 1960s.[119] But this did not mean that DePaul and other nonprofit hospitals failed to provide outpatient services. Instead, the hospital emergency room (ER) became the favored option. Almost 90 percent of nonprofit hospitals provided outpatient care in the ER by 1977, DePaul included.[120] ERs were not the solution to the problem, however. Large numbers of poor people used them for nonurgent reasons.[121] According to a 1970 study of New York City area hospitals, only 8 percent of ER patients at urban hospitals were true emergencies, while 68 percent of those at suburban hospitals required emergency treatment.[122]

Responding to the lack of nonurgent, primary care facilities for the indigent, several local health departments expanded their services. By 1969, health departments in Denver, Washington, DC, New York, Philadelphia, and several other cities operated "comprehensive health centers" or planned for them.[123] In 1965, the federal government joined the effort when the Office of Economic Opportunity revitalized the neighborhood health centers movement. Though a few medical societies still resisted, much of the hostility by this time had dissipated.[124] By 1971, almost one hundred centers, the majority of them in inner cities, received federal assistance.[125]

The Daughters recognized the need for community health centers and sought to promote them. Their attempt to convert DePaul Hospital into a comprehensive healthcare facility was a good example. In addition, they pursued similar initiatives in other parts of the country. Among the earliest and best-organized efforts occurred at Boston's Carney Hospital. In 1962, members of Carney's ER committee recommended expansion because of "an increase in the number of [nonurgent] patients."[126] Though the Daughters made some adjustments and planned to construct a new facility, they realized that expanding the ER was not a panacea. Unlike DePaul, Carney had a robust outpatient department that oversaw twenty-six specialty clinics. From 1960 to 1967, clinic visits at Carney increased from 13,028 to 22,785 (74 percent), while ER visits rose from 17,800 to 35,094 (97 percent).[127] Demand for healthcare services, the Daughters observed, had "far outstripped . . . medical manpower" because of enhanced insurance coverage and the diminishing number of general practitioners. In 1968, they announced the formation of a "Sixth Major Division" at Carney, the "Division of Ambulatory and Community Services." Henceforth, they would strive to bring services to the patient and not simply "beckon the needy" to come to the hospital.[128]

After giving serious consideration to starting a mobile clinic, the Daughters at Carney decided that permanent facilities located in outlying areas were better. By 1974, they had established two satellite clinics and had reached formal agreements with two free-standing community health centers.[129] Staffing and financial resources were among the factors the Daughters considered in site selection and affiliation. For purposes of economy and to prevent "isolation," hospital outpatient departments, clinics, and health centers shared nurses and physicians. Doctors assigned to the clinics and health centers "spent at least one half-day per week" at one of Carney's outpatient departments. They had "full admitting privileges" at the hospital and actively participated in its "teaching programs."[130]

The formation of satellite clinics and the promotion of freestanding neighborhood health centers at Carney Hospital and elsewhere in the early 1970s signaled a change in strategy. The provision of primary care services to the indigent outside the hospital setting expanded, given the extensive changes occurring in healthcare finance and delivery, the shifting racial composition of urban areas, the surge of illegal drugs, and the proliferation of chronic diseases among poor people in the inner cities and in rural parts of the country. Ambulatory care was becoming more portable, physician group practice and other innovative forms of healthcare delivery were advancing, and data collection and communications technology were progressing. At the same time, however, managing a hospital was becoming a very complex undertaking, requiring a large staff of highly trained administrators who could handle the growing needs and interests of internal and external stakeholders. A 1976 report from Carney Hospital noted that costs were mounting, that health insurance coverage "varied greatly from area to area and even from neighborhood to neighborhood," and that retention of professional staff was a problem.[131]

THE DAUGHTERS CONSOLIDATE THEIR ASSETS

Escalating healthcare costs in the 1970s and 1980s forced third-party payers (governments and private insurers) to initiate stringent cost containment measures. With the insolvency of the Medicare Part A (Part A covered hospital expenses) trust fund looming, Congress in 1983 changed the traditional manner of hospital reimbursement from retrospective to prospective payment. Under the new arrangement, hospitals received payment in advance based on a patient's diagnosis rather than retrospectively for services rendered. But instead of receding, hospital margins grew before the federal government, in 1986, lowered the annual percentage increase for prospective payments.[132]

Encountering declining revenues, hospitals increased their rates to private insurers, an approach known as cost-shifting.[133] Private insurers in turn raised their premiums, forcing numerous employers, particularly small ones, either to drop health insurance altogether or provide marginal coverage. Meanwhile, many large employers switched from traditional indemnity insurance to more cost-effective managed care plans, which big commercial insurers began to offer in the mid-1980s. As the percentage of employees in managed care plans increased from 27 percent in 1988 to 73 percent in 1995, bargaining leverage shifted from providers to payers, that is, from hospitals and physicians to large insurance companies.[134]

Seeking to combat the enhanced bargaining power of insurers, numerous hospitals responded by forming multihospital systems. Physicians also banded together in group practices. Some even joined the new hospital systems. Catholic hospitals were particularly well-suited to system formation because sisterhoods often sponsored more than one hospital. In 1978, as nurse historian Barbra Mann Wall noted, there were forty-five Catholic congregations in the United States with four or more healthcare facilities.[135] Obstacles to system formation were easier to overcome in such circumstances. Common goals, norms, values, and philosophies were already in place, as was the sponsoring entity, the religious community.

For the Daughters, the integration of their hospitals and other healthcare facilities to achieve economies of size and scale was not an insurmountable challenge. By this time, the community had several outstanding leaders with strong business acuity who, with assistance from skilled laypersons, worked together on several occasions to surmount local and regional barriers. Indeed, the Daughters had already established central purchasing departments in the Eastern and Western Provinces before the 1969 division. In 1982, under the leadership of Sister Bernice Coreil, DC, visitatrix of the West Central Province, the Daughters founded a national purchasing service to centralize procurement. Two years later, in 1984, the three western provinces (East Central, West Central, and West) founded Daughters of Charity Health Systems Inc.[136] And in 1986, the Northeast Province and the Southeast Province joined them to form the Daughters of Charity National Health System (DCNHS).[137]

Upon its incorporation on July 18, 1986, DCNHS became the umbrella organization for forty-three healthcare facilities (forty acute-care hospitals and three nursing homes) in seventeen states and the District of Columbia.[138] Through eight corporate offices in different regions of the country, DCNHS provided the means for coordinating and consolidating purchasing, data processing, risk management, insurance, pension, and financial services.[139] DCNHS's corporate structure maximized the Daughters' control over key functions. A majority of the DCNHS board of directors had to be Daughters, as well as the corporate president or chief executive officer; so did the governing boards of the regional corporations that oversaw the hospitals in that region. Though governance of local hospitals did not change (laypersons might outnumber Daughters on individual hospital boards, for instance), the new arrangement afforded the Daughters veto and appointment powers, subject to "local law and/or regional preferences."[140]

When established in 1986, DCNHS became the fourth largest multihospital chain in the country measured by the number of licensed acute-care beds (13,228).[141] Only three systems surpassed it—Hospital Corporation of America, Humana, and American Medical International—all of them for-profit entities. DCNHS also was among the leaders in total assets and annual revenues. Its combined assets in 1986 totaled $2.4 billion, while annual income topped $2.6 billion, making DCNHS the fifth largest multihospital system in terms of revenue generation.[142]

At a June 1986 meeting, the five provincial superiors chose Sister Irene Kraus, DC, for DCNHS president and Sister Theresa Peck, DC, for executive vice president. Having entered the community in 1941 at age seventeen, Kraus taught in Catholic schools in Richmond, Virginia, for seven years before receiving a degree in nursing from the Catholic University of America. Initially an operating room nurse, Kraus excelled as a hospital administrator, serving as president/CEO at seven different hospitals, including Providence Hospital in Washington, DC (1975–83). Before becoming president at DCNHS, she already had chaired the boards of both the CHA (1971–74) and the American Hospital Association (1979–81). In 1986, the same year she took over at DCNHS, Kraus received the American Hospital Association's Distinguished Service Medal and, five years later in 1991, the Gold Medal for Excellence in Hospital Administration from the American College of Health Care Executives.[143]

Sister Theresa Peck also was an experienced hospital administrator at the time of her appointment. After entering the community in 1956, she obtained her degree in nursing from Marillac College before serving at St. Mary's Help Hospital in San Francisco, Hôtel Dieu in El Paso, and St. Vincent's Medical Center in Los Angeles. Upon receiving a master's degree in business administration in 1969 from George Washington University, Peck became chief executive officer at St. Joseph Hospital in Chicago. Several more top assignments at hospitals followed, including CEO at St. Mary Medical Center in Evansville and St. Vincent Hospital in Indianapolis.[144]

Kraus and Peck were examples of the "more active, visible, and vocal" Daughters the community sought to foster. By the end of the 1960s, several Daughters were in leading positions at national organizations. They were policymakers, not passive bystanders. As board chair at the CHA, Kraus worked alongside Sister Mary Maurita Sengelaub, RSM, the CHA's first female chief executive officer.[145] Together with Sengelaub in the early 1970s, Kraus helped to develop the framework for Catholic-sponsored multihospital systems.[146] In 1973, Sengelaub established a "Study Committee" and directed its members to assess and define the CHA's future role in Catholic healthcare delivery. With assistance from industry consultants, the Study Committee issued several recommendations that the association largely implemented. The recommendations included "developing alternatives for sponsorship, with an emphasis on building systems, . . . [and] strengthening the association's advocacy and government efforts."[147] In 1979, the CHA changed its name from the Catholic Hospital Association to the Catholic Health Association in recognition of the increasing importance of outpatient care and the growing prevalence of new types of healthcare facilities to deliver it.

When Sengelaub resigned for health reasons in 1977, Sister Helen Kelley, DC, succeeded her. Similar to Kraus and Peck, Kelley had a master's degree in health administration and had served as an administrator at several of the Daughters' hospitals, including Sisters of Charity in Buffalo, St. Agnes in Baltimore, and Carney in Boston, before becoming the CHA's top executive. During her brief tenure at CHA (1977–79), Kelley continued and completed the work of the Study Committee.[148]

Clearly, the CHA and the Daughters were closely aligned in the 1970s and 1980s, exchanging ideas and information. Just as Kelley's experience as chair of the Work Study Commission for the Northeast Province in the early 1970s influenced the findings of the CHA's Study Committee, so Kraus's work on systems formation at the CHA guided her efforts as DCNHS president. The working relationship between the Daughters and the CHA developed and flourished in the following years and decades. They had several common interests. One of them concerned governmental challenges to the tax-exempt status of nonprofit hospitals.[149] The other was federal legislation to expand insurance coverage.

SIX

RECONCILING DIVISIONS OVER ACCESS TO REPRODUCTIVE SERVICES

Before Vatican II, the Daughters' contests with bishops largely occurred within the church, such as the rift with Bishop John Hughes over their refusal to take in older male children at their New York City orphanages. But the Vatican II pronouncements, coupled with the broader cultural changes occurring in 1960s America, brought internal church divisions into the public forum. This was particularly the case in the healthcare industry, where government and private insurers set the parameters in the final decades of the twentieth century for healthcare delivery. These parameters sometimes conflicted with church prohibitions on certain reproductive services—contraception, sterilization, and abortion.

The resulting conflicts among church prelates, public health officials, community activists, and politicians over access to reproductive services often required the Daughters and other hospital-owning sisterhoods to navigate between two polar and frequently irreconcilable positions. When the Daughters sought to merge, affiliate, or sell their hospitals to non-Catholic facilities that performed artificial contraception, sterilizations, and abortions, they had to find ways to distance their facilities from these practices or face recrimination from the bishops. And when they sought to increase access to care for poor people through legislation that provided insurance coverage for such services, they faced opposition from the clergy.

MERGERS, SALES, AND ACQUISITIONS

While Catholic prelates and theologians were united in their opposition to elective abortions, there was widespread disagreement concerning the church's long-standing proscriptions on artificial contraception and sterilization. Several "revisionist" Catholic theologians, including Charles Curran, Albert Jonsen, John Courtney Murray, SJ, and Richard McCormick, SJ, believed that church doctrine should be more flexible, that it should accommodate America's shifting cultural norms governing reproductive matters. Vatican II, they argued, called for a more nuanced position on contraception and sterilization. The church's traditional "absolutist" proscriptions, they claimed, failed to embrace Vatican II teachings.[1] Such views gained acceptance within the nascent field of bioethics, which emerged in the 1960s at several universities, including the Kennedy Institute at Georgetown University and other church-sponsored institutions.[2]

At the close of Vatican II, the Catholic hierarchy seemed receptive to the "revisionist" thesis. In 1965, Boston Archbishop Richard Cushing, for instance, did not oppose a bill in the Massachusetts legislature allowing doctors to prescribe contraceptives.[3] Father John Courtney Murray, SJ, an articulate spokesperson for religious liberty, agreed with Cushing's position. He asserted that Catholic religious principles should not inhibit civil legislation.[4] Two years after the US Supreme Court's 1965 decision in *Griswald v. Connecticut*[5] striking down a Connecticut law criminalizing the sale of contraceptives, a papal commission recommended that the church should end its ban on artificial contraception. Considering the groundswell of opinion within the church supporting liberalization, many anticipated that Pope Paul VI would relax the prohibition. But in a 1968 papal encyclical, *Humanae Vitae*, the pope retained it.[6]

Before 1971, there were no uniform guidelines or standards governing the provision of reproductive services at Catholic-owned or -administered healthcare facilities. Though the CHA had promulgated *Ethical and Religious Directives for Catholic Health Facilities* (the *Directives*) in 1949, they had no force and effect unless the local bishop applied them to hospitals located in his diocese. The 1949 *Directives* received disparate treatment depending on the particular location, a situation known as "geographic morality."[7] While some bishops prohibited artificial contraception and sterilization, others allowed it, such as Archbishop Robert J. Dwyer of Portland, Oregon. Declaring that "nothing in Catholic doctrine prevents the practice of good medicine," Dwyer approved sterilization for birth control purposes at Sacred Heart Hospital in Eugene, Oregon, on February 26, 1970.[8]

Only a few weeks after Dwyer's decision, the issue surfaced again in Waterville, Maine, where the Daughters owned and operated Elizabeth Ann Seton Hospital. A relatively small town with a population of just over eighteen thousand, Waterville had three local hospitals—Thayer Hospital, Northern Light Inland Hospital, and Elizabeth Ann Seton Hospital. Constructed in 1965, the 140-bed Seton Hospital was the largest of the three.[9] Sometime in the early 1970s, Thayer's administrator approached Seton's sister servant, Sister Lorraine O'Brien, DC, seeking a merger between the respective hospitals' obstetrical departments. Thayer's obstetrical facilities did not meet standards for accreditation, and, hoping to avoid departmental closure or renovation, it sought a partner.[10] There is no indication that the merger of the obstetrical departments went forward in 1970, however. In 1973, the Daughters withdrew from Seton, citing a shortage of sisters, and in 1975, Seton and Thayer merged their facilities, forming Mid-Maine Medical Center.[11]

At the CHA's urging, the National Conference of Catholic Bishops issued a new set of *Directives* in 1971 in an effort to end "geographic morality." The revisionists were disappointed. The new *Directives* contained blanket prohibitions or "moral prescriptions" that left little room for more nuanced and scientific applications in concrete situations. Two of the proscriptions concerned artificial contraception and sterilization. In addition, the 1971 *Directives* made local bishops the sole arbiters in medical and ethical decision-making, notwithstanding their lack of expertise in these areas.[12]

Not every bishop agreed with the 1971 *Directives*. Bishop Peter L. Gerety of Portland, Maine, whose diocese included Seton Hospital, was among the dissenters. On June 20, 1972, Sister Mary Walter Boyle, DC, Seton Hospital's administrator (Boyle succeeded O'Brien), wrote to Bishop Gerety notifying him that the hospital board had adopted the *Directives*.[13] Gerety opposed the board's decision. At a meeting of the hospital board, Gerety's representative, Father Robert Lee, told the board members that the *Directives* were "inadequate for today's problems," that they had been "cut to pieces by the Catholic Hospital Association" before their publication, and that "because [Seton] is a community hospital, [the board] can't impose [its] morality on others."[14] Clearly, Gerety had embraced the revisionist argument. Yet, on January 31, 1973, Gerety changed his position. "We are going to promulgate the [*Directives*] for Catholic Hospitals in the Diocese of Portland," he wrote Boyle. The US Supreme Court's January 22 decision in *Roe v. Wade*,[15] recognizing a woman's constitutional right to an abortion, was the reason. "The recent Supreme Court decision has made this particularly urgent, at least psychologically," Gerety stated.[16]

After the Supreme Court announced the *Roe* decision, much of the political and social discourse on human reproduction and sexuality centered on abortion. Catholic bishops reacted swiftly, calling the *Roe* decision "wrong and entirely contrary to the fundamental principles of morality."[17] So did the CHA, which issued a statement deploring the decision and announcing that its member hospitals "would continue their tradition of not performing abortions despite the high court ruling."[18] Medical associations representing Catholic physicians joined the criticism. The president of the National Federation of Catholic Physicians' Guilds, for instance, declared that the Supreme Court had ignored "indisputable evidence . . . that life begins at the moment of conception."[19]

Responding to the public outcry, Congress passed the Church Amendment, the first in a series of laws intended to protect the religious and moral beliefs of healthcare providers from adverse actions of government agencies and public officials, such as withholding public funds for refusing to perform abortions.[20] Pro-choice groups countered, suing Catholic hospitals for failing to provide tubal ligations and pressing state legislature to pass laws mandating insurance coverage for contraceptives.[21] Catholic sisters who owned hospitals increasingly found themselves in challenging situations as disputes over abortion subsumed discussions over emergency contraception, residency programs in obstetrics and gynecology, and other matters related to human reproduction and family planning.[22] Hospital mergers, sales, and acquisitions between Catholic and non-Catholic hospitals garnered close attention.

For much of the 1980s, the bishops did not closely examine hospital mergers to see if they violated the *Directives* because many of them, the formation of DCNHS, for example, involved Catholic-owned facilities. But mergers or affiliations between sister-owned hospitals and non-Catholic facilities offering reproductive services were a different matter altogether. Bishops scrutinized such mergers and affiliations in order to determine the extent to which the Catholic hospital was involved in the delivery of prohibited services by the non-Catholic entity. Approval hinged on whether the Catholic hospital indirectly or directly participated. "Indirect participation" was permissible, but "direct participation" was not.[23]

Several of the Daughters' ventures passed careful scrutiny. Their investment in the Middle Tennessee Medical Center in Murfreesboro, Tennessee, received the local bishop's endorsement, for instance, even though a women's clinic located on the first floor of the medical center provided artificial contraception and sterilization. The clinic, known as the "Baptist Women's Pavilion," rented the space from the medical center and had its own sign and its own entrance.[24] The formation of Western Maryland Health System in Cumberland, Maryland, involving Memorial Hospital and Daughter-owned Sacred Heart Hospital, also passed inspection, as did a joint venture between the Daughters and a chain of Baptist hospitals in Jacksonville, Florida. In both situations, the non-Catholic hospitals continued to provide artificial contraception and sterilization under their own auspices. The purpose of the joint ventures was to increase market share and eliminate the duplication of services, not to give the Daughters' direct oversight of the affiliated institutions or the services they provided.[25]

Because the distinction between indirect and direct participation was subject to the local bishop's interpretation, the outcome was uncertain. The 1971 *Directives* provided little guidance in close situations, prompting revisions in 1994, 2001, 2009, and 2018 to account for changing circumstances and advancing technology.[26] The stakes were high. Should a merger go forward without the bishop's endorsement, the Daughters' hospital faced loss of church sponsorship. Loss of church sponsorship, though an infrequent occurrence in the 1970s, became more prevalent in the 1980s and 1990s. Between 1984 and 1999, sixty-seven Catholic hospitals lost church sponsorship when they acted without clerical authority.[27]

One of the reasons, if not the main reason, for the higher rate of disapprovals toward the end of the twentieth century was the increase in mergers between Catholic hospitals and financially distressed public hospitals in urban areas. By the late 1990s, several inner-city public hospitals were faltering and needed outside assistance in order to stay open. Catholic health systems and their affiliated hospitals, on the other hand, had stabilized their finances following their consolidation in the late 1980s and early 1990s. Though the Daughters (and other sisterhoods) sought to help the distressed facilities, they struggled to meet the standard for indirect participation.[28] Unlike mergers and affiliations between equal partners such as those in Cumberland and Jacksonville, Catholic health systems and hospitals were the dominant parties in many of these transactions. They had to find ways to distance themselves from offering prohibited services, notwithstanding their controlling interest in these undertakings.

In 1997, for example, Niagara Falls Memorial Hospital sought the Daughters' financial and managerial assistance. Negotiations stalled when a local citizens' group, fearing the loss of women's reproductive services, resisted. The Daughters were caught in the middle, between the local ordinary, Bishop Henry Mansell of Buffalo, and the community activists who wanted the services to continue. Following further discussions, Bishop Mansell granted a "temporary" exception. Niagara Falls Memorial could not provide the prohibited services while under the Daughters' auspices, but an affiliated outpatient clinic under separate management in a building located a few blocks from the hospital could furnish them.[29] The contemplated merger between the Daughter-owned hospital in the area, Mount St. Mary's, and Niagara Falls Memorial did not materialize, however, and the parties went their separate ways in 2007. Yet, for ten years, the initial partnership provided a temporary solution to Niagara Memorial's financial problems.[30]

Negotiations between Daughter-owned Seton Medical Center and city-owned Brackenridge Hospital in Austin, Texas, led to a similar outcome, though the process was more lengthy and contentious. Debt-ridden Brackenridge Hospital needed financial support, and Seton Medical Center was willing to give it. In May 1995, Seton and Brackenridge reached an agreement in which Seton would lease Brackenridge and take over its management. The terms of the lease provided that Brackenridge could continue to deliver contraceptive and sterilization services on the leased premises.

Though Bishop John McCarthy, the local prelate, approved the undertaking, the Vatican instructed McCarthy to reverse his decision after a group of Catholic laity wrote to the Congregation for the Doctrine of the

Faith (the conclave of cardinals at the Vatican responsible for religious discipline) voicing their objections.[31] Unless the Daughters could find a solution that satisfied the Catholic hierarchy, they would have to dissolve the partnership with Brackenridge. During another round of negotiations, the parties reached an acceptable solution. Under the new arrangement, city employees provided sterilization and contraceptive services in a separately licensed facility on the fifth floor of Brackenridge, "a hospital within a hospital."[32]

The events at Niagara Falls and Austin illustrate the wide-ranging dynamics surrounding the delivery of reproductive services at Catholic-administered or Catholic-affiliated healthcare facilities. In both situations, city officials were persistent and the local bishops were willing to consider the options. Had the bishops opposed the ventures, the Daughters would have had to terminate discussions or face the loss of Catholic sponsorship. Though the Daughters could move forward in Niagara Falls and Austin, that was not the case at Carney Hospital in Boston.

THE SAD SAGA OF BOSTON'S CARNEY HOSPITAL

In 1997, the Daughters sold Carney Hospital to Caritas Christi Heath System, which the Boston Archdiocese owned and operated. The Daughters did not want to sell Carney to Caritas; they had better options, but Boston Archbishop Bernard Cardinal Law thwarted their objectives.

A mainstay of the greater Boston community, Carney encountered many of the problems facing small community hospitals bordering low-income neighborhoods—declining utilization and decreasing insurance reimbursements. Carney needed assistance. Law wanted to help, but only if the Daughters sold Carney to Caritas. Formed in 1986, one year after Law arrived in Boston, Caritas comprised six hospitals, a hospice, and several other healthcare facilities. St. Elizabeth's Medical Center, located in Brighton, Massachusetts, was the largest of the six hospitals.[33]

In May 1994, the Daughters "entered into discussions" with Partners HealthCare Systems, which included Massachusetts General and Brigham and Women's Hospitals, two of the leading academic medical centers in the country with ties to Harvard University.[34] Carney's board of directors strongly supported an affiliation with Partners; so did Carney's medical staff. "Carney Hospital's only real chance for survival and its chance to continue to do . . . great work [for] this community . . . is for it to join The Partners," board member Cyril Mazansky advised Sister Louise Gallahue, DCNHS president for the Northeast region.[35] "It is [the medical staff's] collective judgment that an open and vital relationship with Partners provides the *best* opportunity to accomplish this goal," Edward Reardon, medical staff president, informed Gallahue (emphasis in original).[36]

Despite these endorsements, Archbishop Law adamantly opposed the venture, noting that in 1994 Brigham and Women's Hospital performed about two thousand abortions.[37] Speaking before an audience of hospital administrators and trustees on May 5, 1995, Law claimed that an "alliance" with Brigham and Women's would "compromise" Carney's Catholic identity and create a "scandal."[38] When Michael Lasalandra, a reporter from the *Boston Herald*, asked Law to clarify his position given the large numbers of joint ventures between Catholic and non-Catholic hospitals in other parts of the country, Law indicated that the situation was unusual because Brigham and Women's performed a large number of abortions. "Alliances might be able to be formed between Catholic and non-Catholic hospitals that performed limited numbers of abortions," Law told Lasalandra, "but it would be wrong for a Catholic hospital to enter into an affiliation with an institution where the incidence of abortion is the highest in the commonwealth."[39]

Those who favored Carney's sale to Partners claimed that the number of abortions was an excuse, that Law was deliberately blocking Carney's sale to Partners because he wanted Carney to join Caritas.[40] "Contrary to what" Law has claimed, Mazansky wrote Gallahue, he opposes an affiliation with Partners "primarily" for "business," not "religious and ethical" purposes.[41] It is the "strong consensus" of Carney's medical staff, Reardon added, that "Caritas Christi's model of health care delivery . . . has little, if any chance of long term success. Except for Cardinal Law and the leadership of Caritas, no one we know views such a network as viable in the competitive environment of Boston."[42]

While discussions were ongoing with Partners, the Daughters sought advice from canon law experts concerning Law's ability to prevent the transaction. On October 14, 1994, Michael Riley, senior vice president for DCNHS's East Central region, contacted Father John G. Nugent, CM, asking about the "role of the local Ordinary." Riley wanted to know if the

Daughters needed Law's permission to join Partners. Technically, they did not, Nugent told him. The Daughters were "exempt" from diocesan approval concerning the "alienation of property" valued at over three million dollars because the community was a "pontifical right society." Under canon law, the Daughters needed approval from "the Holy Father . . . the Superior General of the Congregation of the Mission . . . and the Superioress General," but not Cardinal Law, Nugent advised Riley.[43] From a practical standpoint, however, the Daughters required Law's support in order to gain the Vatican's endorsement. The Vatican "would most probably want to hear from [Law]" before deciding, Nugent indicated. Given Law's close ties to prominent clerics at the Vatican, as well as several US congressmen, senators, and even US presidents, the Daughters terminated negotiations with Partners.[44]

Still, the Daughters continued to search for allies other than Caritas. In June 1995, they approached nearby Quincy Hospital, a small public facility the City of Quincy owned and operated.[45] As a public hospital, Quincy had to provide certain reproductive services, including sterilizations and abortions, but the number of abortions was quite small, only two in all of 1994.[46] If Law's main objection to the alliance with Partners was the number of abortions, then Quincy should not pose a problem. With Law's knowledge and tacit approval, Carney and Quincy worked toward a network affiliation that involved the creation of a subsidiary corporation to provide reproductive services, thereby separating Carney from the prohibited undertaking.[47]

The enterprise appeared to be moving toward completion. But on May 22, 1996, after the parties had reached an agreement and had forwarded several documents to Law for his review and examination, Law told Carney's president, Mattias Maguire, that the arrangement was "unacceptable." The attempt "to isolate [certain immoral] practices . . . by forming a subsidiary of Quincy [was] inadequate to [prevent] real scandal," Law told Maguire. "While there may be a separation of assets through the use of a subsidiary," Law asserted, "the location of such an entity on the Quincy Hospital premises and the continued responsibility for it by the Quincy Hospital Corporation is not sufficient to allay the justified reservations of Catholics that Catholic identity is being compromised."[48]

The aborted arrangement with Quincy bolstered the view that Law would thwart any attempt to sell Carney to an entity other than Caritas.[49]

Lacking further options and in desperate need of a partner, the Daughters sold Carney to Caritas on December 4, 1996, for several million dollars below market value.[50] John Nuveen, the company that the Daughters engaged to perform the market analysis, labeled the transaction "a distressed sale" because of adverse publicity from the "failed affiliation with Partners" and the failed "merger with Quincy."[51] Though Carney stayed open for the next twenty-eight years, it struggled financially for much of that period, aided by millions of dollars from the State of Massachusetts for facilities that handled a disproportionate share of poor patients.[52]

In January 2002, the child sexual abuse scandal involving Catholic priests unfolded in Boston. Over the next several months, details emerged about Law's role in transferring pedophile priests from one location to another without informing parishioners or law enforcement officials. Facing declining donations to the diocese and hundreds of lawsuits seeking damages, Law resigned as Boston's archbishop in December.[53] Appointed to succeed Law in 2003, Archbishop Sean P. O'Malley initiated several changes.[54] Though Caritas "rebounded" in 2005, the hospital system soon deteriorated as management turnovers accelerated.[55] By 2006, "Caritas was struggling financially," the Massachusetts attorney general reported. "It had outdated facilities, significant debt, and a significant shortfall in funding its pension plans."[56] St. Elizabeth's and Carney were "among the worst-performing hospitals in the Boston area," the Massachusetts Division of Health Care Finance and Policy indicated.[57]

Beginning in late 2006, Archbishop O'Malley sought an affiliation with a national, nonprofit Catholic health system. Ironically, the leading prospect was Ascension, the successor to DCNHS. Following a five-month review, Ascension abandoned the effort, citing "large unfunded pension liabilities and a rapid decrease in the number of patients."[58] Discussions with other nonprofit health systems also faltered, and in April 2008, at the urging of Massachusetts Attorney General Martha Coakley, O'Malley turned the management of Caritas over to an independent board of governors.[59] Soon thereafter, the board hired cardiac surgeon Ralph de la Torre as president and chief executive officer.[60] Called a "charismatic driver" by a Caritas board member, de la Torre recruited a new management team and initiated a "complete operational restructuring" of the organization.[61]

Though Caritas's earnings subsequently increased, its pension obligations and outstanding debts failed to diminish. Caritas required a large cash infusion in order to remain viable.[62] Unable to find a nonprofit health system willing to assume its outstanding liabilities, Caritas turned to Cerberus Capital Management, a large private equity firm. On March 19, 2010, Caritas's board of governors entered into an asset purchase agreement with Steward Health Care System, a Cerberus affiliate.[63] After the transaction, de la Torre became president and chief executive officer of Steward.[64] Under de la Torre, Steward significantly expanded, acquiring thirty-six hospitals in ten different states across the country.[65] But in the process, Steward became overextended. Refusing to commit additional capital to sustain the enterprise, Cerberus sold its controlling interest in Steward to a group of physicians that de la Torre represented.[66]

On May 6, 2024, Steward filed for Chapter 11 bankruptcy protection amid numerous allegations involving financial mismanagement.[67] Four months later, in September, the office of Massachusetts Senator Edward J. Markey issued a report citing several deficiencies at Steward-owned facilities. "At Carney Hospital in Dorchester," the Markey report stated, "the quality of care fell so steeply that some workers began referring to the hospital as 'Carnage' Hospital."[68] Between 2014 and 2024, Steward closed eight of its hospitals. Carney was among the casualties. Unable to find a qualified buyer, the US bankruptcy court announced that Carney would close on August 31, 2024, an ignominious end to a once-venerable institution that had served with distinction the Dorchester community and the greater Boston area for over 150 years.[69]

THE QUEST FOR UNIVERSAL HEALTH INSURANCE

The political will to engage in comprehensive healthcare reform coalesced in the early 1990s. US healthcare spending, while double that of the leading industrialized nations, failed to provide health insurance coverage to a significant portion of the population. Job layoffs resulting from corporate restructuring contributed to the problem.[70] President William Clinton, at the start of his first term in office in 1993, launched a bold initiative that ultimately faltered. Though Clinton made more headway during his second term (the Children's Health Insurance Program [CHIP] Act of 2000), the number of uninsured persons continued to mount, rising to 44.9 million or 14.9 percent of the population in 2009 when Barak Obama became president.[71] Obama's efforts to pass a comprehensive health insurance program were more successful than Clinton's. On March 23, 2010, he signed the Affordable Care Act (ACA) into legislation.

On each occasion, the US bishops opposed the legislative initiative, claiming that it would foster abortion. The bishop's disapproval was politically damaging, a substantial barrier to congressional passage. Presidents Clinton and Obama needed support from religious leaders in order to counter the bishops. They received it from several Catholic sisters, including two highly placed Daughters at the Catholic Health Association—Sisters Bernice Coreil, DC, and Carol Keehan, DC. Coreil and Keehan used their respective positions to endorse the Clinton and Obama proposals. Both Daughters faced harsh criticism for their efforts.

Born and raised in New Orleans, Sister Bernice Coreil, DC, had significant experience and expertise in healthcare finance and delivery. Possessing a master's degree in health administration, Coreil was a strong proponent of health system integration. She was a member of the CHA's Task Force on the Health Care of the Poor, which in 1986 touted "integration" and "collaboration" between hospitals and primary care clinics to improve the health of indigent persons.[72] After the report's release, Coreil continued to advance her strongly held views and positions. "Our system is no longer adequately accountable to the individuals and communities it serves," Coreil wrote in 1993 while chairing the CHA's Leadership Task Force. "It is built on an irrational mix of skewed financial incentives that accentuate institutional, acute care services; encourage inappropriate levels of care; and deemphasize preventive and primary care."[73]

Two major components of universal healthcare systems in other countries—finance and delivery—were out of sync in America.[74] Lack of convergence between the two was an important reason why costs exploded following the enactment of the Medicare and Medicaid programs, and why efforts to contain spending reduced services to poor people.[75] Coreil captured the essence of the problem when she wrote that "skewed financial incentives" accentuated the division. Rather than focus on finance, however, Coreil stressed healthcare delivery. "A financing plan that ignores delivery issues will only reinforce an unnecessarily costly system characterized by fragmentation, duplication, and uneven access," she contended.[76]

In March 1992, Coreil's Leadership Task Force launched the CHA's proposal for healthcare reform at the start of the Clinton administration.

The proposal called for the formation of "Integrated Delivery Networks," comprising "doctors, care givers, hospitals, nursing homes, and other healthcare providers."[77] When finally announced in September 1993, the Clinton Plan mirrored the CHA's initiative. "If you look at [the president's plan]," Hillary Rodham Clinton, First Lady and chair of the President's Health Care Task Force, observed, "it is remarkably similar to the plan put forward by the Catholic Health Association." CHA members, she noted, "worked for two years before my husband was even elected President, [yet they] arrived at so many overlapping conclusions and proposed solution[s]."[78]

Most features of the Clinton Plan did not trouble the bishops. Voluntary hospitals were firmly entrenched by this time, and the bishops largely had reconciled their fears about government financing. What piqued the bishops was the plan's mandated benefit package, which included coverage for elective abortions.[79] Notwithstanding the bishops' objections, Coreil testified in support of the Clinton Plan before two subcommittees of the House Energy and Commerce Committee. She also spoke on the South Lawn of the White House, praising the president for his efforts.[80] Coreil's vocal support for the plan triggered several recriminations. "I resent your speaking for me and the majority of Catholics in this country who are opposed to abortion," wrote a detractor.[81] "Doesn't Sister Bernice realize she is being used by this very anti-life administration?" complained Bishop Thomas J. Welsh in a letter to Visitatrix Gallahue.[82] "I believe the Catholic Health Association has a most serious responsibility to disown [Coreil's] presentation" on the South Lawn of the White House, Bishop Edward T. Hughes of Metuchen, New Jersey, told CHA President Jack Curley.[83]

In the years following the failure of the Clinton Plan, the number of uninsured persons mounted. An emergency room nurse before she became a Daughter, Sister Carol Keehan, DC, witnessed firsthand the perils of those who lacked insurance coverage. "I could give you a million examples," she told a reporter. "There's the pregnant woman who comes to the emergency room ready to deliver who hasn't had an ounce of prenatal care. Or there's the woman who has a tumor so large that it is actually coming through her breast. . . . We see people with ulcers on their legs that have become so grotesquely infected, which could have been easily addressed much sooner."[84]

Using her platform as CHA president and chief executive officer, Keehan backed the ACA, President Obama's legislative initiative. The

ACA comprised many of the Clinton Plan's former features. "Insurance exchanges" replaced the "regional health alliances," and "Affordable Care Organizations" replaced the Integrated Delivery Networks.[85] But there was one big difference, and that was the standard benefit package. Unlike the Clinton Plan, the ACA eschewed abortion coverage largely because of the lobbying efforts of Keehan, the CHA, and others.[86] While Keehan and her colleagues at the CHA believed that the law's language was sufficient to preclude abortion coverage, the bishops were unrequited. They claimed that the law contained too many loopholes.[87] So did the Catholic Medical Association, which through its president asserted that the ACA "fails to respect fundamental ethical, constitutional, and social principles."[88]

Contingent on the vote of a few key congressional members, the debate in the weeks preceding the ACA's 2010 passage was highly contentious. The bishops and their spokespersons targeted the CHA and Keehan, accusing them of opening a "wound to Catholic unity." Attacks against Keehan were often personal, direct, and pointed. "Keehan ignores, intentionally or otherwise," certain sections of the bill "which provide federal subsidies for health plans that cover abortions," claimed Cathy Ruse, senior fellow at the Family Research Council and former chief spokesperson on human-life issues for the US Conference of Catholic Bishops (USCCB, successor to the National Conference of Catholic Bishops).[89] "Keehan is either incredibly naïve or disingenuous," Kansas City Archbishop Joseph Nauman contended.[90] Distressed by such accusations and the recriminations, Keehan staunchly defended her efforts and those of her colleagues.[91] "For us as Catholics," Keehan responded, "it's very hard to be pro-life when we don't give care to many mothers who are pregnant or when we don't provide pediatric care and well-baby care and sick-baby care to children. We have 9 million uninsured children in this country. That's not pro-life."[92]

President Obama praised Keehan for her steadfast support and efforts. "We would not have gotten the Affordable Care Act done had it not been for her," he stated in a speech before the Catholic Health Association.[93] In succeeding years, the ACA's opponents made several attempts to overturn it.[94] These attempts largely failed, though Congress in 2017 struck some important features, such as the individual mandate, which required all persons to have health insurance coverage. Ironically, the bishops altered their stance when a Republican Congress threatened to repeal it. Writing on behalf of the USCCB on January 18, 2017, Bishop Frank Dewane of Venice,

Florida, urged Congress to retain it. "A repeal of key provisions of the [ACA] ought not to be undertaken without the concurrent passage of a replacement plan that ensures access to adequate health care for the millions of people who now rely upon it for their wellbeing," he asserted.[95]

Dewane's statement vindicated Keehan. The protections against the use of federal funds for abortion contained in the legislation had proven adequate.[96] In addition, the ACA substantially increased health insurance coverage for many Americans who previously lacked it. The joint efforts of the Daughters, the CHA, and many other sisterhoods and organizations made a big difference. Though not intended as a compliment, the remarks of Francis Cardinal George, OMI, Chicago's archbishop, recognized the significance of Keehan's efforts. "Sister Carol and her colleagues are to blame" for the bill's passage, he stated.[97] Unfortunately, there were fewer than 750 Daughters around to savor the victory, the vast majority of them over sixty.[98] By the time of the ACA's enactment, the Daughters no longer owned or managed any hospitals.

SEVEN

"TIME TO LEAVE"

During the 1990s and early 2000s, the number of Daughters in the United States continued to plummet. In 2000, there were 1,051 Daughters left in America.[1] By 2024, there were only 308, almost all of them over the age of sixty-five.[2] A rapidly changing and increasingly complex healthcare environment in the final decades of the twentieth century had stretched their resources, forcing provincial leaders to consolidate. But these efforts, though momentous for the future prosperity of their enterprise and Catholic hospitals in general, could only delay their departure. Dwindling numbers of Daughters with expertise in healthcare administration was unsustainable.

In the 1990s, the Daughters sold, merged, or otherwise transferred several financially distressed hospitals to more robust local partners. After the formation of Ascension Health in 1999, which the Daughters cosponsored with another religious community, their work in healthcare was almost over.[3] Between 1999 and 2011, they continued to serve on corporate boards or in other leadership positions. But lacking younger replacements for the majority of sisters who were in their seventies and eighties, they tendered control of Ascension Health in 2012 to a lay-sponsored entity, a nonprofit holding company named Ascension.[4] "It was time to leave healthcare," veteran hospital administrator Sister Theresa Peck, DC, reflected. Some Daughters "remained on boards or worked in clinics," but there were simply "not enough sisters" to continue our hospital-based ministry.[5]

Leaving their hospitals was a difficult and painstaking process.[6] During the transition, the Daughters gradually shifted their focus to the sponsorship of freestanding community clinics. They returned to their roots in America: the provision of primary care and social services to the indigent, many of them Hispanic immigrants.

THE SALE AND TRANSFER OF SEVERAL OF THE DAUGHTERS' HOSPITALS

Because healthcare delivery was primarily local in nature, even those hospitals affiliated with national health systems needed local partners. Absent local partners, individual hospitals could not compete for managed care contracts, absorb the loss of inpatients to outpatient facilities, and offset declining insurance reimbursements. Facing stiff competition and falling revenue in several local markets, the Daughters began to sell, transfer, or otherwise relinquish control of several of their hospitals in the early 1990s. Six of the Daughters' long-standing hospitals mentioned throughout this book were among those they sold or transferred. They included Hôtel Dieu in New Orleans, DePaul Health Center (formerly DePaul Hospital) in St. Louis, St. Joseph Hospital in Chicago, DePaul Medical Center (formerly DePaul Hospital) in Norfolk, St. Mary's Hospital in Rochester, and Carney Hospital in Boston.

The Daughters began searching for a partner for Hôtel Dieu in the mid-1980s. The New Orleans market was oversaturated ("overbedded" is the term used in the healthcare industry). On August 22, 1988, a management team cited several deficiencies. Hôtel Dieu "has been in a constant state of uncertainty with a freeze on capital expenditures, layoffs of personnel, and reduction of some services," the management team discovered.[7] Two opportunities for joint partnership arose in the mid-1980s, the first with the Sisters of Mercy and the second with the State of Louisiana. In 1985, the Daughters approached the Sisters of Mercy, who owned nearby Mercy Hospital.[8] The Daughters proposed several joint ventures, including a mobile clinic for the "poor elderly."[9] But the mobile clinic and the other "joint projects" failed to materialize. In the meantime, negotiations between the Daughters and the State of Louisiana moved forward.[10] In 1992, the Daughters sold Hôtel Dieu to the state government.[11] Renamed University Hospital, Hôtel Dieu became part of the Louisiana State University System.[12]

Conditions in the local St. Louis market in the early 1990s were similar to those in New Orleans—overbedded and highly competitive. Indeed, St. Louis was "one of the most over-bedded communities in the country," according to a 1993 assessment. DePaul Health Center, which the Daughters established in 1978 after relocating from the inner city to the suburbs, "has experienced a significant deterioration in inpatient volumes over the last five years, much of it related to the lack of participation in managed care contracts," the assessment indicated.[13] DePaul needed a partner in order to compete with other large health systems in the area.[14] After considering various options, including a merger with the Sisters of St. Mary (SSM), DePaul's board of trustees sold the facility to SSM on April 28, 1995, for about $32 million.[15] The Daughters used the sale's proceeds to establish a foundation, the Daughters of Charity Foundation of St. Louis. In 2019, the Daughters changed the name of the Foundation to the Marillac Mission Fund.[16]

The frenzied consolidation of hospitals also occurred in Chicago in the mid-1990s. In 1993, 43 percent of the hospitals in the Chicago area were in multihospital systems; only two years later, 71 percent of the city's hospitals had joined a network. The largest systems included Northwestern Health Network, Advocate Network, and Rush-Presbyterian-St. Luke's Medical Center.[17] Fearing that Catholic hospitals in his diocese might not survive without local partners, Chicago's archbishop, Joseph Cardinal Bernadin, urged them to consolidate.[18] In 1995, soon after Bernardin issued his warning, most of the Catholic hospitals in the Chicago area came together, forming Catholic Health Partners and Unified Health Care. Daughter-owned St. Joseph Hospital merged with Catholic Health Partners.

Network formation continued in Chicago. In 1998, Resurrection Health Care approached Catholic Health Partners, but negotiations stalled because one of the hospitals, St. Anthony's, "was too far South," the *Chicago Tribune* reported. "We're interested in markets contiguous or adjacent to us," Robert Barrigar, a senior vice president at Resurrection stated.[19] St. Joseph Hospital, on the other hand, was on Chicago's North Side, within the vicinity of Resurrection's four hospitals, nine nursing homes, and affiliated clinics. On September 28, 2000, Resurrection announced plans to purchase St. Joseph.[20] Following several more mergers involving Resurrection and other Catholic health systems, St. Joseph later became part of Ascension, the successor to DCNHS.[21]

In 1993, the Daughters and the Sisters of Bon Secours entered into negotiations for the purchase of DePaul Medical Center located in Norfolk,

Virginia. When discussions began, DePaul was in financial difficulties. Three years later, however, DePaul's finances had improved; expenses had declined and revenues had increased. "Now was the appropriate time," DePaul's President and CEO Kevin Conlan stated, "to get ourselves aligned with another strong local Catholic health-care organization."[22] On November 1, 1996, Bon Secours Health System bought DePaul Medical Center. Unfortunately, DePaul's financial problems resumed in the early 2000s. "Citing extremely low patient volume and empty beds," Bon Secours closed DePaul in 2021.[23]

St. Mary's Hospital in Rochester merged with Park Ridge Hospital in the town of Greece, a suburb of Rochester, forming Unity Health System in 1997. Though St. Mary's transferred all of its operations to Park Ridge after the merger, DCNHS remained a stakeholder in Unity.[24] Unity initially "performed well" but then faltered. DCNHS advanced "cash loans" in 1988 to help sustain the enterprise, but Unity's financial condition continued to worsen. At the end of 1999, DCNHS withdrew from Unity.[25]

THE FORMATION OF ASCENSION

The sale or transfer of the Daughters' hospitals to other hospital systems in New Orleans, St. Louis, Chicago, Norfolk, Rochester, and Boston was often episodic and reactive, reflecting lack of foresight and planning for what transpired. Absent a national strategy, DCNHS continued to fracture. Though the national office in St. Louis oversaw purchasing, data processing, risk management, and insurance, it did not exercise decision-making authority in local markets. The regional corporations did that. As a result, CEOs and bishops negotiated directly with the regional corporations, not with the national office.

By the mid-1990s, several DCNHS leaders recognized that the original configuration was no longer working, that a new approach was needed to address the rapidly changing healthcare environment.[26] In April 1997, a task force comprising the visitatrixes and the regional executives, among others, approved a "unified sponsorship model" that eliminated the regional corporations. "This model will enable simpler and more expeditious decision-making and, thereby, result in a more nimble organization," task force members maintained. Our intention is to advance "system-level cosponsorship with other religious institutes," they stated. "By moving to a unified Daughters of Charity sponsorship of the entire system, we are in a stronger position to participate in both co-sponsored regional health care systems and creating or participating in a co-sponsored national health care system."[27]

Soon after the DCNHS restructure, two sisterhoods approached the Daughters about a joint venture, the Sisters of Charity of the Incarnate Word and the Sisters of St. Joseph Health System, headquartered in Kalamazoo, Michigan.[28] In May 1998, the Daughters reached a decision. They wanted a cosponsorship arrangement with the Sisters of St. Joseph.[29] For the Daughters, this was their first involvement in shared sponsorship at the national level with a different group of Catholic sisters.

Though the Sisters of St. Joseph initially were interested, they hesitated following closer inspection of the Daughters' record. "In reviewing your *Essential Elements of Catholic Identity*," Sister Janet Fleischhacker, SSJ, wrote to Sister Xavier Balance, DC, on May 15, 1998, "we find areas of discomfort," particularly your focus on "history and heritage."[30] Fleischhacker feared that the Daughters' traditions might inhibit the transition to "full lay partnership" that the Sisters of St. Joseph strongly favored. "While lay sponsorship in the future will build on the heritage of the past, it will need to transcend all individual religious traditions and charisms. We feel you need to know how strongly we believe in this theology," Fleischhacker told Balance.[31]

Facing stiff competition from other hospital systems in their service area, the Sisters of St. Joseph overcame their apprehension and entered into negotiations.[32] On September 15, 1999, four of the five visitatrixes (the West Province did not participate) announced the decision to sign an agreement with the Sisters of St. Joseph. The terms of the agreement indicated that both sides had made some concessions. Attempting to address the concerns of the Sisters of St. Joseph, the arrangement opened the door to lay sponsorship and "focused on a ministry of the Church and not on [the Daughters' history and heritage]."[33]

After the merger and the creation of Ascension Health on November 1, 1999, the Daughters largely exited the US healthcare industry. As cosponsors of Ascension-owned hospitals, they retained some oversight authority, but this waned as laypersons increasingly filled the top corporate positions.[34] Ascension Health continued to expand as other Catholic health systems joined the network. These included Carondelet Health System in 2002, Alexian Brothers Health System in 2012, certain health ministries of the former Marian Health System in 2013, and Wheaton Franciscan Healthcare in 2016.[35] As of October 2023, Ascension Health owned 3,055 healthcare facilities in sixteen states. The heaviest concentrations were in Michigan, Illinois, Indiana, Tennessee, Florida, Texas, Wisconsin, Kansas, Oklahoma, and New York.[36]

The addition of new hospital systems dramatically altered the cosponsorship arrangement between the Daughters and the Sisters of St. Joseph.[37] The original agreement called for a Sponsors Council comprising four Daughters (one from each of the four provinces), four Sisters of St. Joseph, and two laypersons.[38] But the inclusion of the other hospital networks made cosponsorship untenable. Under US civil law, a legal mechanism was readily available that would secure the respective interests of each participant—the parent or holding company. But under canon law, the sisterhoods had to relinquish control to a lay entity. "A health system composed of many traditions cannot be a blend of charisms," canon law expert David J. Nygren, CM, instructed. "It may have a culture, an operating environment, and be in the lineage of charismatic traditions, [but] its end and inspiration is Jesus, not the founders of the congregations, however important they may be to the spiritual history," Nygren indicated.[39]

The canon law counterpart for the civil law corporation was the public juridic person or PJP.[40] As a 2014 publication of the Catholic Health Association explained, "A juridic person is to canon law what a corporation is to civil law. It is an entity within the Roman Catholic Church that enables a ministry to relate directly to the church."[41] During the 1990s, the concept gained a foothold. By 2009, ten lay-sponsored Catholic health systems or PJPs existed in America—Catholic Health Care Federation (1991), Covenant Health Systems (1995), PeaceHealth (1997), Catholic Health Ministries (2000), Bon Secours Ministries (2006), St. Joseph Health Ministry (2006), CSA Health System Ministries (2007), Mercy Health Ministry (2008), Leaven Ministries (2008), and Providence Ministries (2009).[42] Created in 2012, Ascension became the eleventh.

At the time Ascension formed, Catholic prelates and hospital executives more often used the term "ministerial juridic person" as opposed to "public juridic person" to indicate that under church auspices healthcare was a ministry and not a business.[43] Still, it was difficult to separate the two, as the

Daughters' lengthy history of hospital administration reflected. When Ascension began to place its name before each of the Daughters' former hospitals, some of the Daughters expressed their dissatisfaction.[44] Sisters from other communities also had misgivings about the direction of lay-sponsored networks. "We put lots of businessmen with financial expertise on boards. They leave the 'mission' to the sisters and make all the real decisions," a sister protested.[45]

COMMUNITY HEALTH MINISTRIES

When the Daughters sold or transferred control of their hospitals in the 1990s, they sometimes shifted personnel to community health centers in locations where poor people resided. In some instances, proceeds from the sales of the Daughters' hospitals produced the funds to start new ventures.[46] Before the formation of Ascension Health, much of this activity occurred in the West Central Province, where provincial leadership organized to address the lack of healthcare services in certain areas. The decision to start a community health center typically depended on the availability of Daughters, physicians, and nurse practitioners who had the necessary wherewithal and training. Community clinics or health centers that the Daughters established were largely freestanding, unattached to a particular hospital.

Among the principal movers in the West Central Province was Sister Mary Walz, DC, a licensed and trained social worker. Walz had worked at DePaul Family Health Center in San Antonio from 1971 to 1975 and Marillac Social Center in Dallas from 1975 to 1987. In 1987, the West Central Province tasked Walz and Sister Joan Pytlic, DC, a family nurse practitioner, to conduct a needs assessment of the province's underserved communities.[47] In their needs assessment, Walz and Pytlic targeted El Paso, Texas; New Orleans, Louisiana; and Gould, Arkansas, for additional resources. The first two were logical choices. The sales of Hôtel Dieu Medical Center in El Paso and Hôtel Dieu Hospital in New Orleans created a gap in services at both locations. Seeking to address the needs of the local populations, provincial leaders used some of the money gained from the sales to finance new community clinics, including the San Vincente Family Health Center in El Paso and Daughters of Charity Health Center in New Orleans' Carrollton Plaza.[48]

Gould, Arkansas, on the other hand, seemed an unlikely candidate for the Daughters' attention. They did not own or manage any facilities in southeast Arkansas, let alone in rural parts of the country where few Catholics resided. The main reason Walz and Pytlic selected Gould was because three Vincentian priests had alerted them to the town's lack of resources. There was no local doctor and no local pharmacy for Gould's population of 1,200. Responding to the priests' call for assistance, Walz and Pytlic co-founded St. Elizabeth Health Center in 1990.[49] Two years later, the West Central Province established a second clinic in Dumas, Arkansas, ten miles from Gould. Both clinics, St. Elizabeth in Gould and DePaul Health Center in Dumas, were "free and charitable clinics," that is, they charged a minimal fee on a sliding-scale basis and obtained most of their funds from grants and private donations.[50]

Daughter-sponsored free clinics appeared elsewhere in the early to mid-1990s, in places such as Evansville, Indiana, and Fayetteville, North Carolina. Founded in 1993, the CARE Clinic in Fayetteville emerged largely because of the organizational skills of Sister Jean Rhodes, DC, a registered nurse with a masters' degree in health services administration. CARE's medical director, Tinsley Rucker, described the difficulties involved in establishing the free clinic. There were no government funds for start-up, Rucker noted. Money came from nonprofit organizations and individual donors. Organizers had to recruit volunteer healthcare providers such as physicians, dentists, and nurses to work certain hours. In addition, they had to establish a support network of "readily available ancillary services, such as laboratory, X-ray, an onsite pharmacy and specialty backup."[51] In 1994, Rhodes received the North Carolina Governor's Award for organizing the CARE Clinic, and in 1997 the city of Fayetteville made Rhoads its Citizen of the Year "for her dedication to improve the health of the working poor."[52]

Following the formation of Ascension Health in 1999, the Daughters' work in healthcare became more sporadic. Ascension Health and later Ascension expanded the provision of clinic services at New Orleans and El Paso, but only a small handful of Daughters were able to participate in these endeavors. Still, the Daughters remained vigilant to the health and social welfare needs of the poor, many of them Hispanic immigrants. Sister Christine Mura, DC, a pastoral care worker at St. Mary's Hospital in Amsterdam, New York, for example, helped Hispanic farmers obtain access to health and social services.[53] Sister Isabel Fierro, DC, a former nurse midwife who was eighty-five years old in 2022, worked in New Orleans as a medical office translator for Spanish-speaking patients.[54] And in 2021, the Daughters sent three sisters to Charleston, South Carolina, where they provided spiritual and social services to migrant laborers.[55]

In 2004, Walz left Gould, Arkansas, and joined the leadership council of the West Central Province.[56] For the next seven years, the first three as a council member (2004–7) and the next four as visitatrix (2007–11), Walz participated in two epic changes: (1) Ascension's transition from a sister-sponsored to a lay-sponsored organization, and (2) the consolidation of the Northeast, East Central, Southeast, and West Central Provinces into the Province of Saint Louise on July 31, 2011 (the West Province was not part of the merger). Marillac Provincial House became the headquarters of the new province, and Sister Louise Gallahue, DC, was voted its first visitatrix. Gallahue continued as visitatrix until Sister Catherine (Katie) Mary Norris succeeded her in 2017. Walz meanwhile stayed in St. Louis, serving on the first Sponsors Council for Ascension and the first leadership council for the Saint Louise province.[57]

In 2017, Walz returned to the rural Mississippi Delta, this time as a social worker at a doctor-run clinic located in Holmes County, Mississippi, one of the poorest counties in America.[58] Walz arrived at the Lexington Medical Clinic in Holmes County with two other sisters, Sister Medeline Kavanaugh, DC, and Sister Sheila Conley, SC. They came following the deaths of Sister Paula Merrill, SC, of the Sisters of Charity of Nazareth, Kentucky, and Sister Margaret Held, OSF, of the School Sisters of St. Francis in Milwaukee. Merrill and Held had worked for over a decade in Holmes County, six of those years at the Lexington Clinic as nurse practitioners, before a person living near their home in Durant, Mississippi, killed them. At the sentencing, members of the deceased sisters' respective communities asked the judge to forego the death penalty. So did Walz. "I believe [that Merrill's and Held's] last breath was a prayer for forgiveness," she told the judge. Looking at the defendant, she said, "God still has plans for you. Our prayer is that you will use the rest of your life to do good."[59]

Sister Mary Walz's actions and attitude toward her work largely encapsulate the Daughters' two-hundred-year history of service to the sick poor in America. Walz is a doer, an organizer, and a leader. She is ready and willing to do just about anything the community asks of her, whether that means delivering food and medicine in poverty-stricken areas of Arkansas and Mississippi, teaching and counseling persons with diabetes, or serving on Ascension's Sponsors Council. While Walz's actions attest to her individual abilities, she functions as part of a group, a community of like-minded women with an established mission, rules, and values. Neither Walz nor any of her predecessors or contemporaries such as Sisters Ursala Mattingly, Matilda Coskery, Bertrande Meyers, or Bernice Coreil has operated independently of the community. Their accomplishments are group accomplishments. They neither sought nor received the public notoriety granted to Clara Barton, Florence Nightengale, Jane Addams, or other talented and resourceful individuals.

Group action, resolve, and cohesion built on rules, norms, values, and mission are a big reason why the Daughters were so successful in the healthcare arena. Group action, resolve, and cohesion helped to withstand the vicissitudes of wars, epidemics, technological changes, economic recessions, social movements, and political upheavals. Group action, resolve, and cohesion helped to overcome challenges from bishops, priests, doctors, bureaucrats, military leaders, and politicians. Group action, resolve, and cohesion helped the Daughters navigate societal and political divisions over anti-Catholicism, "socialized medicine," race relations, women's liberation, and abortion. Group action, resolve, and cohesion sustained the Daughters' hospitals, the centerpiece of their US healthcare apostolate.

The Daughters' governing framework also was important. Based on the motherhouse model, the Daughters' form of governance combined central oversight with decentralized administration. Having a central location that operated independently of diocesan bishops fostered uniformity, standardization, and coordination. Still, the Daughters would not have owned a large number of hospitals absent America's unique political, legal, and cultural climate. These distinctive features aided the growth of private, nonprofit institutions, of which Catholic hospitals were among the most enduring. Pillars of immigrant communities alongside schools and churches, Catholic hospitals and the sisterhoods that owned them significantly contributed not only to the expansion of American healthcare but also to the advancement of American society.

Looking back, the Daughters' contributions and those of other sisterhoods to US healthcare delivery were extensive. The Daughters enhanced the development of nursing as a profession in the 1800s through uniform preparation, through supervised training, through a written code of conduct that stressed the fair and ethical treatment of all patients, and by claiming certain tasks and responsibilities for nursing at their hospitals. They pioneered early forms of health administration by stressing order, discipline, accountability, cleanliness, sanitation, reporting, and hierarchical organization. And they extended healthcare services beyond the inpatient setting through outpatient clinics, community health centers, and alliances with local and regional public health facilities.

The Daughters were a force for moderation, moreover, a bulwark against the excesses of special interests, and a leading player in the nonprofit sector. Further, they were innovators in hospital finance and organizational efficiency, in the coordination and consolidation of certain jobs and functions, in the integration of hospitals and related institutions, and in the promotion of specialized facilities for the elderly, the mentally ill, and women and children.

Today's large corporations, healthcare systems, media outlets, and government agencies stress data-driven outcomes, often for comparative purposes. But such statistical measures were not the main focus of the Daughters' mission throughout their two-hundred-year history of healthcare delivery in America. The Daughters' numerous reports and correspondence consistently emphasize the human element of nursing and hospital administration, the blending of the spiritual and the corporal based on their founders' teachings. These teachings prescribed an approach to healthcare delivery that treated all people as unique human beings, no matter their social position or economic situation.

APPENDIX

Chronological List of Mother Superiors and Visitatrixes

Superiors of the Sisters of Charity of St. Joseph's (1809-1850)

Mother Elizabeth Ann Seton 1809–1821
Mother Rose White 1821–1827, 1833–1839
Mother Mary Augustine Decount 1827–1833
Mother Mary Xavier Clark 1839–1845
Mother Etienne Hall 1845–1850

Visitatrixes of the US Province of the Daughters of Charity (1850-1910)

Mother Etienne Hall 1850–1855
Mother Regina Smith 1855–1859
Mother Ann Simeon Norris 1859–1866
Mother Euphemia Blenkinsop 1866–1887
Mother Mariana Flynn 1887–1901
Mother Margaret O'Keefe 1901–1910

Visitatixes of the Two US Provinces After the 1910 Division (1910-1969)

Eastern Province (Emmitsburg, MD)

Mother Margaret O'Keefe 1910–1923
Sr. Paula Dunn 1923–1944
Sr. Gertrude Eisele 1944
Sr. Isabel Toohey 1944–1962
Sr. Eleanor McNabb 1962–1969

Western Province (St. Louis, MO)

Sr. Eugenia Feely 1910–1936
Sr. Caroline Collins 1936–1952
Sr. Catherine Sullivan 1952–1962
Sr. Mary Rose McPhee 1962–1969

Visitatrixes of the Five US Provinces After the 1969 Division (1969-2011)

Southeast Province (Emmitsburg, MD)

Sr. Eleanor McNabb 1969–1974
Sr. Mary Clare Hughes 1974–1983
Sr. Genevieve Kureth 1983–1989
Sr. Virginia Ann Brooks 1989–1998
Sr. Elyse Staab 1998–2007
Sr. Claire Debes 2007–2011

Northeast Province (Albany, NY)

Sr. Mary Basil Roarke 1969–1981
Sr. Mary Rose McGready 1981–1987
Sr. Margaret John Kelly 1987–1993
Sr. Louise Gallahue 1993–2002
Sr. Mary Francis Martin 2002–2008
Sr. Kathleen Appler 2008–2009
Sr. Louise Gallahue 2009–2011

East Central Province (Evansville, IN)

Sr. Elise Boudreaux 1969–1981
Sr. Gertrude Bastnagel 1981–1990
Sr. Dorothea Huber 1990–1996
Sr. Catherine Madigan 1996–2005
Sr. Honora Remes 2005–2011

West Central Province (St. Louis, MO)

Sr. Mary Rose McPhee 1969–1974
Sr. Mary John Lindner 1974–1983
Sr. Bernice Coreil 1983–1989
Sr. Nanette Gentile 1989–1998
Sr. Marie Therese Sedgwick 1998–2007
Sr. Mary Walz 2007–2011

Province of the West (name changed in 1969 to Province of St. Elizabeth Ann Seton) (Los Altos Hills, CA)

Sr. Rose Collins 1969–1981
Sr. Teresa Piro 1981–1990
Sr. Joyce Weller 1990–1999
Sr. Margaret Keaveney 1999–2008
Sr. Marjory Ann Baez 2008–2014
Sr. Julie Kubasak 2014–2022
Sr. Christina Maggi 2022–

Visitatrixes of the Province of St. Louise After the Unification of Four of the Five Provinces (St. Louis, MO) (2011-)

Sr. Louise Gallahue 2011–2017
Sr. Catherine (Katie) Mary Norris 2017–2023
Sr. Teresa George 2023–

NOTES

Introduction

1. See, e.g., Wall, *Unlikely Entrepreneurs*; Wall, *American Catholic Hospitals*; McGuinness, *Called to Serve*; Hoy, *Good Hearts*; Coburn and Smith, *Spirited Lives*; McCauley, *Who Shall Take Care of Our Sick?*; Nelson, *Say Little, Do Much*; Stepsis and Liptak, *Pioneer Healers*; Risse, *Mending Bodies, Saving Souls;* Kauffman, *Ministry and Meaning*; Casterline, "St. Joseph's and St. Mary's"; Libster and McNeil, *Enlightened Charity*; Oates, *Catholic Philanthropic Tradition*; Richardson, *History of the Sisters of Charity Hospital*; Gunnell, "Daughters of Charity."

2. See, e.g., Starr, *Social Transformation of American Medicine*; Rosenberg, *Care of Strangers*; Stevens, *In Sickness and in Wealth*; Kisacky, *Rise of the Modern Hospital*; Robinson, *Corporate Practice of Medicine*; Freidson, *Profession of Medicine*; Porter and Teisberg, *Redefining Health Care*; Weissert and Weissert, *Governing Health*; Shi and Singh, *Essentials of the U.S. Health Care System*; Sultz and Young, *Health Care USA*; Bodenheimer and Grumbach, *Understanding Health Policy*; Marmor, *Understanding Health Care Reform*; Patel and Rushefsky, *Health Care Politics and Policy in America*; Budrys, *Our Unsystematic Health Care System*; Kronenfeld, *Changing Federal Role in U.S. Health Care Policy*; Longest, Rakich, and Darr, *Managing Health Organizations and Systems.*

3. "Sisters" refers to an active community of religious women, while "nuns" refers to a cloistered community. This book uses the designation "sisters" because those who provided healthcare in hospitals, homes, or clinics were not cloistered.

4. Tess Solomon, Lois Uttley, Patty HasBrouck, and Yoolim Jung, *Bigger and Better: The Growth of Catholic Health Systems*, Community Catalyst, February 8, 2020, https://www.communitycatalyst.org.

5. Stewart, *Marvels of Charity*, 516–48; John Paul Newport, "Health Care: Mission + Margin: The Nun as C.E.O.," *New York Times Magazine*, June 9, 1991.

6. Hickey, *Local Hospitals in Ancien Régime France*, 137.

7. Local bishops or ordinaries were responsible for enforcing cloister in their respective dioceses. De Lavergnée, *Streets as a Cloister*, 25; Rapley, *The Dévotes*, 23–73.

8. Hickey, *Local Hospitals in Ancien Régime France*, 114; Rapley, *The Dévotes*, 74; de Lavergnée, *Streets as a Cloister*, 36.

9. Fuechtmann, "'There is Great Charity,'" 46; Rapley, *The Dévotes*, 81–82; Hickey, *Local Hospitals in Ancien Régime France*, 139; Flinton, "Louise de Marillac," 12–13.

10. Jones, *Charitable Imperative*, 93.

11. Jones, *Charitable Imperative*, 92–93.

12. O'Donnell, "Vincent de Paul," 26; Sullivan, "Louise de Marillac"; Jones, *Charitable Imperative*, 100–103.

13. O'Donnell, "Vincent de Paul," 31.

14. In 1633, Marguerite died from the plague after "sharing her bed with a poor plague-stricken girl." Rapley, *The Dévotes*, 83–84, 249; de Lavergnée, *Streets as a Cloister*, 141–46.

15. De Lavergnée, *Streets as a Cloister*, 144–45, 192–203, 221–22; Rapley, *The Dévotes*, 85–86; Nelson, *Say Little, Do Much*, 18–19.

16. Quote in Flinton, "Louise de Marillac," 38.

17. Quote in Flinton, "Louise de Marillac," 38.

18. Sullivan, "Louise de Marillac," 45–46.

19. "Rule" encompasses a particular community's governing framework, organization, terms of membership, mission, vows, spiritual practices, habit, and daily regimens.

20. Flinton, "Louise de Marillac," 41.

21. Quote in Flinton, "Louise de Marillac," 42.

22. Kuhns, *The Habit*, 110.

23. In 1649, the French civil authorities sanctioned the arrangement, and eight years later, in 1657, the King of France confirmed it. Letters Patent Approving the Company of the Daughters of Charity, November 1657, in de Lavergnée, *Streets as a Cloister*, 234.

24. De Lavergnée, *Streets as a Cloister*, 213–28.

25. Rapley, *The Dévotes*, 87; Rybolt, "Growth of the Constitutions of the Daughters of Charity."

26. At the time of Vincent's death in 1660, there were twenty-five houses, including mission centers, seminaries, and parishes in France, Poland, and elsewhere. Editorial Staff of the Vincentian Studies Institute, "A Survey of American Vincentian History: 1815–1987," August 2016, http://vincentians.com.

27. De Lavergnée, *Streets as a Cloister*, 226–27.

28. De Lavergnée, *Streets as a Cloister*, 227.

29. Coburn and Smith, *Spirited Lives*, 84.

30. Hickey, *Local Hospitals in Ancien Régime France*, 168; Nelson, *Say Little, Do Much*, 25.

31. Quote in Rapley, *The Dévotes*, 82.

32. De Lavergnée, *Streets as a Cloister*, 327–35; Rapley, *The Dévotes*, 88; O'Donnell, "Vincent de Paul," 30–33.

33. Jones, *Charitable Imperative*, 94.

34. Rapley, *The Dévotes*, 84.

35. Flinton, "Louise de Marillac," 62, 91, 104, 107, 111–12, 123, 138.

36. Rapley, *The Dévotes*, 90.

37. Rapley, *The Dévotes*, 89–94; de Lavergnée, *Streets as a Cloister*, 208–10; Jones, *Charitable Imperative*, 94; Hickey, *Local Hospitals in Ancien Régime France*, 164–69.

38. Rapley, *The Dévotes*, 178.

39. De Lavergnée, *Streets as a Cloister*, 238–39; Ryan and Rybolt, *Vincent de Paul and Louise de Marillac*, 167–68. The management contract with Hôtel-Dieu in Angers served as the precedent for future hospital-based missions. Seeking to maintain the Daughters' group identity (their vows, norms, daily rituals, and attire while working), the Angers contract called for two separate lines of authority—the first spiritual and the second temporal. The Vincentians would oversee spiritual matters, "and no others may interfere," the contract stated; hospital directors "must give them total liberty to live according to their rule." As for temporal affairs, "the service of the sick poor and government of [the] hospital," the contract held that the Daughters would "be totally under the authority [of the hospital's] administrators." De Lavergnée, *Streets as a Cloister*, 208–10.

40. Ryan and Rybolt, *Vincent de Paul and Louise de Marillac*, 184.

41. Wittberg, *The Rise and Fall of Catholic Religious Orders*, 38–39; Nelson, *Say Little, Do Much*, 23–26.

42. O'Donnell, *Elizabeth Seton*, 69–108; Barthel, *American Saint*, 70–88, 127. See also Cummings, *Saint of Our Own*.

43. O'Donnell, *Elizabeth Seton*, 146, 211–29; Barthel, *American Saint*, 88–134.

44. Quote in Hannefin, *Daughters of the Church*, 7.

45. Hannefin, *Daughters of the Church*, 7–8; O'Donnell, *Elizabeth Seton*, 230–34, 240–47.

46. "Sisters of Charity of Saint Joseph," *Vincentian Encyclopedia*, https://famvin.org.

47. Hannefin, *Daughters of the Church*, 11–14.

48. O'Donnell, *Elizabeth Seton*, 297; Hannefin, *Daughters of the Church*, 12–15; Barthel, *American Saint*, 143–46, 153–54.

49. O'Donnell, *Elizabeth Seton*, 304–6.

50. Nelson, *Say Little, Do Much*, 11–12, 16–17, 24–16, 37–38; Jones, *Charity and Beinfaisance*, 49–56, 111–12, 251–52.

51. Quote in McCann, *History of Mother Seton's Daughters*, 58.

52. William J. Stern, "How Dagger John Saved New York's Irish," *City Journal*, Spring 1997, https://www.city-journal.org.

53. Quote in Hannefin, *Daughters of the Church*, 88 (Hughes to Archbishop Eccleston, December 5, 1842). Sister Regina Bechtle points out that Hughes's predecessor, Bishop Dubois, also felt that the missions were ranging too far from the motherhouse. Bechtle, "1846 Separation of the New York Sisters," 67n16.

54. Hannefin, *Daughters of the Church*, 85–89; Nelson, *Say Little, Do Much*, 36–37; Michael Barga, "Sisters of Charity of New York," https://socialwelfare.library.vcu.edu; Encyclopia.com, "Sisters of Charity Federation," https://www.encyclopedia.com.

55. There is some disagreement in the various accounts about the age of male children. See Bechtle, "1846 Separation of the New York Sisters," 63; Hannefin, *Daughters of the Church*, 86.

56. Hannefin, *Daughters of the Church*, 85–89; Bechtle, "1846 Separation of the New York Sisters," 63–73; Nelson, *Say Little, Do Much*, 36–37; McCauley, *Who Shall Take Care of Our Sick?*, 19; Wittberg, *Rise and Fall of Catholic Religious Orders*, 93; Barga, "Sisters of Charity of New York."

57. Hannefin, *Daughters of the Church*, 89, 295n15; Nelson, *Say Little, Do Much*, 37; Barga, "Sisters of Charity of New York."

58. Hannefin, *Daughters of the Church*, 90–92, 296n21.

59. Hannefin, *Daughters of the Church*, 92.

60. Author unknown, "By Their Fruits, You Shall Know Them!," Buffalo, New York/Sisters of Charity Hospital Collection, RG 11-2-2:11(2), APSL.

61. McCann, *History of Mother Seton's Daughters*, 41.

62. McCann, *History of Mother Seton's Daughters*, 41; "Sisters of Charity of Cincinnati," https://www.srcharitycinti.org.

63. Rapley, *The Dévotes*, 87; Rybolt, "Growth of the Constitutions of the Daughters of Charity."

64. Hannefin, *Daughters of the Church*, 92–93; "A History of the Sisters of Charity Federation," https://sistersofcharityfederation.org. Before 2004, provincial directors exercised governmental authority as "major superiors" to whom the Daughters "owed obedience." It is hard to know precisely what a director's duties entailed or how much authority he had since his duties were not defined and often "varied." Revisions to the Daughters' Constitutions and Statutes in 2004 significantly altered this arrangement by removing the director's authority over governmental affairs and defining his role as one of "collaboration and accompaniment to assist [the sisters] in responding to the requirements of their vocation." *Directory of the Provincial Directors of the Daughters of Charity* and accompanying *Constitutions* and *Statutes* (2016), https://dbcm.cmglobal.org.

One. *The Hospital, a Place They Could Call Their Own*

1. Quote in O'Donnell, *Elizabeth Seton*, 304.

2. O'Donnell, *Elizabeth Seton*, 4–7; Barthel, *American Saint*, 211; Caroline Lang, "The Mother of Catholic Education," https://ace.nd.edu; "Seton Catholic Schools," https://www.setoncatholicschools.com.

3. De Lavergnée, *Streets as a Cloister*, 252–55.

4. Fr. John Dubois to Granville Pattison, May 10, 1822, Baltimore, MD/Baltimore Infirmary Collection, RG 11-2-2:1(3), APSL; Lomas, "As It Was in the Beginning," 186–92.

5. Dubois to Pattison, May 10, 1822, APSL; Hannefin, *Daughters of the Church*, 33–34.

6. Quotes from Lomas, "As It Was in the Beginning," 192–93.

7. Quotes from Lomas, "As It Was in the Beginning," 198–200.

8. Kraman, "Women Religious in Health Care," 22, 31; Nelson, *Say Little, Do Much*, 25.

9. Rybolt, "Joseph Rosati, CM," 395–97.

10. Thomas Meehan, "John Mullanphy," *The Catholic Encyclopedia*, 10 (1911), https://www.newadvent.org.

11. Upon their arrival in Baltimore and before heading west, the Vincentian priests were guests of the president of St. Mary's College, Father Simon Bruté, PPS. The encounter was highly fortuitous because twelve years later, when Rosati sought to attract the Sisters to St. Louis, Bruté was in Emmitsburg teaching at Mount St. Mary's. Learning that Bruté was in Emmitsburg, Rosati wrote him in August 1828 asking for his help in persuading the Sisters to come to St. Louis. Trained in medicine before entering the priesthood, Bruté was predisposed toward the mission that Rosati had proposed. O'Donnell, *Elizabeth Seton*, 386–90; McCann, *History of Mother Seton's Daughters*, xiii, 65–68, 97–98, 113, 137–39; Sister Lilliana Owens Account, St. Louis, MO/DePaul Hospital Collection, RG 11-2-2:15(5), APSL.

12. Bishop Joseph Rosati to Fr. Simon Bruté, June 23, 1828, St. Louis, MO/DePaul Hospital Collection, RG 11-2-2:15(3), APSL.

13. Bishop Joseph Rosati to Mother Augustine Decount, November 27, 1828, St. Louis, MO/DePaul Hospital Collection, RG 11-2-2:15(3), APSL.

14. Sr. Francis Xavier letters to Mother Augustine DeCount, October 1828, St. Louis, MO/DePaul Hospital Collection, RG 11-2-2:15(3), APSL.

15. Rosati to DeCount, November 27, 1828, APSL; Rybolt, "Joseph Rosati," 396–98. Another reason for Rosati's absence was poor communication. Rosati apparently had no advance notice of the Sisters' progress and the date they would be arriving.

16. Rybolt, "Congregation of the Mission in the United States."

17. Sister Lilliana Owens Account, APSL; Sr. Henrietta Guyot, "The Sisters of Charity Respond," Special Services: Epidemics Collection, RG 7-6-1:1(1), APSL; "DePaul Sesquicentennial Event," St. Louis, MO/DePaul Hospital Collection, RG 11-2-2:15(1), APSL; Jeannette Cooperman, "Take Care and Don't Take the Cholera," *St Louis Magazine*, July 2010.

18. Sister Lilliana Owens Account, APSL; United States Department of the Interior, National Park Service, *National Register of Historic Places Inventory—Nomination Form*, DePaul Hospital, Item No. 8, https://dnr.mo.gov; Sister Elspeth Ann Gartner, "History of DePaul Hospital with Description of the Development of the Social Service Department," St. Louis, MO/DePaul Hospital Collection, RG 11-2-2:15(5), APSL.

19. Jones, *Charitable Imperative*, 184.

20. Jones, "Sisters of Charity and the Ailing Poor," 343.

21. Jones, "Sisters of Charity and the Ailing Poor," 342.

22. Jones, "Sisters of Charity and the Ailing Poor," 342; Jones, *Charitable Imperative*, 185–91.

23. Jones, *Charitable Imperative*, 199. See also Charpy, "Challenge to Napoleon," 47–89.

24. Abstract of recorded deed, October 29, 1828, St. Louis, MO/DePaul Hospital Collection, RG 11-2-5-1, APSL; John Rothensteiner, "History of the Archdiocese of St. Louis," St. Louis, MO/DePaul Hospital Collection, RG 11-2-2:15(8), APSL.

25. "An Act to Incorporate 'The St. Louis Hospital Association,'" January 25, 1843, St. Louis, MO/DePaul Hospital Collection, RG 11-2-5-1, APSL.

26. Constitutions and By-Laws of the St. Louis Hospital Association, February 20, 1843, St. Louis, MO/DePaul Hospital Collection, RG 11-2-5-1, APSL.

27. O'Melinn, "Neither Contract nor Concession," 201.

28. Frederick County Com'rs v. Sisters of Charity of St. Joseph, 48 Md. 34, 36 (1878).

29. 17 U.S. (4 Wheat) 518 (1819).

30. Trustees of Dartmouth College v. Woodward, 17 U.S. (4 Wheat), at 628, 632–37, 640–41, 645.

31. O'Melinn, "Neither Contract nor Concession," 216–19; Powell and Menendian, "Beyond Public/Private," 53–54.

32. O'Melinn, "Neither Contract nor Concession," 206–9, 233–40; McGarvie, "Creating Roles for Religion and Philanthropy," 549–55; Powell and Menendian, "Beyond Public/Private," 48–62.

33. Charpy, "Challenge to Napolean," 47, 49–50; Weiss, "Origins of the French Welfare State," 47–66; Gunn, "Religious Freedom and Laïcité," 432–40; Stone, "Anticlericals and *Bonnes Soeurs*," 103, 108–12.

34. Weiss, "Origins of the French Welfare State," 51; Archambault, "Historical Roots," 204–11; Gunn, "Religious Freedom and Laïcité," 420–21.

35. Gunn, "Religious Freedom and Laïcité," 439–41; Archambault, "Historical Roots," 210; Stone, "Anticlericals and *Bonnes Soeurs*," 103–5, 116, 127 (more so in schools than in hospitals).

36. Archambault, "Historical Roots," 209–10.

37. The French government's determination in the late 1800s to separate civil society from religious society, known as *laïcité*, did not countenance Vincentian spirituality in public hospitals. McGarvie, "Creating Roles for Religion and Philanthropy," 567.

38. O'Melinn, "Neither Contract Nor Concession," 226.

39. Wall, "Science and Ritual," 58.

40. Stewart, *Marvels of Charity*, 516–18.

41. O'Grady, *Catholic Charities in the United States*, 201; Oates, *Catholic Philanthropic Tradition*, 39.

42. Ryan and Rybolt, *Vincent de Paul and Louis de Marillac*, 167–93; de Lavergnée, *Streets as a Cloister*, 252–65, 313–16, 320–24, 427–29, 445–61.

43. Ryan and Rybolt, *Vincent de Paul and Louis de Marillac*, 168.

44. Hickey, *Local Hospitals in Ancien Régime France*, 169–74.

45. Mother Mary Xavier Clark, "Instructions on the Care of the Sick," circa 1846, Health Apostolate Collection, RG 16-2-1:13(2), APSL.

46. For a textual analysis of the writings of Mother Xavier Clark, see Wall, "Textual Analysis as a Method for Historians of Nursing," 22–42.

47. Libster and McNeil, *Enlightened Charity*, 42–46.

48. Clark, "Instructions on the Care of the Sick," APSL, 46–63.

49. Clark, "Instructions on the Care of the Sick," APSL, 33–34, 71–73.

50. Jones, *Charitable Imperative*, 164, 198.

51. Vincent preferred "sister servant" over "superior" or "superioress." He told the French Daughters at one of his conferences that "the Blessed Virgin" had taken the title and that Madame Goussault had recommended it for the superioress of Hôtel-Dieu. Dirvin, *Louise de Marillac of the Ladies and Daughters of Charity*, 219.

52. Clark, "Instructions on the Care of the Sick," APSL, 58–59.

53. *Lives of Deceased Sisters*, Matilda Coskery, 3, APSL.

54. Sr. Matilda Coskery, *Advices Concerning the Sick*, circa 1850, Health Apostolate Collection, RG 16-2-4, APSL.

55. Libster and McNeil, *Enlightened Charity*, 90–95; Patricia D'Antonio, "History of Psychiatric Hospitals," https://www.nursing.upenn.edu.

56. Coskery, *Advices Concerning the Sick*, APSL, 31.

57. Libster and McNeil, *Enlightened Charity*, 173.

58. Rosenberg, *Care of Strangers*, 218, 270–77.

59. In order to avoid confusion, I will use the designation "Daughters" from here on to encompass both the Sisters and Daughters, unless referring to "Sisters" because of the specific chronological context.

60. Problems with doctors and boards of directors had surfaced in France before the French Revolution. Disputes occurred with some frequency over dissections, the amount of food given to patients, certain types of treatments such as bloodletting, and the mixing and administration of drugs and other remedies. In many of these instances, hospital administrators sided with the nursing sisters, whom Colin Jones characterized as "the fiercest critics of the medical profession." At Montpellier's Hôtel-Dieu, Jones observed, "the hospital board showed itself in full agreement with the nursing sisters that the hospital was a charitable institution before it was a medical one, and that the first priority must always be to the welfare of the inmates rather than the cause of medical science." Jones, *Charity and Bienfaisance*, 127–28.

Clashes between sisters and doctors intensified at the end of the eighteenth century as clinical medicine gained favor in French medical schools and clinics. But though anticlericalism buttressed physicians' criticism of nursing sisters for crossing the line into "medical" treatment, the lack of visible results on their part (death rates were high during hospital operations) sustained the uneasy balance between the two contenders. This was the state of affairs when the Sisters of Charity entered the Baltimore Infirmary. Until medical science began to show concrete results in the second half of the nineteenth century, the Daughters' nursing skills trumped the medical care of most doctors. Jones, *Charitable Imperative*, 15–17, 137, 154–56, 194–95; Jones, "Sisters of Charity and the Ailing Poor," 343–47; Jones, *Charity and Bienfaisance*, 113–30, 127, 128, 203–8. See also de Lavergnée, *Streets as a Cloister*, 488–94; Hickey, *Local Hospitals in Ancien Régime France*, 170–74.

61. Rosenberg, *Care of Strangers*, 272, 279.

62. Jones, *Charitable Imperative*, 15, 137, 194–15; de Lavergnée, *Streets as a Cloister*, 488–93.

63. Coskery, *Advices Concerning the Sick*, APSL, 1, 3–4, 5–6, 67–76.

64. Coskery, *Advices Concerning the Sick*, APSL, 45.

65. Coskery, *Advices Concerning the Sick*, APSL, 49.

66. Cavico and Cavico, "Nursing Profession in the 1990's," 569–70; Armstrong, "Nurse Malpractice in North Carolina," 581–83; Eccard, "Revolution in White," 855–59, 871.

67. Coskery, *Advices Concerning the Sick*, APSL, 45.

68. Coskery, *Advices Concerning the Sick*, APSL, 11.

69. Rosenberg, "From Almshouse to Hospital," 113–14.

70. Buhler-Wilkerson, *No Place Like Home*, 4–7.

71. Quote in Rosenberg, "From Almshouse to Hospital," 134.

72. Rosenberg, *Care of Strangers*, 4, 42–43; Kauffman, *Ministry and Meaning*, 33.

73. Duffy, *The Sanitarians*, 80–81; Carter, "Cincinnatians and Cholera," 33–37.

74. A summary of several reports appears in the *Northern Pennsylvanian* (Dundaff, PA) of June 22, 1832 (all newspaper articles are from https://newspapers.com unless noted otherwise).

75. Pyle, "Diffusion of Cholera in the United States," 60–65.

76. Carter, "Cincinnatians and Cholera," 32–33; Robert McNamara, "The Cholera Epidemic of 1832: As Immigrants Were Blamed, Half of New York City Fled in Panic," February 29, 2020, https://www.thoughtco.com.

77. Watson, "Sisters of Charity," 2.

78. Rutkow, *Bleeding Blue and Grey*, 28–33.

79. Duffy, *The Sanitarians*, 47.

80. Watson, "Sisters of Charity," 6–9.

81. In 1834, the almshouse portion of the hospital relocated to Blockley Township in West Philadelphia and changed its name to Blockley. Rosenberg, "From Almshouse to Hospital," 117.

82. Rosenberg, "From Almshouse to Hospital," 113–24, 127–28.

83. Armiger, "Two Sister-Nurses Claimed by Cholera," 54–55.

84. Watson, "Sisters of Charity," 11.

85. John B. Osborne, "Cholera," *Encyclopedia of Greater Philadelphia*, https://philadelphiaencyclopedia.org; Rosenberg, *Cholera Years*, 59–60.

86. Author unknown, "Noble Work in Caring for Destitute Patients in the Almshouse Here During the Cholera Epidemic of 1832," RG 7-6-1:1(1), APSL.

87. Dr. Jesse Burden, an almshouse director who was also speaker of the Pennsylvania State Senate, was the one who solicited Kenrick. "Communication," *National Gazette*, September 4, 1832; Watson, "Sisters of Charity," 12.

88. Watson, "Sisters of Charity," 12; Hannefin, *Daughters of the Church*, 51–52.

89. Watson, "Sisters of Charity," 12.

90. Watson, "Sisters of Charity," 12–13.

91. Armiger, "Two Sister-Nurses Claimed by Cholera," 54–55.

92. "Noble Work," APSL.

93. "Noble Work," APSL.

94. Watson, "Sisters of Charity," 13.

95. "Noble Work," APSL.

96. "Noble Work," APSL.

97. Casterline, "St. Joseph's and St. Mary's," 302.

98. Population figures are from Gerber, *Making of an American Pluralism*, 6; author unknown, "From Acorn to Oak," Buffalo, NY/Sisters of Charity Hospital Collection, RG 11-2-2:11(4), APSL.

99. Gerber, *Making of an American Pluralism*, 3–21, 121–31, 163–79.

100. "125th Anniversary of Sisters Hospital," Buffalo, NY/Sisters of Charity Hospital Collection, RG 11-2-2:11(2), APSL.

101. "125th Anniversary of Sisters Hospital," APSL.

102. Gerber, *Making of an American Pluralism*, 280–317; Paul E. Lubienecki, "John Timon—Buffalo's First Bishop: His Forgotten Struggle to Assimilate Catholics in Western New York," 2010, https://newyorkhistoryblog.org.

103. "By Their Fruits, You Shall Know Them!," APSL; "Sisters Hospital, Buffalo (Chronology 1848–1995)," Buffalo, NY/Sisters of Charity Hospital Collection, RG 11-2-2:11(1), APSL.

104. Flint, "Original Communications," 313–15.

105. "A Brief History of St. Mary's Infant Asylum and Maternity Hospital," 1937, Buffalo, NY/St. Mary's Infant Asylum/Buffalo Widows Asylum Collection, RG 11-4:1(4), APSL.

106. "Brief History of St. Mary's Infant Asylum," APSL.

107. The accounts concerning the beginning of the Buffalo infant asylum are confusing and frequently contradictory. There is much uncertainty concerning where the Sisters came from (one archival account says "Sisters' Hospital," another the "Central House," and still others say Detroit or elsewhere) and when Brown arrived to assume charge of the mission (one newspaper account says 1848 and another 1850). The best evidence, which is consistent with the events described in Libster and McNeil, has Brown arriving in 1854 to take charge of the asylum. This makes the most sense based on the Detroit material and the beginning of her fundraising efforts on behalf of the asylum. In addition, other archival material confirms this. See Libster and McNeil, *Enlightened Charity*, 149–50.

108. "Brief History of St. Mary's Infant Asylum," APSL.

109. "Special Notices: Asylum for Widows, Lying-in Women and Foundlings," *Buffalo Courier*, June 27, 1854.

110. Sister Rosaline Brown, "Notice," *Buffalo Daily Republic*, September 9, 1857.

111. "Providence Retreat," Buffalo, NY/Sisters of Charity Hospital Collection, RG 11-2-2.1(8), APSL.

112. Statistics from Catholic Directories, Buffalo, NY/St. Mary's Asylum/Buffalo Widows Asylum Collection, RG 11-4:1(4), APSL.

113. "Providence Retreat," APSL.

114. "Providence Retreat," APSL.

115. "Providence Retreat," APSL; "Contributions of the Daughters of Charity to Health Care, 1800–1980," Buffalo, NY/Sisters of Charity Hospital Collection, RG 11-2-2:11(2), APSL.

116. "New Insane Asylum," *Buffalo Currier*, November 3, 1860.

117. "New Insane Asylum," *Buffalo Currier*, November 3, 1860.

118. "Providence Insane Asylum," *Buffalo Courier*, September 14, 1863 (the newspaper excerpted portions of Miner's article from the *Buffalo Medical and Surgical Journal*).

Two. *Immigration, Epidemics, Anti-Catholicism, and Slavery*

1. Daniels, *Coming to America*, 121–29.

2. Daniels, *Coming to America*, 129, 146; Ouimette and Rencher, "Irish Emigration and Immigration to North America," 21; "Irish Potato Famine: Gone to America," History Place, 2000, https://www.historyplace.com.

3. Daniels, *Coming to America*, 126–25; Gleeson, *Irish in the South*, 10–22; Gerber, *Making of an American Pluralism*, 187–99.

4. Haller, *Across the Atlantic*, 203.

5. Kauffman, *Ministry and Meaning*, 69.

6. Desmond, *Know-Nothing Party*, 15–16, 38–42; Billington, *Protestant Crusade*, 67–69, 220–34.

7. Quinn, "Expecting the Impossible?"; Gleeson, *Irish in the South*, 7–8, 139–40; Hannefin, *Daughters of the Church*, 107–8. See also Morrow, *Persons of Color and Religious*, 40, 250–56; Oates, *Catholic Philanthropic Tradition*, 58–67.

8. McGuinness, *Called to Serve*, 9; Kauffman, *Ministry and Meaning*, 79–80.

9. Kauffman, *Ministry and Meaning*, 82–83.

10. Rosenberg, *Cholera Years*, 61–64; Geary, "Epidemic Diseases of the Great Famine"; Kraut, *Silent Travelers*, 27–30.

11. Newspapers often used the terms "ship fever" and "typhus" interchangeably. See, e.g., "Ship Fever," *Glasgow Herald*, September 20, 1847; *Buffalo Courier*, November 19, 1853; *Freeman's Journal* (Dublin, Ireland), January 25, 1848; "Correspondence," *Public Ledger* (Philadelphia, PA), November 16, 1853; *New Orleans Crescent*, March 17, 1848; "Ship Fever," *Washington Union*, July 16, 1847.

12. "Epidemic Typhus," Centers for Disease Control and Prevention, https://www.cdc.gov.

13. Quote in "Review of M. Louis's Researches Upon Typhoid Fever," 214.

14. Gerhard, "Gerhard on Typhus Fever," 38.

15. "Report on Ship Fever," *Middlebury Register* (Middlebury, VT), July 6, 1847.

16. "Emigrant Ships," *Bristol Mercury and Daily Post*, July 3, 1847; "Ship Fever," *Glasgow Herald*, September 20, 1847.

17. Typhus was so widespread in Ireland during the Great Famine that the government added "373 emergency institutions . . . to the hundred or so fever hospitals already in existence." Geary, "Epidemic Diseases of the Great Famine." See also "Epidemic Fever in Ireland," 389–93.

18. "Emigrant Ships," *Bristol Mercury and Daily Post*, July 3, 1847.

19. Castle, "Common-Sense Talk About 'Ship Fever,'" 291–94. See also McManus, "Emigrating Fifty Years Ago," *Boston Globe*, February 4, 1900.

20. *New Orleans Crescent*, March 17, 1848.

21. "Ship Fever," *Washington Union*, July 16, 1847.

22. *Bristol Mercury and Daily Post*, July 3, 1847.

23. "Report of the Superintendents of the Poor of Erie Co.," 446–47; "The Ship Fever in New Orleans," *The Tennessean* (Nashville, TN), February 25, 1848; *New Orleans Crescent*, March 17, 1848; *Brooklyn Evening Star*, May 26, 1847; *Brooklyn Daily Eagle*, June 3, 1847; *Sandusky Clarion* (Sandusky, OH), January 25, 1848; *Public Ledger*, November 16, 1853; *Buffalo Currier*, November 19, 1853; *Evening Courier and Republic* (Buffalo, NY), February 1, 1862; *The Gazette* (Montreal, QC), July 25, 1970.

24. "The Ship Fever in New Orleans," *The Tennessean*, February 25, 1848.

25. In 1847, the price of steerage was much cheaper for ships traveling to Canada than the United States because Canada was a British colony. This explains why many Irish immigrants first came to Canada and then crossed into the United States, often on foot. By early 1848, however, the price of steerage to the United States had fallen to the point that the majority of Irish immigrants traveled by ship directly to US ports. One of the reasons why many came from Liverpool to the United States rather than from an Irish port, such as Dublin, was because there were more ships leaving Liverpool for the United States. Ouimette and Rencher, "Irish Emigration and Immigration to North America," 21, 25; *Freeman's Journal*, January 25, 1848.

26. "The Distressing Condition of the Irish Passengers," *Baltimore Sun*, May 11, 1847.

27. "The Destitute Immigrants," *Baltimore Sun*, May 12, 1847.

28. Williams, *History of the Hibernian Society of Baltimore*, 20–21; "The Distressing Condition of the Irish Passengers," *Baltimore Sun*, May 12, 1847.

29. Williams, *History of the Hibernian Society of Baltimore*, 23–24.

30. The number is a guestimate. The Daughters' account states as follows: "When an epidemic of ship fever, diagnosed as typhus, broke out in June, 1847, one hundred seventy cases were treated at the Infirmary, and less than ten percent

died." "Summary of Works and Deaths of Sisters from Epidemic—first on file," 1919–1932, Special Services: Epidemics Collection, RG 7-6-1:1(1), APSL.

31. *Baltimore Sun*, June 7, June 12, and July 27, 1847; Williams, *History of the Hibernian Society of Baltimore*, 24. Another sister, Ann Barrilia Lynch, died of typhus in 1847 while caring for sick patients at New Orleans' Charity Hospital.

32. Summaries of Works and Deaths of Sisters, APSL.

33. "Hospital of the Sisters of Charity," *Detroit Free Press*, July 28, 1851.

34. Morens, "Commentary: Cholera Conundrums," 43–44.

35. Morens, "Commentary: Cholera Conundrums," 43–44.

36. Rutkow, *Bleeding Blue and Grey*, 31; Rosenberg, *Cholera Years*, 72–74; Kotar and Gessler, *Yellow Fever*, 3; Gaynes, *Germ Theory*, 23–25; Duffy, *The Sanitarians*, 20–22.

37. Rutkow, *Bleeding Blue and Grey*, 31.

38. Duffy, *The Sanitarians*, 67–68; *Burlington Weekly Free Press* (Burlington, VT), June 22, 1832.

39. *National Gazette* (Philadelphia, PA), August 4, 1832.

40. Rosenberg, *Cholera Years*, 57.

41. Morens, "Commentary: Cholera Conundrums," 43.

42. Morens, "Commentary: Cholera Conundrums," 45–49; Pyle, "Diffusion of Cholera," 60.

43. Gaynes, *Germ Theory*, 16–30.

44. Rutkow, *Bleeding Blue and Grey*, 28–34; Gaynes, *Germ Theory*, 23–27.

45. Rosenberg, *Cholera Years*, 154–64; *Buffalo Courier*, May 29, 1849; "Cholera in New York," *Buffalo Weekly Republic*, July 17, 1849.

46. Coskery, *Advices Concerning the Sick*, APSL, 45, 49.

47. Rosenberg, *Care of Strangers*, 212, 217–18.

48. Pyle, "Diffusion of Cholera," 67.

49. Daly, "Black Cholera," 143–53.

50. "St. Louis Mullanphy Hospital," St. Louis, MO/DePaul Hospital Collection, RG 11-2-2:15(3), APSL.

51. Flint, "Original Communications," 319.

52. Flint, "Original Communications," 313–15.

53. In addition to founding and editing the *Buffalo Medical Journal*, Flint cofounded the Buffalo Medical School in 1847 and, years later, pioneered the field of cardiology while working at New Orleans's Charity Hospital. The "Flint murmur" was among his notable achievements. Mehta, Mehta, and Khan, "Austin Flint," 386–89.

54. Flint, "Original Communications," 322–23.

55. Flint, "Original Communications," 323.

56. "From Acorn to Oak," APSL.

57. Flint, "Original Communications," 332.

58. Flint, "Original Communications," 332–33.

59. Dr. Stephen Smith, "Some Recollections of Events on the Establishment of the Sisters Hospital of Charity of Buffalo," Buffalo, NY/Sisters of Charity Hospital Collection, RG 11-2-2:1(2), APSL.

60. Crosby, *American Plague*, 43.

61. Kotar and Gessler, *Yellow Fever*, 7.

62. Crosby, *American Plague*, 70–71.

63. Quote in Kotar and Gessler, *Yellow Fever*, 3.

64. Coskery, *Advices Concerning the Sick*, APSL, 69.

65. Coskery, *Advices Concerning the Sick*, APSL, 69–72.

66. Coskery, *Advices Concerning the Sick*, APSL, 71–76.

67. Joseph Roger Baudier, "Hôtel Dieu—a Century of Service," New Orleans, LA/Hôtel Dieu Hospital Collection, RG 11-2-1:11(5), APSL.

68. Baudier, "Hôtel Dieu—a Century of Service," APSL.

69. Kendall, *History of New Orleans*, 175.

70. This is a ballpark figure. Elizabeth Wisner notes "the lack of adequate mortality statistics in that summer of near chaos." Wisner, "Howard Association," 411. See also Kotar and Gessler, *Yellow Fever*, 198–200, for reported figures from the New Orleans Board of Health.

71. "Lives of Our Deceased Sisters, 1852–1869," 13, APSL.

72. Wisner, "Howard Association," 411.

73. Kotar and Gessler, *Yellow Fever*, 201.

74. "Lives of Our Deceased Sisters, 1852–1869," 13, APSL.

75. Lon Wagner, "The Fever: A Story in 14 Parts," *Virginian-Pilot*, special reprint edition, originally published July 10–23, 2005, https://pilotonline; Albin Trant Butt, "A Century of Service to the Sick: The 100 Year History of the Hospital of St. Vincent De Paul, Norfolk, Virginia, 1856–1956," Norfolk, VA/DePaul Hospital Collection, RG 11-2-2:5(1), APSL. These accounts are largely consistent, with some minor discrepancies. For example, Wagner claims that the crewman's body was buried on the Portsmouth side of the river, while Butt asserts that it was buried on the Norfolk side.

76. Butt, "Century of Service to the Sick," APSL.

77. "History of Yellow Fever in Norfolk," *Richmond Dispatch*, August 31, 1855.

78. Wagner, "Fever: A Story in 14 Parts," 3–8.

79. "Progress of the Fever in Norfolk and Portsmouth," *Richmond Dispatch*, August 20, 1855.

80. T. H. Conaway Jr., "Pertinent Facts About the Role of the Daughters of Charity at the Naval Medical Center, Portsmouth, Virginia," Norfolk, VA/DePaul Hospital Collection, RG 11-2-2:5(2), APSL. Conaway states that "one hundred and

seven doctors came into the area to assist. Many of them were soon stricken with yellow fever and twenty-four succumbed to the disease." Lon Wagner, on the other hand, indicates that "twenty of 87 visiting doctors had died, along with more than half of the local physicians." Wagner, "Fever: A Story in 14 Parts," 27.

81. "Correspondence of the Dispatch," *Richmond Dispatch*, September 4, 1855.

82. Sister Aloysia Dugan, "Service During Epidemics," Special Services: Epidemics Collection, RG 7-7-1:1, APSL.

83. A thirteen-year-old boy died, along with one of the Daughters. "Health at the Catholic College," *Richmond Dispatch*, September 24, 1855.

84. Butt, "Century of Service to the Sick," APSL. Captain Conaway of the US Navy's Medical Service Corps praised the Sisters: "Three Sisters of Charity volunteered their nursing skills and worked untiringly in the wards of the Naval Hospital." Conaway, "Pertinent Facts," APSL.

85. "Progress of the Fever in Norfolk and Portsmouth," *Richmond Dispatch*, September 3, 1855.

86. "Recapitulation of the Dead—Some Reflections," *Richmond Dispatch*, October 16, 1865.

87. Butt, "Century of Service to the Sick," APSL; author unknown, "The Hospital of St. Vincent de Paul," Norfolk, VA/DePaul Hospital Collection, RG 11-2-2:5(2), APSL.

88. Billington, *Protestant Crusade*, 380–99; Desmond, *Know-Nothing Party*, 49–70.

89. Billington, *Protestant Crusade*, 388–89, 423–30; Desmond, *Know-Nothing Party*, 60–70.

90. Mobile's mayor in 1852 was Joseph Seawell, a Democrat. Seawell served in the Alabama legislature in the 1840s before running for mayor of Mobile in 1851. The 1851 mayoral race was hotly contested. Charles Carter (C. C.) Langdon, a Whig, beat Seawell in the initial tally by only eleven votes. Langdon, who had won the previous election, remained in office until the courts resolved the matter in favor of Seawell (Seawell claimed that there were "fraudulent and illegal votes") almost one year later. Seawell's term was short-lived, for in 1852, Langdon won the rematch. Langdon served as mayor of Mobile until 1855 when he lost to Mitchell Withers, a Democrat. *Spirt of the South* (Eufaula, AL), January 14, 1851; *Alabama Beacon* (Greensboro, AL), December 6, 1851; *The Courier* (Butler, AL), September 20, 1883.

91. Fr. James McGarahan to Fr. Francis Burlando, May 15, 1854, Mobile, AL/ Providence Hospital Collection, RG 11-2-2:5(2), APSL.

92. "Daughters of Charity Originating and Withdrawal Dates," Mobile, AL/ Providence Hospital Collection, RG 11-2-2:5(2), APSL; Gleeson, *Irish in the South*, 69, 113.

93. McGarahan to Burlando, May 15, 1854, APSL.

94. McGarahan to Burlando, June 22, 1854, APSL.

95. *Brooklyn Daily Eagle*, July 18, 1854; *Hartford Courant*, July 22, 1854.

96. McGarahan to Burlando, July 3, 1854, APSL. In his letter to Burlando, McGarahan referred to Langdon as a "shrewd Yankee politician" who "could not afford to be honest," because "his re-election to office was at stake." In retrospect, it seems mystifying that the politically experienced McGarahan was "deceived" by the mayor, Charles Carter Langdon. Langdon's political ambitions were widely known. A frequent candidate for state and federal office since the 1830s, Langdon was owner and editor of the *Mobile Daily Advertiser*, a Whig Party newspaper. "Rearin' Up and Kickin' Up," *Weekly Advertiser* (Montgomery, AL), May 28, 1851; *Sumter Democrat* (Livingston, AL), August 23, 1852.

97. "Daughters of Charity Originating and Withdrawal Dates," APSL.

98. "Charity Hospital Welcomes Sister Regina," New Orleans, LA/Charity Hospital Collection, RG 11-2-2:2(7), APSL.

99. Billington, *Protestant Crusade*, 132; Desmond, *Know-Nothing Party*, 26–28; Gleeson, *Irish in the South*, 114–18.

100. "Brief History of Hôtel Dieu," New Orleans, LA/Hôtel Dieu Hospital Collection, RG 11-2-1:11(5), APSL.

101. "Brief History of Hôtel Dieu," APSL.

102. Accounts indicate that the Sisters "open[ed] subscription lists" to secure a portion of the funding. "History of Hôtel Dieu Sisters' Hospital," New Orleans, LA/Hôtel Dieu Hospital Collection, RG 11-2-1:11(5), APSL.

103. "History of Hôtel Dieu Sisters' Hospital," APSL.

104. "History of Hôtel Dieu Sisters' Hospital," APSL. The Know-Nothing movement lasted longer in New Orleans than in most other places. In 1857, the Know-Nothings still maintained control of the city council. But any antagonism against the Daughters, or against all Catholics for that matter, had significantly diminished by then. Weakening hostility stemmed from internal party divisions and class distinctions that fractured New Orleans society. Gleeson, *Irish in the South*, 108, 114–20.

105. Gerber, *Making of an American Pluralism*, 301; O'Driscoll, "Political Nativism in Buffalo," 292–93.

106. Gerber, *Making of an American Pluralism*, 301; O'Driscoll, "Political Nativism in Buffalo," 295.

107. Gerber, *Making of an American Pluralism*, 301–2, 315; Lubienecki, "John Timon."

108. "125th Anniversary of Sisters Hospital," APSL; "From Acorn to Oak," APSL; O'Driscoll, "Political Nativism in Buffalo," 297; Flint, "Original Communications," 313–33.

109. Strum, "To Feed the Hungry," 6; Zwierlein, "Catholic Beginnings in the Diocese of Rochester," 282–98.

110. "Chronology," Rochester, NY/St. Mary's Hospital Collection, RG 11-2-2:14(12), APSL. See also Sr. Delphine Steele, "Historical Sketch of St. Mary's Hospital, Rochester, 1857–c.1952," Rochester, NY/St. Mary's Hospital Collection, RG 11-2-2:14(12), APSL; Betsy C. Corner, "A Century of Medicine in Rochester," Rochester, NY/St. Mary's Hospital Collection, RG 11-2-2:14(1), APSL; "Public Notice," Rochester, NY/St. Mary's Hospital Collection, RG 11-2-5:24(1), APSL; "Brief History of St. Mary's Hospital, Rochester, N.Y.," Rochester, NY/St. Mary's Hospital Collection, RG 11-2-2:14(1), APSL; Joseph P. Henry, "Century of Service, St. Mary's Hospital," Rochester, NY/St. Mary's Hospital Collection, RG 11-2-2:14(9), APSL.

111. Zwierlein, "Know Nothingism in Rochester," 38, 41–48, 52, 59–62, 67.

112. Steele, "Historical Sketch of St. Mary's Hospital," APSL; Corner, "Century of Medicine in Rochester," APSL; "Public Notice," APSL; "Brief History of St. Mary's Hospital," APSL; Henry, "Century of Service," APSL.

113. Quote in Steele, "Historical Sketch of St. Mary's Hospital," APSL, 7.

114. Steele, "Historical Sketch of St. Mary's Hospital," APSL, 5-6.

115. Quote in Steele, "Historical Sketch of St. Mary's Hospital," APSL, 8.

116. St. Mary's financial condition did not measurably improve, however, until the Civil War started and the federal government began paying for convalescing soldiers sent to St. Mary's Hospital. Steele, "Historical Sketch of St. Mary's Hospital," APSL, 7–11.

117. The Erie County Poor House, the Buffalo Protestant Orphanage, and New York City public hospitals barred Catholic clergy. Kauffman, *Ministry and Meaning*, 67–69; Gerber, *Making of an American Pluralism*, 313; Oates, *Catholic Philanthropic Tradition*, 39; Cetina, "In Times of Immigration," 94–95.

118. Libster and McNeil, *Enlightened Charity*, 58.

119. Sr. Mary Ann McAleer, "Letters of Her Experience at St. Agnes Hospital, Baltimore," Baltimore, MD/St. Agnes Hospital Collection, RG 11-2-3:14(1).

120. Rosenberg, *Care of Strangers*, 33.

121. McAleer, "Letters of Her Experience at St. Agnes Hospital," APSL.

122. Sr. M. Virginia Joyce, "Notes of Sr. M. Virginia Joyce," Baltimore, MD/St. Agnes Hospital Collection, RG 11-2-2:13(1), APSL.

123. McAleer, "Letters of Her Experience at St. Agnes Hospital," APSL.

124. Rosenberg, *Care of Strangers*, 22–30.

125. Buhler-Wilkerson, *No Place Like Home*, 1–10.

126. "The History of Nursing Homes," Foundation Aiding the Elderly, https://www.4fate.org.

127. Bates, *Bargaining for Life*, 3–5, 186; McCauley, *Who Shall Take Care of Our Sick?*, 48; Kauffman, *Ministry and Meaning*, 64–65.

128. McAleer, "Letters of Her Experience at St. Agnes Hospital," APSL.

129. McAleer, "Letters of Her Experience at St. Agnes Hospital," APSL.

130. McAleer, "Letters of Her Experience at St. Agnes Hospital," APSL.

131. McAleer, "Letters of Her Experience at St. Agnes Hospital," APSL.

132. Bates, *Bargaining for Life*, 1–8.

133. "Brief History and Description of St. Agnes Hospital," Baltimore, MD/St. Agnes Hospital Collection, RG 11-2-2:13(1), APSL. The full statement contained in the Daughters' archives is as follows: "St. Agnes Hospital is a general hospital opened during the Civil War to serve 'the Catholic poor' of Baltimore in response to the invitation of Archbishop Kenrick."

134. "Notes of Sr. M. Virginia Joyce," APSL.

135. "Account of July 22, 1863," Baltimore, MD/St. Agnes Hospital Collection, RG 11-2-2:13(1), APSL.

136. "History of St. Agnes Hospital, 1862–1992," Baltimore, MD/St. Agnes Hospital Collection, RG 11-2-2:13(1), APSL.

137. Gleeson, *Irish in the South*, 112–20.

138. Quotes from Desmond, *Know-Nothing Party*, 106.

139. *Mobile Daily Advertiser*, July 23, 1844; "Native Americanism," *Mobile Daily Advertiser*, July 27, 1844.

140. Langdon's defeat at the ballot box in 1855 closely tracked Know-Nothing Party losses elsewhere. Southern pro-slavery forces were unrelenting in their zeal to defeat anyone or any party that sided with the "Unionists." Despite Langdon's apparent disavowal of abolitionism—he had stated that slavery was "in harmony with the economy of nature" when running for Congress in 1851—he could not deflect his previous expressions of pro-Union sentiment. "Rearin' Up and Kickin' Up," *Weekly Advertiser* (Montgomery, AL), May 28, 1851; *Sumter Democrat* (Livingston, AL), August 23, 1852.

141. "Hospitals in Alabama," Mobile, AL/Providence Hospital Collection, RG 11-2-2:5(2), APSL. The dates of the Daughters' subsequent work at City Hospital are convoluted. Apparently, they left and returned on more than one occasion in subsequent years and decades. See memorandum of August 2, 2004, from Sr. Mary Elizabeth Cullen to Sr. Catherine Madigan, Mobile, AL/City Hospital Collection, RG 11-2-2:1(4), APSL; "Daughters of Charity Originating and Withdrawal Dates," APSL.

142. Baudier, "Hôtel Dieu—a Century of Service," APSL.

143. Rice and Jones, *Public Policy and the Black Hospital*, 1–4; Gamble, *Making a Place for Ourselves, 47.*

144. Baudier, "Hôtel Dieu—A Century of Service," APSL.

145. Rabinowitz, "From Exclusion to Segregation," 327–54; Rice and Jones, *Public Policy and the Black Hospital*, 8–9; Gamble, *Making a Place for Ourselves*, 5–6.

146. Kauffman, *Ministry and Meaning*, 79.

147. Gamble, *Making a Place for Ourselves*, 5–6. See also Rosenberg, *Care of Strangers*, 301–3.

148. Kauffman, *Ministry and Meaning*, 79.

149. Kauffman, *Ministry and Meaning*, 79.

150. Hannefin, *Daughters of the Church*, 44.

151. Butt, "Century of Service to the Sick," APSL, 12–13.

152. O'Donnell, *Elizabeth Seton*, 263, 290. In contrast, see Dan Stockman, "Early Sisters of Charity Owned Slaves in U.S., Research Shows," Catholic News Service, February 16, 2022, https://catholicphilly.com.

153. "Notes of Sister Paula," New Orleans, LA/Charity Hospital Collection, RG 11-2-2:2(5), APSL.

154. William Fanning, "Plenary Councils of Baltimore," *Catholic Encyclopedia*, vol. 2, https://www.newadvent.org.

155. Alberts, "Black Catholic Schools," 78–87; Plessy v. Ferguson, 163 U.S. 537 (1896).

156. "The St. Euphemia's School Collection," APSL, https://docarchivesblog.org; Morrow, *Persons of Color and Religious at the Same Time*, 21, 201; Scally, "Two Nuns and Old Thad Stevens," 71.

157. Morrow, *Persons of Color and Religious at the Same Time*, 117–18.

158. Morrow, *Persons of Color and Religious at the Same Time*, 20–21, 138–39, 251.

159. Gamble, *Making a Place for Ourselves*, 31–32, 42, 58.

160. "Colored Women as Nurses," 144.

161. Gamble, *Making a Place for Ourselves*, 7, 11.

162. Gamble, *Making a Place for Ourselves*, xi.

Three. *Wartime Service*

1. Accounts differ concerning the precise number of Catholic sisters involved. See Hannefin, *Daughters of the Church*, 110 (570 sisters from 12 communities); Maher, *To Bind Up the Wounds*, 69 (617 sisters from 21 communities); Endres and Kurtz, *Soldiers of the Cross*, xii–xiii ("nearly" 700 from "at least" 20 communities and "over three hundred sister nurses" from the Daughters of Charity); McNeil, *Balm of Hope*, xxiv ("Emmitsburg sent over 300 sister nurses to serve in hospitals and on battlefields").

2. The Dodge Commission counted twelve Sisters of Mercy, fourteen Sisters of the Holy Cross, twelve Sisters of St. Joseph, and five from the Congregation of American Sisters (Native Americans from South Dakota). United States

Commission Appointed by the President to Investigate the Conduct of the War Department in the War with Spain, *Report of the Commission* (hereafter *Dodge Commission Report*), 9. Sister Gertrude Fenner's account is more complete, most likely because she also included communities that did not sign army contracts. Her tally was twenty-one Sisters of the Holy Names of Jesus and Mary, twenty Sisters of St. Joseph, seventeen Sisters of Mercy, twelve Sisters of the Holy Cross, eleven Sisters of St. Francis of Philadelphia, eight Sisters of Charity of Nazareth, and four from the Congregation of American Sisters. Fenner, "Daughters of Charity in the Spanish-American War," 36.

3. Dock, *History of American Red Cross Nursing*, 666.

4. Stanley B. Burns, "Disease," Mercy Street, https://www.pbs.org.

5. American Battlefield Trust, "Civil War Casualties," https://www.battlefields.org. More recent estimates place the death toll even higher, close to 750,000 men. Guy Gugliotta, "New Estimate Raises Civil War Death Toll," *New York Times*, April 2, 2012, https://www.nytimes.com.

6. American Battlefield Trust, "Civil War Casualties."

7. Rada, *Battlefield Angels*, 5, 24, 32.

8. Giesberg, *Civil War Sisterhood*, 31–43; Wormeley, *United States Sanitary Commission*, 1–9.

9. Giesberg, *Civil War Sisterhood*, 43–44; Maher, *To Bind Up the Wounds*, 51–57, 128–29.

10. Schultz, *Women at the Front*, 15.

11. Giesberg, *Civil War Sisterhood*, 118, 120.

12. Schroeder-Lein, *Encyclopedia of Civil War Medicine*, 234; Cunningham, *Doctors in Grey*, 72; Hilde, *Worth a Dozen Men*, 149–54; Maher, *To Bind Up the Wounds*, 46.

13. Cumming, *Kate*, 65.

14. Cunningham, *Doctors in Grey*, 72.

15. Massey, *Women in the Civil War*, 47; Schultz, *Women at the Front*, 18; Cunningham, *Doctors in Grey*, 73.

16. Hilde, *Worth a Dozen Men*, 38–51.

17. Maher, *To Bind Up the Wounds*, 109; Schultz, *Women at the Front*, 3.

18. Wormley, *United States Sanitary Commission*, 246–47.

19. Cumming, *Kate*, 178.

20. Quote in Rutkow, *Bleeding Blue and Gray*, 127.

21. Massey, *Women in the Civil War*, 47.

22. Schultz, *Women at the Front*, 113, 100–101; Maher, *To Bind Up the Wounds*, 27, 38.

23. Pfanz, *Clara Barton's Civil War*, 46; Maher, *To Bind Up the Wounds*, 51.

24. Pfanz, *Clara Barton's Civil War*, 46; Maher, *To Bind Up the Wounds*, 51.

25. Maher, *To Bind Up the Wounds*, 100.

26. This chain of care began with the evacuation of wounded soldiers in ambulances or wagons to makeshift hospitals where the majority of emergency surgeries (typically amputations) transpired. Sick and wounded soldiers who could travel went by trains or boats to military hospitals in major cities such as Philadelphia, New Orleans, and Washington. Varon, *Armies of Deliverance*, 167–68; McGaugh, *Surgeon in Blue*, 124, 130–34.

27. Rutkow, *Bleeding Blue and Gray*, xv–xvi, 233; McGaugh, *Surgeon in Blue*, 85–86; Devine, *Learning from the Wounded*, 202–9.

28. Devine, *Learning from the Wounded*, 101–31.

29. McNeil, *Balm of Hope*, 426 (Sr. Euphemia Blenkinsop to Mother Elisabeth Montcellet, August 16, 1862).

30. Peter W. Houck, "A Prototype of a Confederate Hospital Center in Lynchburg, Virginia," Military Services by American Sisters/Civil War Collection, RG 7-5-1(3), APSL.

31. "Ladies' Hospitals for the Soldiers of the Confederate Army, at Richmond," *Richmond Enquirer*, October 4, 1861.

32. Rada, *Battlefield Angels*, 10–11, 46–47.

33. Houck, "Prototype of a Confederate Hospital Center," APSL.

34. McNeil, *Balm of Hope*, 520 (appendix F, "Daughters of Charity Missions—Hubs for Sending Sisters to Nurse Sick and Wounded Soldiers, 1861–1865").

35. American Battlefield Trust, "10 Facts: Harpers Ferry," https://www.battlefields.org; McNeil, *Balm of Hope*, 38 (Recollections of Sr. Matilda Coskery, Harpers Ferry, Virginia).

36. McNeil, *Balm of Hope*, 35–37.

37. McNeil, *Balm of Hope*, 39, 43–44.

38. McNeil, *Balm of Hope*, 45.

39. Robert M. Browning Jr., "The Union Blockade of the Southern States," https://www.essentialcivilwarcurriculum.com.

40. "Blockage Blocked," *Times-Picayune* (New Orleans, LA), August 16, 1861.

41. McNeil, *Balm of Hope*, 420 (Sr. Regina Smith to Mother Elisabeth Montcellet, New Orleans, Louisiana, August 11, 1862).

42. McNeil, *Balm of Hope*, 425 (Sr. Euphemia Blenkinsop to Mother Elizabeth Montcellet).

43. McNeil, *Balm of Hope*, 291 (Memories of 1861).

44. McNeil, *Balm of Hope*, 292.

45. Gallagher et al., *Civil War: Fort Sumter to Appomattox*, 118.

46. McNeil, *Balm of Hope*, 175–76.

47. Gallagher et al., *Civil War*, 119; Varon, *Armies of Deliverance*, 119–20.

48. McNeil, *Balm of Hope*, 422–23.

49. Gallagher et al., *Civil War*, 52–61.

50. Varon, *Armies of Deliverance*, 78–83.

51. McNeil, *Balm of Hope*, 81 (W. A. Hammond, *Telegraphic Dispatch*, June 17, 1862).

52. McNeil, *Balm of Hope*, 83 (Fr. Francis Burlando to Mother Ann Simeon Norris, June 23, 1862).

53. McNeil, *Balm of Hope*, 87 (Recollections of Sister Matilda Coskery, White House Landing, Virginia).

54. Caulfield, "History of Providence Hospital," 232, 234; McNeil, *Balm of Hope*, 265n484.

55. Schroeder-Lein, *Encyclopedia of Civil War Medicine*, 330–31.

56. "Civil War Era Cliffburne Army Hospital," http://kaloramahistory.blogspot.com.

57. McNeil, *Balm of Hope*, 439 (Sr. [Helen] Ryan to [Mother Elisabeth Montcellet], Cliffburn Hospital, September 22, 1862).

58. Hilde, *Worth a Dozen Men*, 18.

59. McNeil, *Balm of Hope*, 61, 137 (Recollections of Sr. Rose Noyland, Central Virginia, Richmond General Hospital [#1]; Recollections—the Infirmary of St. Francis de Sales, Richmond, Virginia). The name "Louisiana" did not refer to the location of the hospital but rather to the state that sponsored it on behalf of troops who hailed from that state. Other Southern states also had hospitals in Richmond and the surrounding area that they supported through public and private funds. Such hospitals gave priority to soldiers from their respective states but did not exclude soldiers from other states.

60. McNeil, *Balm of Hope*, 164–65 (Sr. Ann Louise O'Connell to Mother Euphemia Blenkinsop, Recollections—Virginia).

61. Hilde, *Worth a Dozen Men*, 25–26.

62. William A. Carrington, "Inspection Report of Louisiana Hospital, 15 November 1862," William A. Carrington Papers, National Archives, Washington, DC, https://www.civilwarrichmond.com.

63. Wormeley, *United States Sanitary Commission*, 112–14. See also McGaugh, *Surgeon in Blue*, 134–51.

64. Varon, *Armies of Deliverance*, 268. See also Maher, *To Bind Up the Wounds*, 83–84. Maher notes that after the first two years of the war, there were fewer Daughters available to send, that most were already serving in hospitals or other designated locations. But she also acknowledges that many of the Daughters were at Satterlee or other large military hospitals. The Daughters' administration of these hospitals was closely linked to the institutional and organizational progress the North had made in the care of sick and wounded soldiers.

65. McNeil, *Balm of Hope*, 445 (Sr. Camilla Bowden to Mother Elizabeth Montcellet).

66. Nightingale, *Notes on Hospitals*, 56.

67. Rutkow, *Bleeding Blue and Gray*, 114.

68. Rutkow, *Bleeding Blue and Gray*, 114.

69. McNeil, *Balm of Hope*, 340–41 (Recollections, Satterlee Hospital).

70. McNeil, *Balm of Hope*, 340–41.

71. *Dictionary of Canadian Biography*, "Isaac Israel Hayes," https://www.biographi.ca.

72. McNeil, *Balm of Hope*, 302 (Recollections, Opening of Satterlee Hospital, Philadelphia Pennsylvania, June 9, 1862).

73. McNeil, *Balm of Hope*, 516–19 (appendices D and E); Hannefin, *Daughters of the Church*, 125. A more modest figure for soldiers served was "upwards of forty-eight thousand under their care." McNeil, *Balm of Hope*, 342 (Recollections, Satterlee Hospital).

74. On August 1, 1863, the federal government built a prisoner-of-war camp about one-half mile northeast of the hospital. Named Camp Hoffman, the prison eventually held as many as twenty-two thousand Confederate soldiers. The conditions at the prison camp were grim. Fresh water and food were scarce. The prisoners were confined to tents and shacks, exposing them to extreme heat in the summer and cold and wet weather in the winter. Approximately three thousand prisoners died at Point Lookout during the war's final two years. "Point Lookout Prisoner of War Camp," https://www.mycivilwar.com.

75. Susan C. Lawrence, "Military Hospitals in the Department of Washington," https://civilwardc.org; William T. Campbell, "The Pavilion-Style Hospital of the American Civil War and Florence Nightingale," https://www.civilwarmed.org.

76. Rada, *Battlefield Angels*, 56–57.

77. Gallagher et al., *Civil War*, 64–79, 167–75; Varon, *Armies of Deliverance*, 242–50.

78. McNeil, *Balm of Hope*, 349–56 (Recollections of Sr. Marie Louise Caulfield).

79. McNeil, *Balm of Hope*, 368–69 (Recollections, Pennsylvania College).

80. McNeil, *Balm of Hope*, 120–21 (Recollections, "Gettysburg Doings").

81. "Medal" refers to the Medal of the Immaculate Conception or the "Miraculous Medal" because of numerous accounts of miracles associated with it. The medal was quite small, not even an inch long and about half an inch wide. "The Miraculous Medal Shrine," https://miraculousmedal.org.

82. Hannefin, *Daughters of the Church*, 123.

83. Varon, *Armies of Deliverance*, 168–69; Gallagher et al., *Civil War*, 127–28, 136–37; Michael B. Ballard, "Vicksburg During the Civil War (1862–1863): A Campaign; a Siege," https://www.mshistorynow.mdah.ms.gov.

84. McNeil, *Balm of Hope*, 431–32 (Sr. Regina Smith to Mother Elisabeth Montcellet, after August 27, 1862).

85. Gallagher et al., *Civil War*, 201–25.

86. McNeil, *Balm of Hope*, 465 (Sr. [Helen] Ryan to [Mother Elisabeth Montcellet], Washington, Lincoln Hospital, October 5, 1864).

87. Senn, *Medical-Surgical Aspects of the Spanish American War*, 194; "Surgeon Senn Reviews the Work of the Hospital Corps," *Courier-Journal* (Louisville, KY), November 20, 1898.

88. Kalisch, "Heroines of '98," 413.

89. Graf, "Women Nurses in the Spanish-American War," 2.

90. Graf, "Women Nurses in the Spanish-American War," 2.

91. "Biography of Dr. Anita Newcomb McGee," https://cfmedicine.nlm.nih.gov.

92. "End of Conflict over Women Nurses: Red Cross Society Candidates Will Get Ample Recognition," *Brooklyn Daily Eagle*, July 23, 1898.

93. "End of Conflict over Women Nurses," *Brooklyn Daily Eagle*, July 23, 1898.

94. Sr. Beatrice Duffy to Mother Mariana Flynn, July 22, 1898, Military Services by American Sisters/Spanish-American War Collection, RG 7-5-2-1, APSL.

95. "Nursing the Sick," *Baltimore Sun*, August 24, 1898.

96. "Nursing the Sick," *Baltimore Sun*, August 24, 1898.

97. "Errand of Mercy: Fifteen Sisters of Charity Going to Santiago de Cuba," *Tampa Tribune*, November 11, 1898; author unknown, "Historical Account," October 10–11, 1898, Military Services by American Sisters/Spanish-American War Collection, RG 7-5-2-1, APSL.

98. *Dodge Commission Report*, 114, 115.

99. *Dodge Commission Report*, 111.

100. "Many Sick Sleep on Floor: Montauk Has Not Sufficient Hospital Accommodations," *Beatrice Evening Times* (Beatrice, NE), August 30, 1898.

101. "Sisters of Charity Leave for Puerto Rico," *Times-Picayune* (New Orleans, LA), September 3, 1898; "Sisters of Charity," *Times-Democrat* (New Orleans, LA), August 11, 1905.

102. Sr. Blanch Hooper to Mother Mariana Flynn, August 31, 1898, Military Services by American Sisters/Spanish-American War Collection, RG 7-5-2-1, APSL.

103. Sr. Adelaide D'Aunoy to Mother Mariana Flynn, August 31, 1898, Military Services by American Sisters/Spanish-American War Collection, RG 7-5-2-1, APSL.

104. Hooper to Flynn, August 31, 1898, APSL.

105. Hooper to Flynn, August 31, 1898, APSL.

106. "A Priest Visits Wickoff," *Pittsfield Sun* (Pittsfield, MA), September 8, 1898.

107. "President at Camp," *Meriden Daily Journal* (Meriden, CT), September 3, 1898.

108. "Dr. Senn Protests: Against Keeping the Soldiers at Camp Wickoff," *Wichita Daily Eagle*, August 31, 1898.

109. "McKinley to Visit Wickoff: Cutting Short His Western Trip on That Account," *Wichita Daily Eagle*, August 31, 1898; "Mr. McKinley at Montauk: He Will Personally Inspect Camp Wickoff," *Democrat and Chronicle* (Rochester, NY), September 3, 1898.

110. "President at Camp," *Meriden Daily Journal* (Meriden, CT), September 3, 1898; Sr. Adelaide D'Aunoy to Mother Mariana Flynn, September 3, 1898, Military Services by American Sisters/Spanish-American War Collection, RG 7-5-2-1, APSL.

111. "President at Camp," *Meriden Daily Journal* (Meriden, CT), September 3, 1898; "President at Wickoff," *Des Moines Register*, September 4, 1898.

112. Noel G. Harrison, "Findings of the Typhoid Board: Disease Spread by Civilians and Members of the Military," https://exhibits.hsl.virginia.edu.

113. In addition to Camp Wickoff, these included Camp Thomas at Chickamauga Park, Georgia; Camp Alger at Falls Church, Virginia; Camp Poland at Knoxville, Tennessee; Camp Wheeler at Huntsville, Alabama; and Camp Cubra Libre at Jacksonville, Florida.

114. Reed et al., *Report on the Origin and Spread of Typhoid Fever*; Harrison, "Findings of the Typhoid Board"; "Report of the Typhoid Fever Board—War with Spain."

115. During July, the number of soldiers diminished. A volunteer division went to Puerto Rico in July. Many other soldiers were either sent home or to other camps. By the end of August, only 13,161 remained. Camp Thomas shut down at the end of September. *Dodge Commission Report*, 98–101.

116. "Soldiers at School: Volunteers at Chickamauga Being Taught the Art of Modern War," *Champaign Daily Gazette* (Champaign, IL), May 25, 1898.

117. *Dodge Commission Report*, 103–5.

118. "Should Move the Camp: The Rev. Chrysostom Schreiner Writes of Discomforts Experienced by Men at Chickamauga," *Brooklyn Daily Eagle*, August 7, 1898.

119. "Field Work Reports from the Red Cross: Interesting Details of the Hospital Operations," *Brooklyn Daily Eagle*, August 14, 1898.

120. Sr. Blanche Foye to Mother Mariana Flynn, August 26, 1898, Military Services by American Sisters/Spanish-American War Collection, RG 7-5-2-2, APSL.

121. Sr. Stella Boyle to Mother Mariana Flynn, September 3, 1898, Military Services by American Sisters/Spanish-American War Collection, RG 7-5-2-2, APSL.

122. Sr. Stella Boyle to Mother Mariana Flynn, September 20, 1898, Military Services by American Sisters/Spanish-American War Collection, RG 7-5-2-2, APSL.

123. "Sister Caroline Dead," *Baltimore Sun*, October 18, 1898; "Sister Mary Agnes Sweeney, an Army Nurse, Dies from Typhoid Fever," *Philadelphia Inquirer*, October 24, 1898; "Death of Sister Anastasia," *Baltimore Sun*, November 28, 1898; "Died in Puerto Rico," *Detroit Free Press*, November 11, 1898.

124. "Blind Men Guides: Mayor Ramsdell of Lynn Goes to See Men of 8th and Makes an Inspection," *Boston Globe*, September 14, 1898.

125. "Noble Sisters in Army Camps," n.d., Military Services by American Sisters/Spanish-American War Collection, RG 7-5-2-3, APSL.

126. *Dodge Commission Report*, 105.

127. Sr. Teresa Carlin to Mother Mariana Flynn, October 11, 1898, Military Services by American Sisters/Spanish-American War Collection, RG 7-5-2-3, APSL.

128. *Dodge Commission Report*, 3.

129. *Dodge Commission Report*, 6.

130. *Dodge Commission Report*, 65–79.

131. *Dodge Commission Report*, 67, 84–85.

132. Dock, *History of American Red Cross Nursing*, 325, 1443–54 (the appendix contains a list of base hospital units and their parent institutions). See also US Army Medical Department, Office of Medical History, "Base Hospitals," https://history.amedd.army.mil.

133. Donna Bingham Munger, "Base Hospital 21 and the Great War," Washington University School of Medicine, https://beckerexhibits.wustl.edu; Dock, *History of American Red Cross Nursing*, 334.

134. Dock, *History of American Red Cross Nursing*, 313–14, 334–35, 356–60.

135. Dock, *History of American Red Cross Nursing*, 333–34, 339–40, 1443–45; US Army Medical Department, Office of Medical History, "Base Hospitals."

136. Dock, *History of American Red Cross Nursing*, 666.

137. "Our Sisters in the American Red Cross," *Catholic Advance* (Wichita, KS), June 30, 1917; "The Red Cross," *Catholic Union and Times* (Buffalo, NY), December 27, 1917; *The Tablet* (Brooklyn, NY), June 9, 1917.

138. Sr. Catherine O'Rourke, "Historical Account of United States Base Hospital Unit 102," 1942, Military Services by American Sisters/World War I Collection, RG 7-5-3:8(1), APSL, 7–8, 10; Salvaggio, *New Orleans' Charity Hospital*, 91, 125; Dock, *History of American Red Cross Nursing*, 665, 668.

139. O'Rourke, "Historical Account of United States Base Hospital Unit 102," APSL, 9.

140. O'Rourke, "Historical Account of United States Base Hospital Unit 102," APSL, 9, 14–17, 84–85; Dock, *History of American Red Cross Nursing*, 665–67.

141. O'Rourke, "Historical Account of United States Base Hospital Unit 102," APSL, 50.

142. Sr. Angela Drendle, "Diary of Sister Angela Drendle," 1918–1919, 2 vols., Military Services by American Sisters/World War I Collection, RG 7-5-3:9(4), APSL.

143. Sr. Catherine Coleman, "Diary of Sister Catherine Coleman," 1918, Military Services by American Sisters/World War I Collection, RG 7-5-3:9(2), APSL.

144. Vanda Wilcox, "Italian Front," *International Encyclopedia of the First World War*, https://encyclopedia.1914-1918-online.net; David Hunt, "About World War I: Brief Overview of the Italian Front," *Owlcation*, https://owlcation.com/humanities; "U.S. Army Base Hospital No. 102," United States World War I Centennial Commission, https://www.worldwar1centennial.org.

145. An American infantry regiment in World War I comprised 112 officers and 3,720 men. Doughboy Center, "The Story of the American Expeditionary Forces: Basic Fighting Unit," http://www.worldwar1.com.

146. Mathew J. Seelinger, "'Viva l'America!': The 332d Infantry on the Italian Front," Army Historical Foundation, https://armyhistory.org.

147. O'Rourke, "Historical Account of United States Base Hospital Unit 102," APSL, 73–75, 79–81; Drendle, "Diary of Sister Angela Drendle," vol. 2, APSL, 12–14; Coleman, "Diary of Sister Catherine Coleman," APSL, 12–13; Sr. Florence Means, "Notes on the Italian Unit," 1918, Military Services by American Sisters/World War I Collection, RG 7-5-3:9(6), APSL, 19, 20; Dock, *History of American Red Cross Nursing*, 671.

148. Drendle, "Diary of Sister Angela Drendle," vol. 2, APSL, 12.

149. Means, "Notes on the Italian Unit," APSL, 17.

150. Means, "Notes on the Italian Unit," APSL, 18.

151. Drendle, "Diary of Sister Angela Drendle," vol. 2, APSL, 15.

152. Means, "Notes on the Italian Unit," APSL, 21.

153. Coleman, "Diary of Sister Catherine Coleman," APSL, 14.

154. Coleman, "Diary of Sister Catherine Coleman," APSL, 14–15.

155. Coleman, "Diary of Sister Catherine Coleman," APSL, 15–16.

156. Drendle, "Diary of Sister Angela Drendle," vol. 2, APSL, 39, 40.

157. Berry, *Great Influenza*, 396–97; Fincher, "America's Deadly Rendezvous," 132.

158. Goldsmith and Miller, "Modern Uses of Electron Microscopy," 552–63; Desselberger, "Emerging and Re-Emerging Infectious Diseases," 3–15.

159. Kauffman, *Ministry and Meaning*, 49; Libster and McNeil, *Enlightened Charity*, 319–24.

160. Berry, *Great Influenza*, 95–97, 169–92, 371–77; Fincher, "America's Deadly Rendezvous," 134–35; Hannefin, *Daughters of the Church*, 211–12.

161. Sr. Raphael Jones, "Epidemic of Spanish Influenza, City of Boston 1918," October 1, 1918, Epidemics/Spanish Influenza Collection, RG 7-7-1-3, APSL.

162. "Dr. Leen, Carney Hospital, Dies Fighting Influenza," *Philadelphia Inquirer*, September 17, 1918.

163. Sr. Madeline Hanigan to Mother Margaret O'Keefe, October 11, 1918, Epidemics/Spanish Influenza Collection, RG 7-7-1-3, APSL.

164. Sr. (name unknown) to Mother Margaret O'Keefe, October 15, 1918, Epidemics/Spanish Influenza Collection, RG 7-7-1-3, APSL.

165. *Evening Star* (Washington, DC), October 25, 1918.

166. *Evening Journal* (Wilmington, DE), October 10, 1918 (quotation is from Anders letter dated September 28 to the *Philadelphia Public Ledger*).

167. *Evening Public Ledger* (Philadelphia, PA), October 10, 1918; *Catholic Advance* (Wichita, KS), November 8, 1918. For a detailed narrative of the various Catholic sisterhoods' work in and near Philadelphia, see Tourscher, "Work of the Sisters During the Epidemic of Influenza," 193–226.

168. "How the A.R.C. Fights 'Flu,'" *New Castle Herald* (New Castle, PA), October 22, 1918.

169. Sr. Elizabeth Boyle to Mother Margaret O'Keefe, October 14, 1918, Epidemics/Spanish Influenza Collection, RG 7-7-1-3, APSL.

170. Sr. Clarisse Bresnan to Mother Margaret O'Keefe, October 8, 1918, Epidemics/Spanish Influenza Collection, RG 7-7-1-3, APSL.

171. Sr. Lizzie Patterson to Mother Margaret O'Keefe, October 13, 1918, Epidemics/Spanish Influenza Collection, RG 7-7-1-3, APSL.

172. Sr. Blanche Summers to Mother Margaret O'Keefe, October 19, 1918, Epidemics/Spanish Influenza Collection, RG 7-7-1-3, APSL.

173. Sr. Camilla to Mother Margaret O'Keefe, October 21, 1918, Epidemics/Spanish Influenza Collection, RG 7-7-1-3, APSL.

174. Sr. Regina Fowler to Mother Margaret O'Keefe, October 30, 1918, Epidemics/Spanish Influenza Collection, RG 7-7-1-3, APSL.

175. Jones, "Epidemic of Spanish Influenza, City of Boston 1918," APSL.

176. "Summary of Works and Deaths of Sisters from Epidemics," 1919–1932, Special Services: Epidemics Collection, RG 7-6-1:1(1), APSL.

177. John O. McReynolds, "Work Done for the Soldiers During the War at St. Paul's Sanitarium, Dallas, Texas," n.d., Epidemics/Spanish Influenza Collection, RG 7-6-2:1(4), APSL; Sr. Stanislaus Malone, "Spanish Influenza—1918, Providence Hospital, Waco, Texas," Epidemics/Spanish Influenza Collection, RG 7-6-2:1(4), APSL; Sr. M. Berchmans to Mother Margaret O'Keefe, October 10 and October 20, 1918, Epidemics/Spanish Influenza Collection, RG 7-7-1-3, APSL; Sr. Lizzie

Patterson to Mother Margaret O'Keefe, October 21, 1918, Epidemics/Spanish Influenza Collection, RG 7-7-1-3, APSL; Camilla to O'Keefe, October 21, 1918, APSL; Hannefin, *Daughters of the Church*, 211.

178. Berry, *Great Influenza*, 370–75.

179. Adding a word of caution, Sister Lizzie Patterson stated that "so many of the old cases have turned to pneumonia which causes the number of deaths to be as great as ever." Patterson to O'Keefe, October 21, 1918, APSL.

180. "Health Officials Much Encouraged," *Morning News* (Wilmington, DE), October 21, 1918.

181. Berry, *Great Influenza*, 372–73.

Four. *Daughters, Doctors, and Outpatient Clinics*

1. Gaynes, *Germ Theory*, 17, 27.

2. Gaynes, *Germ Theory*, 143–234; "Medicine in the 20th Century," *Britannica*, https://www.britannica.com.

3. Kisacky, *Rise of the Modern Hospital*, 103–44; Rosenberg, *Care of Strangers*, 136–50.

4. Rosenberg, *Care of Strangers*, 261–67, 271–82; Stevens, *In Sickness and in Wealth*, 20–39; Richardson, *History of the Sisters of Charity Hospital*, 141–44.

5. Starr, *Social Transformation of American Medicine*, 177–79; Longest et al., *Managing Health Organizations*, 174–77.

6. Starr, *Social Transformation of American Medicine*, 177–79; Longest et al., *Managing Health Organizations*, 174–77.

7. Rosenberg, *Care of Strangers*, 272; Richardson, *History of the Sisters of Charity Hospital*, 142–44.

8. Numbers, *Almost Persuaded*, 97–109; Fishbein, "Present-Day Trends," 2041; Garceau, *Political Life of the American Medical Association*, 132; Campion, *The AMA and U.S. Health Policy*, 175; Fishbein, "History of the American Medical Association," 605.

9. Lomas, "As It Was in the Beginning," 206.

10. Rosenberg, *Care of Strangers*, 175–79.

11. Richardson, *History of the Sisters of Charity Hospital*, 144–51.

12. Richardson, *History of the Sisters of Charity Hospital*, 153.

13. Medical Staff Minutes, November 14, 1900, Buffalo, NY/Sisters of Charity Hospital Collection, RG 11-2-1:4(6), APSL.

14. Richardson, *History of the Sisters of Charity Hospital*, 153.

15. Reverby, *Ordered to Care*, 39.

16. "Patients' lives continued to depend on the food they ate, care in the cleanliness of their dressings, careful watching for dangerous hemorrhaging, and provision of ice bags or baths to control their fevers," historian Susan Reverby wrote in summarizing Nightingale's teachings. Reverby, *Ordered to Care*, 48.

17. University of Pennsylvania School of Nursing, "American Nursing: An Introduction to the Past," https://www.nursing.upenn.edu; Libster and McNeil, *Enlightened Charity*, 302.

18. Reverby, *Ordered to Care*, 47, 52–54, 60–65, 75; Zerr, "Beyond the Bricks and Mortar," 210–12.

19. Hannefin, *Daughters of the Church*, 168–69.

20. Quote in Richardson, *History of the Sisters of Charity Hospital*, 129–30.

21. "Disturbance at the Charity Hospital," 616.

22. Hannefin, *Daughters of the Church*, 170–71; Richardson, *History of the Sisters of Charity Hospital*, 135–36; Salvaggio, *New Orleans' Charity Hospital*, 89; "Management of the Charity Hospital," *Times-Picayune* (New Orleans, LA), April 4, 1882; Wall, *Unlikely Entrepreneurs*, 178.

23. Salvaggio, *New Orleans' Charity Hospital*, 88–89; Fossier, *Charity Hospital of Louisiana*, 44.

24. "The Organization of the Society of the Training School for Nurses Perfected," *Times Democrat* (New Orleans, LA), January 31, 1882.

25. "Management of the Charity Hospital," *Times-Picayune*, April 4, 1882.

26. "Management of the Charity Hospital," *Times-Picayune*, April 4, 1882.

27. Litigation ensued over money that the board had appropriated. The parties eventually resolved their differences. "The Training School," *Times-Picayune* (New Orleans, LA), October 24, 1882.

28. *Provincial Annals*, 1892–1899, APSL.

29. Nursing schools opened at Carney Hospital in Boston (1892), St. Vincent's Hospital in Norfolk (1893), Providence Hospital in Washington, DC (1894), St. Joseph's Hospital in Philadelphia (1894), and Charity Hospital in New Orleans (1894).

30. *Provincial Annals*, 1897, APSL.

31. Salvaggio, *New Orleans' Charity Hospital*, 89–90, 150; Eleonore Villarrubia, "Sister Stanislaus—Winged Angel of New Orleans," https://catholicism.org; Fossier, *Charity Hospital of Louisiana*, 45–46; Henrietta, "Famous New Orleans Hospital," 254–55.

32. Salvaggio, *New Orleans' Charity Hospital*, 89–90, 150; Villarrubia, "Sister Stanislaus"; Fossier, *Charity Hospital of Louisiana*, 45–46; Henrietta, "Famous New Orleans Hospital," 254–55.

33. Sr. Gonzaga McCormick to H. L. Burrell, April 25, 1903, Boston, MA/ Carney Hospital Collection, RG 11-2-3:14(1), APSL; Sr. Delphine Steele, "Carney

Hospital, South Boston, Massachusetts," ca. 1950, Boston, MA/Carney Hospital Collection, RG 11-2-2:13(2).

34. Apparently, the *Boston Globe* never discovered the underlying reason for the change in surgical staff. "Entire Change," *Boston Globe*, June 2, 1903; "Meaning of the Changes in the Carney Hospital Surgical Staff," *Boston Post*, June 3, 1903.

35. Reverby, *Ordered to Care*, 121–27; University of Pennsylvania School of Nursing, "Nursing Through Time," https://www.nursing.upenn.edu.

36. Over eighty medical schools closed between 1906 and 1922. Many accounts attribute the closures to the famed Flexner report of 1910. In truth, the AMA had begun inspections in 1904, six years before the Flexner report was issued. Though the Flexner report enhanced the pace of the closures, the process had already started under AMA sponsorship. Ameringer, *US Health Policy and Health Care Delivery*, 23–24.

37. Starr, *Social Transformation of American Medicine*, 118. See also Bonner, *Becoming a Physician*, 309–20.

38. Rosen, *Structure of American Medical Practice*, 66–69; Rosenberg, *Care of Strangers*, 178; McCauley, *Who Shall Take Care of Our Sick?*, 94–95; Rubin, "Immigration, Quotas and Its Impact on Medical Education," 30–31.

39. Richardson, *History of the Sisters of Charity Hospital*, 107–20, 144–49; Sulmasy, "Can Medical Schools Be Catholic?"

40. "Specialism in Medicine," 379–80.

41. Stevens, *American Medicine and the Public Interest*, 46, 49, 53–54, 85–97, 111–31; Rosen, *Structure of American Medical Practice*, 38–39, 61–66.

42. Rosen, *Structure of American Medical Practice*, 32–36.

43. Rosen, *Structure of American Medical Practice*, 93.

44. Libster and McNeil, *Enlightened Charity*, 317; Kauffman *Ministry & Meaning*, 38.

45. Rosenberg, *Care of Strangers*, 141, 207, 323.

46. See Wall, "'Definite Lines of Influence,'" 317. Researching the role of chaplains in the Civil War, historian William Kurtz discovered that Protestant ministers "repeated[ly]" acknowledged that Catholic sisters "were primarily devoted to physical suffering." Kurtz, *Excommunicated from the Union*, 85.

47. Weitzman, *One Hundred Years of Catholic Charities*; Richardson, *History of the Sisters of Charity Hospital*, 111.

48. Annual Reports of Carney Hospital, 1890 and 1895, Boston, MA/Carney Hospital Collection, RG 11-2-2:3(3), APSL.

49. Gail Farr Casterline, "Twice as Irish: A History of St. Joseph's Hospital, Philadelphia, 1849–1900," 1982, Philadelphia, PA/St. Joseph's Hospital Collection, RG 11-2-2:1(6), APSL. By way of perspective, Johns Hopkins Hospital, widely known for hiring the world's leading specialists, did not even open until May 7,

1889. Flexner and Flexner, *William Henry Welch and the Heroic Age of American Medicine*, 159.

50. Butt, "Century of Service to the Sick," APSL.

51. Wall, *Unlikely Entrepreneurs*, 191.

52. Johnson, *Daughters of Charity in Milwaukee*, 120–22.

53. Starr, *Social Transformation of American Medicine*, 169.

54. Stewart, *Marvels of Charity*, 516-48.

55. Thomas E. Getzen, "The Growth of Health Spending in the USA: 1776 to 2026," 11, https://www.soa.org.

56. Daniels, *Coming to America*, 124.

57. O'Grady, *Catholic Charities in the United States*, 201. See also Oates, *Catholic Philanthropic Tradition*, 39.

58. Sr. Eugenia Fealy to unnamed donor, October 20, 1927, Provincial Correspondence/Eugenia Fealy (1910–1936), APSL ("While we are trying to repair [Mullanphy] temporarily . . . we shall be obliged to begin at once to erect another building"); Treasurer's Report of December 31, 1931 for the Western Province calling attention to limited resources on hand to meet demands, Corporation Minutes, December 31, 1931, Normandy, MO/Marillac Seminary (1817–1945), RG 9-7-0-3:6(2), APSL (Fr. John J. Cronin, Western Province director, suggests that the sister servant "be told to economize and to refrain from making any but absolutely necessary improvements").

59. Corporation Minutes, February 6, 1917; October 14, 1919; September 30, 1920; October 28, 1926; June 6, 1927; October 14, 1927; August 18, 1928; September 4, 1928; and November 12, 1929, Normandy, MO/Marillac Seminary (1817–1945), RG 9-7-0-3:6(2), APSL.

60. Corporation Minutes, September 30, 1920; January 12, 1921; and March 28, 1929, Normandy, MO/Marillac Seminary (1817–1945), RG 9-7-0-3:6(2), APSL.

61. Corporation Minutes, February 6, 1917; October 14, 1919; and September 30, 1920, Normandy, MO/Marillac Seminary (1817–1945), RG 9-7-0-3:6(2), APSL.

62. Corporation Minutes, October 28, 1926; June 6, 1927; October 14, 1927; August 18, 1928; September 4, 1928; and November 12, 1929, Normandy, MO/Marillac Seminary (1817–1945), RG 9-7-0-3:6(2), APSL.

63. Congress appropriated $6,000 annually to Providence beginning in 1864, doubled the appropriation to $12,000 in 1866, raised it to $15,000 in 1873, to $17,000 in 1877, to $19,000 in 1890, and to $23,000 in 1900. Besides these annual appropriations, Congress partially funded certain construction projects at Providence. These included $30,000 in 1866 for the completion of the hospital's west wing, $30,000 in 1868 for completion of the east wing, $30,000 in 1897 for the construction of two isolation buildings, and $130,626.67 in 1907 for the retire-

ment of the hospital's long-standing debt. Board of Directors Minutes, July 25, 1895, Washington, DC/Providence Hospital Collection, RG 11-2-5:65(2), APSL; Congressional Appropriations, 1864–1913, Washington, DC/Providence Hospital Collection, RG 11-2-5:62(1), APSL; Caulfield, "History of Providence Hospital," 234, 240, 242.

64. The Daughters' initial champion was Thaddeus Stevens, a prominent Pennsylvania congressman and an ardent abolitionist. After Stevens's death, Providence received assistance from Samuel J. Randall, House Speaker from 1876 to 1881, and James A. Garfield, who in 1881 briefly served as US president. Caulfield, "History of Providence Hospital," 234. In the early 1900s, the Daughters worked closely with several leading legislators, including Nevada Senator William Morris Stewart, Maryland Senator Arthur Pue Gorman, and Iowa Senator William Boyd Allison. Senator Allison and House Speaker Joseph Cannon helped the hospital retire its debt in 1907. Arthur Pue to Archbishop James Gibbons, n.d., Washington, DC/Providence Hospital Collection, RG 11-2-3:61(1), APSL.

65. Sr. Beatrice Duffy to Secretary of the Interior, June 22, 1876, Washington, DC/Providence Hospital Collection, RG 11-2-3:61(1), APSL.

66. The US Surgeon General's Office handled the distribution of funds for Providence until 1920. Correspondence between Sister Beatrice Duffy, DC, and the surgeon general showed that the federal government, beginning in the 1890s, slowly increased the amount of information required. Duffy had to provide information on patient admissions, discharges, length of stay, and "the daily cost per patient of maintenance." Charles R. Greenleaf to Sr. Beatrice Duffy, April 9, 1891, Washington, DC/Providence Hospital Collection, RG 11-2-3:61(1), APSL; Surgeon General to Sr. Mary Berchmans, July 26, 1912, Washington, DC/Providence Hospital Collection, RG 11-2-5:64(1), APSL. She also had to comply with requests from the District of Columbia's superintendent of charities. Apparently, Duffy failed to provide the superintendent with sufficient information on at least one occasion. In a tersely worded letter, the superintendent stated, "The high standing of your admirable institution renders the omission of statistics . . . a very grave defect in the general Report." John Tracy to Sr. Beatrice Duffy, June 6, 1895, Washington, DC/Providence Hospital Collection, RG 11-2-3:61(1), APSL.

67. Bradfield v. Roberts, 175 U.S. 291, 297-9 (1899).

68. Oates, *Catholic Philanthropic Tradition*, 89.

69. In several of the dioceses, including Pittsburgh, Boston, New York City, Chicago, and Baltimore, the bureaus conducted comprehensive "social surveys" to assess the needs and practices of orphanages and other welfare institutions. Though the professed aim in most instances was to reorganize and redirect resources for dependent children, healthcare facilities were sometimes included in the surveys. Oates, *Catholic Philanthropic Tradition*, 87–97; Brown and McKeown, *Poor Belong to Us*, 51–77.

70. Oates, *Catholic Philanthropic Tradition*, 91–92.

71. Fr. John Cronin to unnamed Sister, March 13, 1937, Director's Correspondence (1915–1947), RG 8-3-2:1(9), APSL.

72. Stevens, *In Sickness and in Wealth*, 49.

73. The request for this data came from the Paris motherhouse. It applied to all provinces. Correspondence from Sister Betty Ann McNeil, DC, May 14, 2022.

74. Statistics of St. Joseph's Hospital, Philadelphia, 1880–1893, Philadelphia, PA/St. Joseph's Hospital Collection, RG 11-2-4-3, APSL; Statistics of Carney Hospital, Boston, 1887–1899, Boston, MA/Carney Hospital Collection, RG 11-2-4-3, APSL.

75. Sr. Elspeth Ann Cartner, "History of De Paul Hospital with Description of the Development of the Social Service Department," 1952, St. Louis, MO/DePaul Hospital Collection, RG 11-2-2:15(4), APSL

76. Joseph S. Wall, "Report of the Work Being Carried On by Providence Hospital, Washington, D.C.," 1911, Washington, DC/Providence Hospital Collection, RG 11-2-1-2:48(10), APSL.

77. Roemer, *Ambulatory Health Services in America*, 31.

78. Davis and Richardson, *New Clinics for Old*, 6; Rosenberg, "Social Class and Medical Care," 34–36; Roemer, *Ambulatory Health Services in America*, 17–21.

79. Buhler-Wilkerson, *No Place Like Home*, 98–110.

80. Rosenberg, *Care of Strangers*, 316–22.

81. Casterline, "Twice as Irish," APSL.

82. Hannefin, *Daughters of the Church*, 165.

83. Carney Hospital Annual Reports for 1883, 1890, 1895, and 1899, Boston, MA/Carney Hospital Collection, RG 11-2-4:3(3,4), APSL.

84. Salvaggio, *New Orleans' Charity Hospital*, 94.

85. Butt, "Century of Service to the Sick," APSL, 18.

86. Sr. Lucia James to Mother Mariana Flynn, September 5, 1894, Baltimore, MD/St. Agnes Hospital Collection, RG 11-2-2:1(1), APSL.

87. Carney Hospital Annual Report for 1899, Boston, MA/Carney Hospital Collection, RG 11-2-4:3(4), APSL.

88. United States Department of Commerce, *Hospitals and Dispensaries*, 6. Michael Davis estimated that the number was much higher. The census figures, he noted, were understated; the "probable number in existence, allowing for those from whom reports have not yet been received, is over 4,000." Davis, "Boom in Dispensary Work," 334.

89. Of the 2,526 dispensaries the Census Bureau reported, 993 or 39.3 percent were outpatient departments of hospitals, while 1,533 or 60.7 percent were freestanding. United States Department of Commerce, *Hospitals and Dispensaries*, 6.

90. Davis, "Boom in Dispensary Work," 85.

91. Seem, "Organization of the Dispensary of Johns Hopkins Hospital," 33.

92. Lambert, "The Real Significance of the Dispensary," 281.

93. Lambert, "Tentative Standards in Organization and Management," 192.

94. Walker, "Social Service Problems in the Hospital," 265.

95. By 1920, the Daughters operated outpatient clinics at St. Joseph's Hospital in Philadelphia, St. Mary's Hospital in Rochester, St. Mary's Hospital in Milwaukee, Carney Hospital in Boston, Charity Hospital in New Orleans, St. Vincent's Hospital in Norfolk, St. Agnes Hospital in Baltimore, Sisters of Charity Hospital in Buffalo, and Providence Hospital in Washington, DC.

96. Cartner, "History of DePaul Hospital," APSL, 41–44.

97. Supervisor, social service department, "Providence Hospital," April 20, 1970, Washington, DC/Providence Hospital Collection, RG 11-2-2:60(11), APSL.

98. Polak, "Relation of the Dispensary to the Community," 154.

99. Boas, "Chronic Diseases," 139.

100. Bluestone, "Aims and Tendencies of Out-Patient Service," 15.

101. Cumming, "Developing a Community Health Program," 1.

102. Rosenberg, *Care of Strangers*, 320; Reverby, *Ordered to Care*, 140.

103. "Points and Principles of Out-Patient Building," 227.

104. Davis, "Dispensary Progress in 1922," 49–50; Davis, "Dispensary Progress in 1924," 27; Davis, "'Clinic' or 'Dispensary'—Which?," 119.

105. Billings, "Relations of Hospitals to Public Health," 4.

106. Ross, "Committee on the Costs of Medical Care," 129.

107. Numbers, *Almost Persuaded*, 106–9.

108. Blasingame, *Digest of Official Actions*, 123–24, 130, 131, 313–18. For the first time, the AMA defined contract practice, a prohibited form of medical practice, to mean "the carrying out of an agreement between a physician *or* a group of physicians, as principals or agents, and a corporation, organization or individual, to furnish partial or full medical services to a group or class of individuals for a definite sum or fixed rate per capita." While stating that "contract practice per se is not unethical," the code made any group activity contingent on state medical society "approval."

109. Shadid, *Doctor for the People*, 115, 124, 133–42, 152–57, 161–63; "American Medical Association: Power, Purpose, and Politics," 953. The US Supreme Court's 1975 decision in *Goldfarb v. Virginia State Bar* (421 U.S. 773 [1975]) struck down the exemption for the "learned professions," such as law and medicine, and opened the door to federal prosecution for antitrust violations. Before 1975, federal and state antitrust authorities had limited success against organized medicine. See, e.g., United States v. American Medical Ass'n, 317 U.S. 519 (1943); United States v. Oregon State Medical Society, 343 U.S. 326 (1952).

110. Kauffman, *Commitment to Healthcare*, 13–14; Peter A. Corning, "The Evolution of Medicare . . . from Idea to Law," Social Security History, https://www.ssa.gov.

111. Kauffman, *Commitment to Health Care*, 4, 7–8, 13–14; Flynn, "Franklin D. Roosevelt and American Catholicism," 61–107; Michael Barga, "Monsignor John Augustine Ryan (1869–1945): Economist, Theologian, Writer, Social Reformer," https://socialwelfare.library.vcu.edu.

112. "Committee on the Costs of Medical Care Presents Its Final Report," 23; Ross, "Committee on the Costs of Medical Care," 130; "Final Report of the Committee on the Costs of Medical Care," 996–97.

113. Ross, "Committee on the Costs of Medical Care," 129.

114. "Committee on the Costs of Medical Care Presents Its Final Report," 21.

115. Falk, "Medical Care in the USA," 3.

116. "Committee on the Costs of Medical Care Presents Its Final Report," 27–30; Ross, "Committee on the Costs of Medical Care," 131, 132.

117. "'Final Report' of the Committee on the Costs of Medical Care," 395.

118. Flynn, "Franklin D. Roosevelt and American Catholicism," 61–107; Corning, "Evolution of Medicare."

119. Schwitalla, "Catholic Viewpoints," 24–25.

120. United States Congress, Senate, 1939 (Testimony of Rev. A. M. Schwitalla); Kauffman, *Ministry and Meaning*, 226.

121. Schwitalla, "Catholic Viewpoints," 27.

122. Schwitalla is quoting here from the minority report, a portion of which he likely wrote. Schwitalla, "Basic Considerations in Minority Report," 865.

123. "Doctors Meet in Kansas City," *Greenville Daily Advocate* (Greenville, OH), October 1, 1934; "Fishbein Warns American Medics," *Wichita Evening Eagle*, October 2, 1934; "Medical Profession Does Not Need Legislation but Understanding by Public: Fishbein, Schwitalla Say," *Daily Times* (Davenport, IA), September 30, 1937.

124. "Community Medical Center Idea Criticized by Fr. Schwitalla," *St. Louis Globe-Democrat*, January 4, 1933.

125. United States Congress, Senate, 1939 (Testimony of Rev. A. M. Schwitalla), 639.

126. Kauffman, *Ministry and Meaning*, 218; "News from the Field," 549.

127. A lengthy search of the Daughters' and the CHA's archives did not produce any documentation to indicate the Daughters' position concerning Schwitalla's opposition to the CCMC's recommendations or federal legislation.

128. Coburn, "Crossing Boundaries and Cultural Barriers," 13–14.

129. Coburn, "Crossing Boundaries and Cultural Barriers," 13–14; Gabow, *Catholic Church and Its Hospitals*, 33.

130. O'Grady, *Catholic Charities in the United States*, 348.

131. Kauffman, *Commitment to Healthcare*, 2.

132. Sr. Mary Delores to Sr. Eugenia Fealy, April 10, 1915, Milwaukee, WI/ St. Mary's Hospital Collection, RG 11-2-3, APSL.

133. "Registered at the First Annual Conference, Milwaukee, Wis., June 24, 25, 26, 1915," CHA Archives.

134. Sr. Eugenia Fealy to Archbishop Sebastian Messmer, January 21, 1915, Provincial Correspondence/Eugenia Fealy (1910–1936), APSL. A search of the Daughters' archives in Emmitsburg and the CHA's archives in St. Louis did not reveal any correspondence or other specific documentation concerning the position of the Eastern Province. Yet the actions of the Eastern Province closely tracked those of the Western Province. The Eastern Province also did not send Daughters to CHA meetings (though it did send lay representatives), and it held its own training sessions, separate and apart from the CHA, in preparation for hospital inspections.

135. Quote in Kauffman, *Ministry and Meaning*, 173.

136. Kauffman, *Ministry and Meaning*, 170.

137. "Registered Attendance at the 1916 Meeting," CHA Archives; "To Attend Convention," *Bismarck Tribune*, June 4, 1916.

138. Shanahan, *History of the Catholic Hospital Association*, 77–78.

139. "Banquet Is Attended by 150 Persons from 20 Catholic Hospitals of State," *Times* (Hammond, IN), October 23, 1935; "Convention Is Closed Today," *Daily Chronicle* (De Kalb, IL), April 30, 1931; "Better Understanding Between Hospital and Public Is Urged," *Catholic Advance* (Wichita, KS), September 15, 1928; "Catholic Hospital Association Here Re-Elects Officers," *Hartford Courant*, October 1, 1926: "Catholic Hospital Association Meets," *Wilkes-Barre Record*, April 14, 1925; "Representatives of Catholic Hospitals Meet at Convention," *Star-Phoenix* (Saskatoon, SK), April 24, 1935; "Catholic Hospital Group Holds Annual Conference," *Baltimore Sun*, April 25, 1925.

140. "Catholic Hospital Group Holds Annual Conference," *Baltimore Sun*, April 25, 1925.

141. Fr. John Cribbins to unnamed Sister, June 27, 1924, Director's Correspondence (1915–1947). The content of Cribbins's letter is similar to that of Sr. Eugenia Fealy's, giving support to the inference that the positions of the Western and Eastern Provinces were in alignment. See Sr. Eugenia Fealy to Archbishop Sabastian Messmer, January 21, 1915, Provincial Correspondence/Eugenia Fealy (1910–1936), APSL.

142. See issues of *Health Progress*, the Catholic Hospital Association's journal, for the years 1915 to 1941. Information contained in these issues shows that certain communities and their representatives took an active role in the association, serving as officers and board members. The most active among them were the Misericordia Sisters, the Sisters of Mercy, the Franciscan Sisters of Mary, and the Religious Hospitallers of St. Joseph.

143. Shanahan, *History of the Catholic Hospital Association*, 193; Kauffman, *Ministry and Meaning*, 219.

144. "Health Insurance Plan Criticized," *St. Louis Post-Dispatch*, June 15, 1933. Before and during his time as CHA president, Schwitalla worked closely with Puppendahl to organize the "University Hospital" system at St. Louis University (today's SSM Health St. Mary's Hospital). University Hospital comprised three sister-owned hospitals—St. Mary's Infirmary, St. Mary's Hospital, and Mount St. Rose Sanatorium. In 1933, the newly completed Firmin Desloge Hospital, a joint undertaking of Schwitalla and Puppendahl, became the teaching hospital for St. Louis Medical School, replacing St. Mary's Infirmary. "Biography of Alphonse M. Schwitalla, SJ," St. Louis University Archives, https://www.archives.slu.edu.

145. Starr, *Social Transformation of American Medicine*, 275–77; Wilson, *Compulsory Health Insurance*, 6–7.

146. Starr, *Social Transformation of American Medicine*, 277.

147. At the Senate hearing, Schwitalla claimed that the CHA had "given its most careful attention and study to the [matter]." United States Congress, Senate, 1939 (Testimony of Rev. A. M. Schwitalla), 635, 643.

148. Fr. Alphonse Schwitalla, "A Proposed Pronouncement of the Catholic Hospital Association on the National Health Program," with cover letter, October 5, 1938, Provincial Correspondence (1915–1947), RG 9-3-2:1(3), APSL. The enclosure was not with the letter. Neither DC nor CHA archivists could locate it.

149. Brown, "To the Public a Hospital Is a Hospital," 611.

Five. *"More Active, Vocal, and Visible"*

1. Schneider, "American Sisters and the Roots of Change," 57; Dries, "Living in Ambiguity," 479; Coburn, "Ahead of Its Time . . . or, Right on Time?," 28; Koehlinger, *New Nuns*, 30; Kauffman, *Ministry and Meaning*, 272.

2. "Plan for the Health Care Apostolate, 'An Active, Visible, and Vocal Witness,'" 1981, rev. 1984, Health Apostolate—East Central Province Collection, RG 16-2, APSL.

3. Robinson, *Corporate Practice of Medicine*, 16–42; Ameringer, *Health Care Revolution*, 42–77, 155–57.

4. Nako, "Nuns in the Newsroom."

5. Sr. Catherine Sullivan to Sr. Mary Meehan, March 24, 1940, Sr. Catherine Sullivan Visitatrix Collection, RG 9-3-3:2(3), APSL; Hannefin, *Daughters of the Church*, 213, 222. The Daughters' pioneering work among patients with Hansen's disease at Carville is the subject of several studies and a full-length book by journalist Pam Fessler. Fessler, *Carville's Cure*, 106.

6. Sr. Catherine Sullivan to Sr. Mary Meehan, September 5, 1940, Sr. Catherine Sullivan Visitatrix Collection, RG 9-3-3:2(3), APSL.

7. Meyers, *Education of Sisters*, xxxi.

8. Meyers, *Education of Sisters*, 53.

9. Coburn, "Ahead of Its Time . . . or, Right on Time?," 28; Meyers, *Sisters for the 21st Century*, 26–37.

10. Meyers, *Sisters for the 21st Century*, 32, 33.

11. Meyers, *Education of Sisters*, 211–12.

12. Meyers, *Education of Sisters*, 212.

13. Coburn, "Ahead of Its Time . . . or, Right on Time?," 28–29.

14. Schneider, "American Sisters and the Roots of Change," 63, 64.

15. Coburn, "Ahead of Its Time . . . or, Right on Time?," 28–32; Schneider, "American Sisters and the Roots of Change," 61–65; Hoy, *Good Hearts*, 128–29; Koehlinger, *New Nuns*, 29–35.

16. Coburn, "Ahead of Its Time . . . or, Right on Time?," 36.

17. Meyers, "Place of Religious in Social Work," 61.

18. Meyers, *Sisters for the 21st Century*, 269–87.

19. "Second Vatican Council: Roman Catholic History (1962–1965)," *Encyclopaedia Britannica*, https://www.britannica.com; Jordan G. Teicher, "Why Is Vatican II So Important?," *NPR Newsletter*, October 10, 2012, https://www.npr.org.

20. "Maria Climbs a Mountain: Mother Suzanne Guillemin and the Vatican II 'Revolution,'" http://www.mariasmountain.net.

21. Carey, *Sisters in Crisis*, 43–44; Koehlinger, *New Nuns*, 43–48.

22. Mother Suzanne Guillemin, Circular Letter, February 2, 1968, RG 6-50.1:3, APSL.

23. Dolan et al., *Transforming Parish Ministry*, 309.

24. Koehlinger, *New Nuns*, 43.

25. "Women's Rights Movement," *Encyclopaedia Britannica*, https://www.britannica.com.

26. Suenens, *Nun in the World*, 45. Suenens's arguments for ending traditional constraints on Catholic sisters received support from social scientists such as Erving Goffman, who in 1961 argued that "total institutions," comprising prisons, asylums, religious orders, and convents, isolated and restricted the "moral autonomy" of their "inmates." Goffman, *Asylums*.

27. Quote in McCormack, "Nun in the World," 744.

28. Carey, *Sisters in Crisis*, 28–34; Koehlinger, *New Nuns*, 47; Dolan et al., *Transforming Parish Ministry*, 165–66.

29. "45,000 Sisters of Charity Doff Old Habit for a Modern Dress," *New York Times*, September 21, 1964.

30. Dolan et al., *Transforming Parish Ministry*, 166–67.

31. Berrelleza et al., "Population Trends Among Religious Institutes of Women," 1–8.

32. Center for Applied Research in the Apostolate (Thomas Gaunt), personal communication, January 18, 2024.

33. Robert Blair Kaiser, "The Nuns That Quit," *Ladies Home Journal*, April 1967.

34. Russell Shaw, "Where Have All the Sisters Gone?," *Catholic Answers Magazine*, December 1, 2006, https://www.catholic.com.

35. Johnson et al., *New Generations of Catholic Sisters*, 7–11; Berrelleza et al., "Population Trends Among Religious Institutes of Women," 3.

36. Johnson et al., *New Generations of Catholic Sisters*, 10–11; Neal, *Catholic Sisters in Transition*, 72–73.

37. Hannefin, *Daughters of the Church*, 256, 261, 271, 279. There are some discrepancies in the archival records. See, for example, "Summary of Five Provinces in the United States," March 1968, Health Apostolate—East Central Province Collection, RG 16-2, APSL.

38. Sr. DeChantal LaRow, "20th Anniversary Report, Health Care Ministry in the Northeast Province," 1989, Health Apostolate—NE Province Collection, RG 16-2:3(5), APSL. From 1977 to 1979, Kelley served as the Catholic Hospital Association's president, among the first in a long line of Daughters to hold a leading position in that organization. Kauffman, *Ministry and Meaning*, 298–99.

39. "Evaluation of the Works: West Central Province," Health Apostolate—WC Province Collection, RG 15-11-1:19(5), APSL.

40. "Evaluation of the Works: West Central Province," APSL; *West Central Province Newsletter*, December 8, 1972, APSL; Ross and Ross, *Walking to New Orleans*, 181n166.

41. *West Central Province Newsletter*, December 8, 1972, APSL.

42. Center for Applied Research in the Apostolate (Thomas Gaunt), personal communication, January 18, 2024.

43. Sr. Ann William Bradley, "Apostolic Assessment, Sisters of Charity Hospital," 1983, Health Apostolate—NE Province Collection, RG 16-2:2(7), APSL.

44. Sr. Marilyn Perkins, "Apostolic Assessment, Carney Hospital," 1983, Health Apostolate—NE Province Collection, RG 16-2:2(7), APSL.

45. Brown v. Board of Education, 347 U.S. 483 (1954).

46. See Smith, "Population Ecology," 561–96; Washington et al., "Segregation, Civil Rights, and Health Disparities," 513–27; Smith, "Racial Integration of Medical and Nursing Associations," 387–401.

47. Smith, "Population Ecology," 561–62; Newman, "Catholic Church in Arkansas," 293–319; Osborne, "Church and the Negro," 129–50; Newman, "'Ra-

cial Discrimination Can in No Way Be Justified,'" 665–98; Alberts, "Black Catholic Schools," 77–98.

48. "Racial Attitude Depends Principally on Location," *Evansville Courier* (Evansville, IN), March 4, 1956.

49. "Racial Attitude Depends Principally on Location," *Evansville Courier*, March 4, 1956.

50. Newman, "Catholic Church in Arkansas," 299, 319.

51. Sager, "Why Urban Voluntary Hospitals Close," 454.

52. Stevens, *In Sickness and in Wealth*, 230.

53. Sager, "Why Urban Voluntary Hospitals Close," 455.

54. Cornely, "Trend in Racial Integration," 8–10; United States Commission on Civil Rights, *Title VI, One Year After*, 1, 6–14.

55. United States Commission on Civil Rights, *Title VI, One Year After*, 14.

56. Washington et al., "Segregation, Civil Rights, and Health Disparities," 516.

57. Washington et al., "Segregation, Civil Rights, and Health Disparities," 516.

58. Washington et al., "Segregation, Civil Rights, and Health Disparities," 515–16, 522–24; Smith, "Racial Integration of Medical and Nursing Associations," 394; Cornely, "Trend in Racial Integration," 8–9.

59. "Hope, Encouragement and Aid from Sisters in the Catholic Hospitals," *Kansas City Times*, May 25, 1953.

60. "Dallas Hospital Admits Five Negro Physicians to Staff," 367.

61. "Three Negro Doctors Admitted to Staff of Providence Hospital," *Evening Star* (Washington, DC), February 27, 1955.

62. "Progress Report of Research of Racial Discrimination in Employment by the University of Kansas and Community Studies," 1964, Kansas City, MO/St. Vincent's Hospital Collection, RG 11-2-1-2:1(3), APSL.

63. "Dallas Catholic Hospital to Admit Negro Doctors," *The Tidings* (Los Angeles, CA), July 2, 1954.

64. "Progress Report of Research of Racial Discrimination in Employment," APSL.

65. "Black History: Black Doctors in Montgomery," *Montgomery Advertiser*, February 23, 1999; "Old St. Margaret's Was Once the City's Finest Facility," *Montgomery Advertiser*, April 16, 1999.

66. Robert M. Browne to Sr. Catherine Fink, April 7, 1965, Montgomery, AL/St. Margaret's Hospital Collection, RG 11-2-2:7(7), APSL.

67. Browne to Fink, APSL.

68. John Leo, "Segregated Sickness," *Commonweal*, December 18, 1964.

69. Sr. Catherine Fink to John Leo, 1964, Montgomery, AL/St. Margaret's Hospital Collection, RG 11-2-2:7(7), APSL.

70. The Sisters of St. Joseph of Rochester, New York, tended to the Black victims of the violence, including John Lewis, at Selma's Good Samaritan Hospital. Wall, "Catholic Sister Nurses in Selma," 91–102; "Martin Luther King, Jr. Biography," Biography.com, https://www.biography.com.

71. Chelsey Parrott-Sheffer, "16th Street Baptist Church Bombing," *Encyclopaedia Britannica*, https://www.britannica.com.

72. "Women Deplore Church Bombing," *Birmingham News*, September 18, 1963.

73. Africa Studies Center, University of Pennsylvania, "Letter from a Birmingham Jail," https://www.africa.upenn.edu.

74. "Problems of Life-and-Death in Birmingham," *Birmingham News*, March 25, 1951; B. Denise Hawkins, "University Hospital Recalls Its Civil Rights Journey on 50th Anniversary of Birmingham Bombing," https://www.diverseeducation.com. St. Vincent's and Jefferson-Hillman Hospital (renamed "University Hospital" in 1955) frequently turned Black patients away if segregated beds for them were not available. "St. Vincent's Birmingham," https://www.bhamwiki.com.

75. United States Department of Health, Education, and Welfare, *Compliance with Antidiscrimination Provision*, 32.

76. Leonard Chamblee, "Negro Woman Proud of Her RN," *Birmingham Post-Herald*, February 21, 1968.

77. Smith, "Racial Disparities in Care," S66; United States Commission on Civil Rights, *Title VI. One Year After*, 6.

78. Smith, "Racial Disparities in Care," S66.

79. Clay Dean to Frank Ahn, December 28, 1967, Mobile, AL/Providence Hospital Collection, RG 11-2-2:5(4), APSL.

80. Smith, "Racial Disparities in Care," S66.

81. Frank Ahn to Sr. Anita Doyle, December 29, 1967, Mobile, AL/Providence Hospital Collection, RG 11-2-2:5(4), APSL.

82. Rappaport, "U.S. Urban Decline," 16.

83. Rappaport, "U.S. Urban Decline," 17.

84. Rappaport, "U.S. Urban Decline," 23–24.

85. Taeuber and Taeuber, *Negroes in Cities*, 2–3.

86. Richard Rothstein, "Modern Segregation," presentation, Atlantic Live Conference: Reinventing the War on Poverty, March 6, 2014, Washington, DC, 5–8, https://www.epi.org.

87. Sager, "Why Urban Voluntary Hospitals Close," 453–55.

88. McNeil and Williams, "Wide Range of Causes Found," 76–81.

89. Mullner, "Closed U.S. Community Hospitals," 357.

90. Hernandez and Kaluzny, "Hospital Closure," 420–22.

91. Sager, "Urban Hospital Closings," 170. Relocating a hospital from an inner-city Black neighborhood to a suburban White community potentially violated Title VI of the Civil Rights Act of 1964 if those opposed to the relocation could show discriminatory impact, such as evidence of a substantial and disproportionate decrease in healthcare services to racial minorities. But even if opponents could establish discriminatory impact, hospital owners could still justify their actions through proof of "important non-race related goals," such as "financial necessity" and cost savings. Because most hospital boards could support their decisions and provide bus service or satellite clinics as alternatives, litigation was not particularly fruitful. Zall, "Maintaining Health Care in the Inner City," 271–302; DiChristina, "'So Sue Me.'"

92. A disproportionate number of hospitals that closed were relatively small in size (fewer than one hundred beds). Mullner, "Closed U.S. Community Hospitals," 357.

93. "Sisters of Charity Hospital Emergency Room History," Chronologies, Buffalo, NY/Sisters of Charity Hospital Collection, RG 11-2-2:11(1), APSL. Had SOC remained at its original site, it would have been in a Black community. By 1980, SOC's former neighborhood was 81 percent Black, while its new location north of the Kensington Expressway was 15 percent Black. United States Department of Commerce, Bureau of the Census, Population Division, *1980 Census of Population and Housing*, table P-3.

94. "Characteristics of the Population in the Hospital Service Area," 1960–1967, Boston, MA/Carney Hospital Collection, RG 11-2-2:39(2), APSL.

95. The old building on Capitol Hill had become "completely worn out" and "taxed beyond [its] capacity," according to an excerpt in the *Congressional Record*. US Congress, House of Representatives, "Providence Hospital," *Congressional Record*, June 6, 1961.

96. Both locations were mostly middle- to upper-class White. Planning for a new hospital began in the early 1950s and reached fruition in the late 1950s with support from Samuel Cardinal Stritch. Construction commenced in May 1961 and finished in December 1963. "The History of Saint Joseph Hospital: Where Diversity Meets Lake Shore Drive," 1964, American Hospital Association Archives, 19.

97. Though the acreage for the new facility was meager, making parking a problem, it was in close proximity to major thoroughfares, including Claiborne Avenue. Interdisciplinary Team Report for Hôtel Dieu, "Background History, the Mission, the Master Plan," 1972, Interdisciplinary Team Reports/West Central Province Collection, RG 15-11:11(1), APSL.

98. Madeline Blackburn, "Rochester's Nineteenth Ward: A Brief History," February 24, 2020, https://digrocreligions.org; Daniel Gorman Jr., "Roman Catholic Church of Ss. Peter and Paul," August 12, 2020, https://digrocreligions.org.

99. Hannefin, *Daughters of the Church*, 255.

100. Gorman, "Roman Catholic Church of Ss. Peter and Paul."

101. Blackburn, "Rochester's Nineteenth Ward"; Gorman, "Roman Catholic Church of Ss. Peter and Paul"; Sara Youngerman, "Agency Approves Renovations at St. Mary's," *Democrat and Chronicle* (Rochester, NY), September 28, 1979.

102. Wendell Cox Consultancy, "Living Wage, Dying St. Louis," *Public Purpose*, no. 40 (December 2000), http://www.publicpurpose.com.

103. Wendy Shaw, "A Tale of Two Cities: The Best of Times, the Worst of Times. Inequality in St. Louis' Metro-East," 1997, https://www.siue.edu.

104. Shaw, "Tale of Two Cities."

105. Board Minutes, November 20, 1968, St. Louis, MO/Depaul Hospital Collection, RG 11-2-5:22(7), APSL.

106. "Planning Report Six," September 19, 1969, St. Louis, MO/Depaul Hospital Collection, RG 11-2-5:22(7), APSL.

107. "Planning Report Six," APSL.

108. "DePaul Also Defies ARCH, Proceeding with Expansion," *St. Louis Post-Dispatch*, March 21, 1972.

109. "Background and Description of the Work," St. Louis, MO/Depaul Hospital Collection, RG 11-2-5:22(7), APSL.

110. Board Minutes, November 20, 1968, APSL.

111. Board Minutes, "Summary Two," December 16, 1968, St. Louis, MO/Depaul Hospital Collection, RG 11-2-5:22(7), APSL.

112. National Center for Health Statistics, *Health, United States, 2004, with Chartbook*, 311.

113. Medical News, "Abandon Internship," 37.

114. Canfield, "Family Medicine," 905–6.

115. Sager, "Why Urban Voluntary Hospitals Close," 458; Sager, "Urban Hospital Closings," 174.

116. Roemer, *Ambulatory Health Services*, 60, 365.

117. "Voluntary Additions to Doctors' Questionnaire," St. Louis, MO/Depaul Hospital Collection, RG 11-2-5:22(7), APSL.

118. Roemer, *Ambulatory Health Services*, 54, 272.

119. "Institutional Self-Evaluation, Section III, Historical Survey of the Institution," January 1972, St. Louis, MO/Depaul Hospital Collection, RG 11-2-1:1(8), APSL.

120. Roemer, *Ambulatory Health Services*, 54.

121. Roemer, *Ambulatory Health Services*, 65.

122. Torrens and Yedvab, "Variations Among Emergency Room Patients," 60–75.

123. Roemer, *Ambulatory Health Services*, 100.

124. Mickey, "Dr. StrangeRove," 38.

125. Mickey, "Dr. StrangeRove," 28–29; Roemer, *Ambulatory Health Services*, 210.

126. Carney Hospital Emergency Room Committee, "Annual Report," 1962, Boston, MA/Carney Hospital Collection, RG 11-2-1-2:50(18), APSL.

127. "Satellite Mobile Clinic: The Need," undated document, Boston, MA/Carney Hospital Collection, RG 11-2-9:39(2), APSL.

128. "Study of a Community Services Division of the Carney Hospital—'Bringing the Services to the Patient,'" undated document, Boston, MA/Carney Hospital Collection, RG 11-2-9:39(2), APSL; "Satellite Mobile Clinic: The Need," APSL; Sr. Helen Kelly, "Preliminary Study: Division of Community Services (Mobile Satellite Clinic)," undated document, Boston, MA/Carney Hospital Collection, RG 11-2-9:39(2), APSL.

129. John Stainton to Sr. Helen Kelly, June 28, 1968, with "Preliminary Report" of planning consultant attached, Boston, MA/Carney Hospital Collection, RG 11-2-9:39(2), APSL; "Sister Helen's Comments on Preliminary Report Prepared by Mr. John Stainton, Planning Consultant Re: Establishment of a Mobile Satellite Clinic by Carney Hospital," undated, Boston, MA/Carney Hospital Collection, RG 11-2-9:39(2), APSL; "Case Study: Carney Hospital Program for Ambulatory Care," April 1, 1976, Boston, MA/Carney Hospital Collection, RG 11-2-9:40(5), APSL; "Financial Participation with Health Centers," undated, Boston, MA/Carney Hospital Collection, RG 11-2-9:40(10), APSL. At Port Norfolk, the location of one of the two freestanding centers, the local "Health Committee" initially examined and then rejected the potential for a mobile clinic. "The use of a mobile unit generated very little enthusiasm," the committee stated. "Health care is an everyday, ongoing process and the Health Committee felt that a mobile unit would not provide adequate health care to the residents it served."

130. "Case Study: Carney Hospital Program for Ambulatory Care," APSL.

131. "Case Study: Carney Hospital Program for Ambulatory Care," APSL.

132. Mayes and Berenson, *Medicare Prospective Payment*, 18, 37, 74.

133. In 1978, the federal and state Medicare and Medicaid programs accounted for 50.3 percent of total hospital income at Sisters of Charity Hospital in Buffalo; by 1982, Medicare and Medicaid dollars comprised 54.2 percent of total gross revenues. Bradley, "Apostolic Assessment, Sisters of Charity Hospital," APSL. In 1978, the share of total gross revenues from Medicare and Medicaid was 54.3 percent at Carney Hospital in Boston; by 1982, the two programs together constituted 57.8 percent of the total. Perkins, "Apostolic Assessment, Carney Hospital," APSL.

134. Jensen et al., "New Dominance of Managed Care," 126–27; Bodenheimer and Sullivan, "How Large Employers are Shaping the Health Care Marketplace," 1004.

135. Wall, *American Catholic Hospitals*, 17.

136. *The Road to Unity: The Origins of the Daughters of Charity Health System, 1960–1986*, RG 29-4-2, APSL.

137. Sr. Marilyn Emminger et al., "Final Report: Task Force for Daughters of Charity National Health System (DCNHS)," June 1986, Health Systems Transitions Collection, RG 29-0-2: (2), APSL.

138. *Road to Unity*, APSL, 44; Emminger, "Final Report," APSL.

139. Emminger, "Final Report," APSL.

140. *Road to Unity*, APSL, 40; Emminger, "Final Report," APSL; Lewis E. Weeks, ed., "Sister Irene Kraus, in First Person: An Oral History," *Hospital Administration Oral History Collection* (Chicago, IL: American Hospital Association and Hospital Research and Education Trust, 1988), 45–50, https://www.aha.org.

141. *Road to Unity*, APSL, 44; "Daughters of Charity Mull National System," *Modern Healthcare*, December 20, 1985.

142. Emminger, "Final Report," APSL.

143. Weeks, "Sister Irene Kraus," iii–v, 10; Robert Thomas Jr., "Irene Kraus, 74, Nun Who Led Big Nonprofit Hospital Chain," *New York Times*, August 27, 1988; "Sister Irene Kraus," *Gettysburg Times*, August 25, 1998; "Sister Irene Kraus Leaves Us a Legacy of Good," *Pensacola News Journal*, October 30, 1995.

144. Author interview of Sr. Theresa Peck, DC, October 17, 2022.

145. Weeks, "Sister Irene Kraus," 10.

146. Kauffman, *Ministry and Meaning*, 296–97.

147. Smith, "Form Follows Function," 52–53.

148. Kauffman, *Ministry and Meaning*, 298–99.

149. See Peck, "Accounting for Charity Care," 50–52.

Six. *Reconciling Divisions over Access to Reproductive Services*

1. Nelson, "God and Woman," 76–77, 105–11; Griffin, "Catholic Bishops," 1414–15.

2. Though few hospitals had ethics committees in the 1960s and 1970s, they became institutionalized in the 1980s. Over 60 percent of hospitals had ethics committees by the late 1980s, and over 90 percent had them at the end of the twentieth century. Aulisio, "Why Did Hospital Ethics Committees Emerge?," 546. Hospital ethics committees largely refuted the church's absolutist positions on reproductive and end-of-life matters. In the words of law professor Leonard Nelson, "the philosophical underpinnings of the secular discipline of bioethics are essentially pragmatic and teleological . . . no one principle trumps the others." Nelson, "God and Woman," 110.

3. Griffin, "Catholic Bishops," 1414.

4. Griffin, "Catholic Bishops," 1415.

5. 381 U.S. 479 (1965).

6. Griffin, "Catholic Bishops," 1413–15.

7. Nelson, "God and Woman," 115–17; O'Rourke et al., "Summary of the Development of the Ethical and Religious Directives," 18–19.

8. Fr. Thomas J. Casey to Sr. Lorraine, Waterville, ME/EA Seton Hospital Collection, RG 11-2-1:1(4), APSL.

9. The Daughters came to Waterville, Maine, in 1913, where they occupied a "small wooden structure," known as Sisters Hospital, to care for the poor. In 1965, they built a "gleaming, six-story facility" and changed the name from Sisters Hospital to Elizabeth Ann Seton Hospital. "Seton Hospital Sponsorship Is Transferred to Diocese," *Central Maine Morning Sentinel* (Waterville, ME), August 1, 1973.

10. Sr. Lorraine O'Brien to Fr. Joseph T. Tinnelly, March 11, 1970, Waterville, ME/EA Seton Hospital Collection, RG 11-2-1:1(4), APSL.

11. "Waterville, Maine," *Maine: An Encyclopedia*, https://maineanencyclopedia.com.

12. Hamel, "Ethical and Religious Directives," 66–67.

13. Sr. Margaret Finnegan to Sr. Virginia Schwager, December 28, 1972, Waterville, ME/EA Seton Hospital Collection, RG 11-2-1:1(4), APSL.

14. Finnegan to Schwager, APSL.

15. 410 U.S. 113 (1973).

16. Bishop Peter L. Gerety to Sr. Mary Walter, January 31, 1973, Waterville, ME/EA Seton Hospital Collection, RG 11-2-1:1(4), APSL.

17. Marjorie Hyer, "Catholic Bishops Condemn Abortion Ruling," *Charlotte Observer*, February 15, 1973.

18. "Diocesan Hospital Group to Continue Abortion Ban," *The Messenger* (Belleville, IL), February 16, 1973.

19. "Diocesan Hospital Group to Continue Abortion Ban," *The Messenger*, February 16, 1973; "Head of Catholic Physicians," *The Messenger*, February 16, 1973.

20. Nelson, "God and Woman," 74–75, 77–79.

21. Taylor v. St. Vincent's Hospital, 369 F.Supp. 948 (D. Mont., 1973); Nelson, "God and Woman," 77–92.

22. Nelson, "God and Woman," 92–101; Hoss and Decker, "When All Roads Lead to Rome," 106–9; St. Anges Hospital of City of Baltimore, Inc. v. Riddick, 748 F.Supp. 319 (D. Md., 1990).

23. Kauffman, *Ministry and Meaning*, 291–93; Gold, "Advocates Work to Preserve Reproductive Health Care Access"; Wall, "Conflict and Compromise."

24. Lucette Lagnado, "Their Role Growing, Catholic Hospitals Must Balance Doctrine with Medicine," *Wall Street Journal*, February 4, 1999; "Murfreesboro in

Rutherford County, Tennessee—the American South (East South Central), Rutherford Hospital/Middle Tennessee Medical Center," Historical Marker Database, https://www.hmdb.org; "Expectant Parents Tour," *Daily News-Journal* (Murfreesboro, TN), February 5, 2002.

25. William Salganik, "Catholic Hospital Chains Are Growing the Fastest," *Baltimore Sun*, March 15, 1998; "Western Maryland Health System Profile and History," https://www.datanyze.com; Gold, "Advocates Work to Preserve Reproductive Health Care Access"; Lagnado, "Their Role Growing."

26. O'Rourke et al., "Summary of the Development of the Ethical and Religious Directives," 20–21; Nelson, "God and Woman," 121–22; Wildes, "Memo from the Central Office," 133–39; United States Conference of Catholic Bishops, *Ethical and Religious Directives*; Hayley Penan and Amy Chen, "The Ethical and Religious Directives: What the 2018 Update Means for Catholic Hospital Mergers," National Health Law Program, 2019, https://healthlaw.org.

27. Singer and Lantz, "Coming Millenium," 301–2. See also Wurdock, "Doctors, Dioceses, and Decisions," 188–92; Wall, "Conflict and Compromise."

28. Kellhofer, "Misperception and Misapplication," 107–8; Singer and Lantz, "Coming Millenium," 313–24; Carlson, "Freedom at Risk," 158–63; Wall, "Conflict and Compromise."

29. Lagnado, "Their Role Growing."

30. Joyce Krysak, "Niagara Falls Hospitals End Merger Talks," Buffalo Toronto Public Media, September 28, 2007, https://www.btpm.org.

31. Wall, "Conflict and Compromise"; "Austin Hospital's Services Criticized by the Vatican," *Fort Worth Star-Telegram*, July 31, 1998; Kim Sue Lia Perkes, "Vatican Dispute Prompts Changes at Brackenridge," *Austin American-Statesman*, August 20, 1998; United States Conference of Catholic Bishops, *Ethical and Religious Directives*.

32. Wall, "Conflict and Compromise"; "Austin Hospital's Services Criticized by the Vatican," *Fort Worth Star-Telegram*, July 31, 1998; Perkes, "Vatican Dispute Prompts Changes at Brackenridge"; United States Conference of Catholic Bishops, *Ethical and Religious Directives*.

33. "Fall River Hospital Is Added to Archdiocese Health System," *Boston Globe*, December 15, 1991.

34. James E. Small to Sr. DeChantal LaRow and Matthias Maguire, "Carney Hospital Market Profile," March 4, 1996, Sr. Louise Gallahue, Visitatrix/NE Province Collection, RG 9-5-4:7(6), APSL.

35. Cyril Mazansky to Sr. Louise Gallahue, October 30, 1995, Sr. Louise Gallahue, Visitatrix/NE Province Collection, RG 9-5-4:7(6), APSL.

36. Edward Reardon to Sr. Louise Gallahue, May 12, 1995, Sr. Louise Gallahue, Visitatrix/NE Province Collection, RG 9-5-4:7(6), APSL.

37. "Cardinal Law Warns of Links with Non-Catholic Hospitals," *Daily Item* (Lynn, MA), May 6, 1995.

38. Richard A. Knox, "Doctors Key to Law's Health Equation," *Boston Sunday Globe*, May 7, 1995.

39. Michael Lasalandra, "Cardinal Eyes Carney for Hospital Alliance," *Boston Herald*, May 6, 1995.

40. Lasalandra, "Cardinal Eyes Carney"; Liz Kowalczyk, "Law: Economy Forcing Ties to Secular Hospitals," *Patriot Ledger* (Boston, MA), May 6–7, 1995; Eileen McNamara, "The Cardinal and Health Care," *Boston Globe*, June 12, 1996.

41. Mazansky to Gallahue, APSL.

42. Reardon to Gallahue, APSL.

43. John G. Nugent to Micheal J. Riley, October 15, 1994, Sr. Louise Gallahue, Visitatrix/NE Province Collection, RG 9-5-4:7(6), APSL.

44. Michael Paulson, "Law Has Little to Say After Rome Trip," *Boston Globe*, February 9, 2002; Eileen McNamara, "The Obituary Bernard Law Deserves," *Boston Globe*, December 21, 2017 ("Admirers thought he might become the first American pope"); Robert D. McFadden, "Bernard Law, Powerful Cardinal Disgraced by Priest Abuse Scandal, Dies at 86," *New York Times*, December 19, 2017.

45. Small to LaRow and Maguire, "Carney Hospital Market Profile," APSL.

46. Richard A. Knox, "Carney Goes Its Own Way," *Boston Globe*, December 17, 1995; McNamara, "Cardinal and Health Care."

47. Small to LaRow and Maguire, "Carney Hospital Market Profile," APSL; James E. Small to Michael Collins, July 3, 1996, Sr. Louise Gallahue, Visitatrix/NE Province Collection, RG 9-5-4:7(6), APSL; Bernard Cardinal Law to Matthias Maguire, May 22, 1996, Sr. Louise Gallahue, Visitatrix/NE Province Collection, RG 9-5-4:7(6), APSL; Knox, "Carney Goes Its Own Way."

48. Law to Maguire, APSL.

49. Stunned by Law's decision, James E. Small, regional executive for DCNHS-NE, wrote Dr. Michael Collins, Caritas's president, expressing his disappointment. "If there was any hint that [the agreement with Quincy] would not have been acceptable to the Cardinal," Small told Collins, "we would have discontinued. . . . We spent a great deal of time and money pursuing these negotiations." Small to Collins, APSL.

50. Sr. Louise Gallahue et al., "Request to Alienate Carney Hospital," December 6, 1996, Sr. Louise Gallahue, Visitatrix/NE Province Collection, RG 9-5-4:7(6), APSL.

51. John Nuveen & Co., "Preliminary Valuation Analysis for Carney Hospital," Sr. Louise Gallahue, Visitatrix/NE Province Collection, RG 9-5-4:7(6), APSL.

52. Christopher Rowland, "Caritas Christi on the Rebound," *Boston Globe*, November 11, 2005; Christopher Rowland, "In Caritas Deal, Fears for Two City Hospitals," *Boston Globe*, February 7, 2007.

53. McFadden, "Bernard Law, Powerful Cardinal"; Sacha Pfeiffer and Matt Carroll, "Voice of the Faithful," *Boston Globe*, July 23, 2002.

54. Liz Kowalczyk and Michael Paulson, "AG Office Seeking Caritas Meeting," *Boston Globe*, April 10, 2004.

55. Rowland, "Caritas Christi on the Rebound"; "Hospitals," *Boston Globe*, December 31, 2006; Christopher Rowland, "Archdiocese Set to End Ownership of Hospitals," *Boston Globe*, February 6, 2007; Office of Attorney General Martha Coakley, *Statement of the Attorney General as to the Caritas Christi Transaction*.

56. Office of Attorney General Martha Coakley, *Statement of the Attorney General as to the Caritas Christi Transaction*, 15.

57. Jeffrey Krasner, "Caritas Christi Chain Collapses," *Boston Globe*, June 29, 2007.

58. Office of Attorney General Martha Coakley, *Statement of the Attorney General as to the Caritas Christi Transaction*, 15; Jeffrey Krasner, "Caritas Christi's Handover Deal Fails: Finances Cloud Talks with Network," *Boston Globe*, June 29, 2007.

59. Office of Attorney General Martha Coakley, *Statement of the Attorney General as to the Caritas Christi Transaction*, 1.

60. Jeffrey Krasner, "AG Urges Change of Course for Caritas: Archdiocese Should Give Up Control of Operations, Coakley Report Says," *Boston Globe*, March 7, 2008.

61. "De la Torre Approved as CEO," *Boston Globe*, April 3, 2008; Office of Attorney General Martha Coakley, *Statement of the Attorney General as to the Caritas Christi Transaction*, 16.

62. Office of Attorney General Martha Coakley, *Statement of the Attorney General as to the Caritas Christi Transaction*, 13.

63. Because the transaction involved the sale of hospitals from a nonprofit to a for-profit entity, the Massachusetts Attorney General's Office had to approve the undertaking. Following an extensive review, the attorney general concluded that "the public is better off with the Transaction than without it." There were certain stipulations. The attorney general conditioned her approval on Steward's commitment to make certain capital expenditures, to "comply with the current Caritas policies concerning indigent and charity care," to "maintain community benefit expenditures at . . . current level[s]," and to "not close, or limit the general purpose of . . . any Caritas Hospital" for a five-year period. Office of Attorney General Martha Coakley, *Statement of the Attorney General as to the Caritas Christi Transaction*, 1, 5, 8, 10, 13–19, 24.

64. Office of Attorney General Martha Coakley, *Statement of the Attorney General as to the Caritas Christi Transaction*, 20, 21.

65. Judith Garber and Imari Daniels, "Steward Implosion Provides Cautionary Tale on Private Equity in Health Care," Lown Institute, March 19, 2024, https://lowninstitute.org.

66. "Statement from Cerberus on Massachusetts Congressional Delegation's Hearing Related to Steward Health Care," April 3, 2024, https://www.cerberus.com; Jonathan Weil, "The CEO Who Made a Fortune While His Hospital Chain Collapsed," *Wall Street Journal*, April 18, 2024.

67. Weil, "CEO Who Made a Fortune."

68. Office of Senator Edward J. Markey, *Steward Health Care Report*; Liz Kowalczyk et al., "They Died in Hallways," *Boston Globe*, September 6, 2024.

69. Office of Senator Edward J. Markey, *Steward Health Care Report*, 2, 3, 18–9, 22; Robert Weisman and Jason Laughlin, "Healey Reveals Deals to Move Six Steward Hospitals to New Owners," *Boston Globe*, August 17, 2024.

70. Johnson and Broder, *The System*, 61–62.

71. Robin A. Cohen and Michael E. Martinez, "Health Insurance Coverage: Early Release of Estimates from the National Health Interview Survey, January–March 2009," Centers for Disease Control and Prevention, September 2009, https://www.cdc.gov.

72. Catholic Health Association, *No Room in the Marketplace*, 20, 21, 25, 26, 27, 28, 38; Coreil, "CHA's Vision of a Redesigned Healthcare System," 12–14.

73. Coreil, "CHA's Vision of a Redesigned Healthcare System," 12.

74. Catholic Health Association, *No Room in the Marketplace*, 21, 27, 33–34.

75. Budrys, *Our Unsystematic Health Care System*, 1–14, 121–39. Before 1983, governments and private insurers paid hospitals retrospectively for services rendered, providing few incentives for hospitals and physicians to control costs. After the Medicare program began to pay hospitals a set amount based on the patient's diagnosis in 1983, however, incentives switched. Under prospective payment, hospital administrators shortened the length of patient stays in order to maintain hospital margins, creating an excess of hospital beds. As a result, many hospitals merged (or downsized) to reduce the number of beds, a process known as "horizontal integration." Linkages between dissimilar entities such as hospitals and physicians, known as "vertical integration," did not gain traction until the late 1980s, when managed care organizations became popular. An early form of managed care organization was the HMO (health maintenance organization). HMOs employed or contracted with primary care physicians who "managed" patients' healthcare, including referrals to specialists. In order to maintain or increase patient referrals, hospitals acquired the practices of primary care physicians. Another type of managed care organization, the preferred provider organization or PPO, appeared around

the mid-1990s after consumer dissatisfaction with HMOs mounted. In a PPO, patients typically could go to any physician, primary care or specialist, so long as the doctor was in the plan "network." Ameringer, *US Health Policy and Health Care Delivery*, 91–114.

76. Coreil, "CHA's Vision of a Redesigned Healthcare System," 12–13.

77. Under the proposal, each IDN would offer an array of services from primary to acute care and from rehabilitative to hospice care. All providers who wanted "to participate" had to belong to "one or more IDNs," which competed for enrollees on the basis of "quality of care, ease of access, and services—but not price." Most localities, the Leadership Task Force anticipated, would have several state-chartered IDNs. Financing for the arrangement was to come from a national trust fund consisting of "current federal healthcare expenditures" and "progressive payroll taxes," which a National Health Board would administer and distribute to IDNs through "risk-adjusted capitated payments." Catholic Health Association, *Setting Relationships Right*, 3–6.

78. Catholic Health Association, *Setting Relationships Right*; Tieman, "Quite a Moment," 5.

79. Dana Priest, "Health Plan Threatened by Abortion Coverage," *Washington Post*, May 19, 1993.

80. Sr. Bernice Coreil Health Reform documents, "CHA Healthcare Reform Update: Past Events and Future Activities," 1992–1994, Health Apostolate/WC Province Collection, RG 16-2:6(3), APSL; Sr. Bernice Coreil Health Reform documents, "Remarks of Sister Bernice Coreil, DC," White House, March 23, 1994, Health Apostolate/WC Province Collection, RG 16-2:6(4), APSL.

81. Mary Janet Kinsella to Sr. Bernice Coreil, April 5, 1994, Health Apostolate/WC Province Collection, RG 16-2:6(4), APSL.

82. Bishop Thomas J. Welsh to Sr. Louise Gallahue, March 24, 1994, Health Apostolate/WC Province Collection, RG 16-2:6(4), APSL.

83. Bishop Edward T. Hughes to Jack Curley, March 31, 1994, Health Apostolate/WC Province Collection, RG 16-2:6(4), APSL.

84. "It's Time to Take Our Medicine," 18–23.

85. Gottlieb, "Clintonian Roots of Obamacare," 53–59; Goldsmith et al., *Integrated Delivery Networks*.

86. Carol Zimmerman, "For Sister Carol Keehan, Faith and Health Care Go Together," *Catholic News Service*, January 25, 2019, https://angelusnews.com; "It's Time to Take Our Medicine," 18–23; Hasstedt, "Abortion Coverage Under the Affordable Care Act"; Salganicoff et al., "Coverage for Abortion Services and the ACA."

87. Barbara Bradley Hagerty, "Catholic Hospitals, Bishops Split on Health Care Bill," NPR News, March 17, 2010, https://www.wbur.org/npr; "Health Care

Debate Exposes Disagreement Among Catholic Church Leaders," *Washington Post*, March 19, 2010.

88. Breschi, "Health Care Reform and the Catholic Perspective," 335.

89. Cathy Ruse, "Catholic Health Association Can't Be Trusted on Obamacare," *National Review*, March 18, 2010, https://www.nationalreview.com.

90. "Health Care Debate Exposes Disagreement Among Catholic Church Leaders," *Washington Post*, March 19, 2010.

91. Zimmerman, "For Sister Carol Keehan."

92. Keehan admitted that the ACA left "a lot of gaps," however. "Even at best," she indicated, "only 32 million of the 47 million American who don't have any health insurance now will get it over the first 10 years. That still leaves 16 million uninsured, and it still leaves immigrants not covered. We've got to continue to address that." "It's Time to Take Our Medicine," 18–23.

93. Zimmerman, "For Sister Carol Keehan"; Michelle Boorstein, "'I Love Nuns': Obama Appeals to Religious Allies as His Landmark Health Care Law Awaits Supreme Court Decision," *Washington Post*, June 9, 2015; Christopher White, "Pope Francis Praises Sr. Carol Keehan, Obamacare Ally, for Her 'Generous Service,'" *National Catholic Reporter*, May 26, 2022.

94. See National Federation of Independent Business v. Sebelius, 567 U.S. 519 (2012).

95. United States Conference of Catholic Bishops, "Letters from the Most Reverend Frank J. Dewane."

96. A major confrontation occurred in 2013 when the Department of Health and Human Services mandated that most employers and their insurers provide coverage for contraceptives, including Catholic schools, universities, and hospitals. Though the Obama administration made some initial concessions, the uproar largely persisted until the Supreme Court upheld President Trump–era regulations expanding the exemption. See Little Sisters of the Poor Saints Peter and Paul Home v. Pennsylvania, 140 S.Ct. 2367 (2020).

97. "Bishops' Conference Blasts Nuns for Health Care Endorsement," CNN, June 16, 2010, https://www.cnn.com.

98. Berrelleza et al., "Population Trends Among Religious Institutes of Women," 2.

Seven. *"Time to Leave"*

1. Center for Applied Research in the Apostolate (Thomas Gaunt), personal communication, January 18, 2024.

2. Davis, "Message from Sr. Teresa George," 2.

3. Author interview of Sister Theresa Peck, DC, October 17, 2022.

4. Ascension Health, comprising the Daughters' hospitals and other health-care facilities, became a subsidiary of lay-sponsored Ascension. Ascension's holdings also included several other subsidiaries, including for-profit corporations in the United States and foreign countries. Srs. Louise Gallahue, Catherine Madigan, Elyse Staab, and Marie Therese Sedgwick to Sisters, September 15, 1999, Health Systems Transitions Collection, RG 29-0-2:5.1(28), APSL; Srs. Louise Gallahue, Catherine Madigan, Elyse Staab, and Marie Therese Sedgwick to Sr. Juana Elizondo, September 15, 1999, Health Systems Transitions Collection, RG 29-0-2:5.1(28), APSL; Jim Doyle, "Ascension: How a St. Louis-Based Health Care System Become One of the Nation's Biggest," *St. Louis Post-Dispatch*, February 3, 2014; Ascension, "History and Sponsorship," https://about.ascension.org.

5. Author interview of Sister Theresa Peck, DC, October 17, 2022.

6. Author interview of Sister Mary Walz, DC, November 11, 2022. See also Wuerl, "Catholic Health Ministry in Transition," 14–16; Wittberg, "Declining Institutional Sponsorship and Religious Orders."

7. Sr. Mary Rose McPhee to Board of Trustees, Hôtel Dieu Hospital, August 22, 1988, New Orleans, LA/Hôtel Dieu Collection, RG 11-2-5-2:30(5), APSL.

8. Sr. Mary Rose McPhee to Don Dreher, June 17, 1985, New Orleans, LA/Hôtel Dieu Collection, RG 11-2-5-2, APSL.

9. Board Minutes, Hôtel Dieu, "DCHS-WC/Sisters of Mercy Task Force Meeting," November 20, 1986, New Orleans, LA/Hôtel Dieu Collection, RG 11-2-5-2:28(2), APSL; Executive Summary, "Collaborative Proposal for a Catholic Mobile Health Service in New Orleans, Louisiana," December 18, 1987, New Orleans, LA/Hôtel Dieu Collection, RG 11-2-5-2:29(7), APSL.

10. There is a reference to the potential sale of Hôtel Dieu to the State of Louisiana in the minutes of the November 20, 1986, meeting between the Daughters and the Sisters of Mercy. "DCHS-WC/Sisters of Mercy Task Force Meeting," APSL.

11. Sr. Mary Rose McPhee to Sr. Seraphine Ferrero, October 16, 1990, New Orleans, LA/Hôtel Dieu Collection, RG 11-2-5:19(3), APSL; Sr. Mary Rose McPhee to Sr. Seraphine Ferrero, November 15, 1990, New Orleans, LA/Hôtel Dieu Collection, RG 11-2-5:19(3), APSL.

12. "Charity Hospital Timeline (1736–2021)," https://www.lcmchealth.org.

13. James S. Kramer to DCNHS Project Review Committee, January 25, 1995, St. Louis, MO/DePaul Hospital Collection, RG 11-2-5-1, APSL; "SSMHCS Acquires DePaul Health Center," press release, October 26, 1994, St. Louis, MO/DePaul Hospital Collection, RG 11-2-5-1, APSL.

14. Judith VandeWater, "University Hospital in Sale Shape," *St. Louis Post-Dispatch*, July 27, 1997.

15. Kramer to DCNHS Project Review Committee, APSL; Sr. Nannette Gentile to Sisters, April 27, 1995, St. Louis, MO/DePaul Hospital Collection, RG 11-2-5-1, APSL.

16. Marillac Mission Fund, "History," https://marillacmissionfund.org.

17. "Hospitals," *Chicago Tribune*, November 15, 1995.

18. "Hospitals," *Chicago Tribune*, November 15, 1995.

19. Bruce Japsen, "Resurrection Health Care Purchasing St. Joseph Hospital on North Side," *Chicago Tribune*, September 29, 2000.

20. Two factors prompted the sale of St. Joseph to Resurrection—the pending merger of competing hospitals on the North Side and the passage of the Balanced Budget Act of 1997, which significantly reduced Medicare payments, causing hospitals to look for more partners in order to spread financial risk and losses. Japsen, "Resurrection Health Care"; Bruce Japsen, "Catholic Hospital Firms May Merge," *Chicago Tribune*, January 27, 2000.

21. Michelle Martin, "St. Joseph Hospital Celebrates 150 Years of Care in Chicago," *Chicago Catholic*, July 24, 2019, https://www.chicagocatholic.com.

22. Jeanne Peck, "DePaul OKs Sale of Medical Center," *Daily Press* (Newport News, VA), July 3, 1996.

23. Elisha Sauers, "Bon Secours Will Close Norfolk's DePaul Hospital Building in April," *Virginian-Pilot*, January 26, 2021.

24. Alan Morrell, "Whatever Happened to . . . St. Mary's Hospital?," *Democrat and Chronicle* (Rochester, NY), August 25, 2017.

25. Sr. Marilyn Perkins to Sisters, November 18, 1999, Sr. Louise Gallahue, Visitatrix/NE Province Collection, RG 9-5-4-2:8(11), APSL; Draft Letter to Sr. Juana (author unknown), December 9, 1999, Sr. Louise Gallahue, Visitatrix/NE Province Collection, RG 9-5-4-2:8(11), APSL.

26. Sponsorship Task Force, "The Future Sponsorship Model for Daughters of Charity Health Ministry," March 20, 1997 (edited April 4, 1997), Health Systems Transitions Collection, RG 29-0-2-5:1(30), APSL.

27. Sponsorship Task Force, APSL.

28. Donald A. Brennan to DCNHS Corporate Members, October 9, 1997, Health Systems Transitions Collection, RG 29-0-2:5.1(3), APSL.

29. Donald A. Brennan to Sr. Xavier Balance, May 14, 1998, Health Systems Transitions Collection, RG 29-0-2:5.1(24), APSL.

30. Janet Fleischhacker to Sr. Xavier, Balance, May 15, 1998, Health Systems Transitions Collection, RG 29-0-2:5.1(24), APSL. See also Lawrence D. Prybil, Memorandum for Record of Discussion with John Lore, May 18, 1998, Health Systems Transitions Collection, RG 29-0-2:5.1(24), APSL.

31. Fleischhacker to Balance, APSL; Prybil, Memorandum for Record of Discussion with John Lore, APSL.

32. Brennan to Balance, APSL.

33. Srs. Louise Gallahue, Catherine Madigan, Elyse Staab, and Marie Therese Sedwick to Sr. Juana Elizando, September 15, 1999, Health Systems Transitions Collection, RG 29-0-2:5.1(28), APSL.

34. Gallahue et al. to Elizando, APSL; Donald A. Brennan to President's Council, "System Organizational Structure," October 12, 1999, Health Systems Transitions Collection, RG 29-0-2:5.1(28), APSL; Moore, "Sponsorship Transformation at Ascension Health," 26.

35. Ascension, "History and Sponsorship."

36. ScrapeHero, "Number of Ascension Health Hospitals in the United States in 2023," https://www.scrapehero.com.

37. Engler et al., "Organizing Healthcare for Changing Markets," 3–15.

38. Gallahue et al. to Elizando, APSL.

39. Nygren, "Effective Governance in Complex Systems," 43.

40. Wuerl, "Catholic Health Ministry in Transition," 14–16.

41. Catholic Health Association, "Ministerial Juridic Person," 61.

42. Catholic Health Association, "Ministerial Juridic Person," 62.

43. Wuerl, "Catholic Health Ministry in Transition," 14–16; Gottemoeller, "Challenges for Sponsorship Today," 13.

44. Based on author interviews and discussions with several sisters, including Srs. Theresa Peck, DC, and Mary Walz, DC, on October 17, 2022, and November 11, 2022, respectively.

45. Wittberg, "Declining Institutional Sponsorship and Religious Orders," 315, 318, 319. Ascension's continuing fidelity to the Daughters' mission is beyond the scope of this book. This book begins and ends with the Daughters' involvement in nursing and hospital administration. As noted, the Daughters' role largely stopped upon the creation of Ascension Health in 1999 and officially ended with the formation of Ascension in 2012. The Ascension system, moreover, is a lay organization combining hospitals and healthcare facilities from several different religious communities. For those interested in a comprehensive discussion of current issues and concerns about lay sponsorship and management of contemporary Catholic health systems, see Gabow, *Catholic Church and Its Hospitals*.

46. McQueary, *Daughters of Charity Community Health Ministries*, 1–33.

47. Author interview of Sr. Mary Walz, DC.

48. McQueary, *Daughters of Charity Community Health Ministries*, 1–33.

49. Author interview of Sr. Mary Walz, DC.

50. St. Elizabeth's eventually gained federal certification as a rural health clinic, which meant that it could bill third parties (Medicare, Medicaid, and private insurers) for services provided. McQueary, *Daughters of Charity Community Health Ministries*, 4. In addition to funding sources, there are other distinctions between

free clinics and those with federal certification. Federally certified rural health clinics have to meet federal law requirements concerning location, range of services, staffing, and hours of operation, while free clinics do not have to meet these requirements. Under the circumstances, free clinics enjoy greater managerial flexibility and lower operating costs. See Rural Health Information Hub, https://www.ruralhealthinfo.org; Jaymie Baxley, "Medicaid Is an 'Expensive Proposition' for Free Clinics," *North Carolina Health News*, May 9, 2023, https://www.northcarolinahealthnews.org.

51. Rucker, "Fanning the Embers," 1–4.

52. Alice Crann, "Pensacola Is Lucky to Have Sister Jean," *Pensacola News Journal*, November 27, 1998.

53. Julie Minda, "St. Mary's Outreach Program Helps Immigrants Overcome Barriers to Health Care," *Catholic Health World*, August 1, 2014.

54. Sister Isabel Fierro, DC, "Being a Daughter of Charity Allows Me to Use My Nursing Gifts," *Clarian Herald* (New Orleans, LA), March 21, 2022.

55. Gustavo Valdez, "New Hispanic Immigrant Ministry in South Carolina," https://charlestondiocese.org.

56. Author interview of Sr. Mary Walz, DC.

57. Author interview of Sr. Mary Walz, DC; Congregation of the Mission, "Four Becomes One—New Province of the Daughters of Charity in the USA," https://cmnewengland.org.

58. In 2016, Holmes County ranked number seven on the list of poorest US counties. Forty-four percent of its residents were indigent. Emily Wagster Pettus, "Nuns Remembered for 'Christian Love in Action,'" *Hattiesburg American*, August 30, 2016.

59. Karen Fioretti, "Mercy: Sanders Admits Guilt," *Star-Herald* (Kosciusko, MS), June 28, 2018; Sisters of Charity of Cincinnati, "Ministry Opening: Prison Ministry, Durant, Mississippi," *Update*, June 8, 2023.

NOTE ON ARCHIVAL SOURCES

Much of the material used in the writing of this book comes from the archives of the Province of St. Louise, located in Emmitsburg, Maryland. Following the merger of four of the five US provinces in 2011, the Daughters consolidated their archival holdings at Emmitsburg. The archives of the Province of St. Elizabeth Ann Seton (formerly Province of the West) were not included in the consolidation. They are located in Los Altos Hills, California. All references in this book to events or occurrences in the Province of St. Elizabeth Ann Seton come from secondary sources or primary materials contained in the Emmitsburg archives.

Though mostly accurate in my estimation, certain of the Daughters' letters, diaries, and reports contain discrepancies and embellishments. When presenting the archival material, I frequently have sought confirmation and context through various sources such as newspaper articles, local histories, government documents, books, journal articles, and materials from other archives. I also have provided further information and explanation in several notes. In some instances, there may be gaps in the description or sequence of events because of partial or selective reporting, lost documents, inaccessible materials, and errors in my research or interpretation.

BIBLIOGRAPHY

Archives

American Hospital Association Archives, Chicago, IL.
Catholic Health Association Archives, St. Louis, MO.
Daughters of Charity, Archives of the Province of St. Louise, Emmitsburg, MD (APSL).
St. Louis University Archives, St. Louis, MO.
William A. Carrington Papers, National Archives, Washington, DC.

Books and Journals

Alberts, John B. "Black Catholic Schools: The Josephite Parishes of New Orleans During the Jim Crow Era." *U.S. Catholic Historian* 12, no. 1 (1994): 77–98.

"The American Medical Association: Power, Purpose, and Politics in Organized Medicine." *Yale Law Journal* 63 (1954): 937–1022.

Ameringer, Carl F. *The Health Care Revolution: From Medical Monopoly to Market Competition*. Berkeley: University of California Press, 2008.

Ameringer, Carl F. *US Health Policy and Health Care Delivery: Doctors, Reformers, and Entrepreneurs*. Cambridge: Cambridge University Press, 2018.

Archambault, Edith. "Historical Roots of the Nonprofit Sector in France." *Nonprofit and Voluntary Sector Quarterly* 30, no. 2 (June 2001): 204–20.

Armiger, Bernadette, DC. "Two Sister-Nurses Claimed by Cholera." *Nursing Outlook* 12 (September 1964): 54–56.

Armstrong, Elizabeth J. "Nurse Malpractice in North Carolina: The Standard of Care." *North Carolina Law Review* 65, no. 3 (1987): 579–97.

Aulisio, Mark P. "Why Did Hospital Ethics Committees Emerge in the US?" *American Journal of Medical Ethics* 18, no. 5 (May 2016): 46–53.

Barthel, Joan. *American Saint: The Life of Elizabeth Seton*. New York: St. Martin's Press, 2014.

Bates, Barbara. *Bargaining for Life: A Social History of Tuberculosis, 1876–1938.* Philadelphia: University of Pennsylvania Press, 1992.

Bechtle, Regina. "The 1846 Separation of the New York Sisters: Conflict over Mission or Clash of Will?" *Vincentian Heritage Journal* 20, no.1 (1999): 63–80.

Berrelleza, Erick, SJ, Mary L. Gautier, and Mark M. Gray. "Population Trends Among Religious Institutes of Women." Center for Applied Research in the Apostolate, Special Report, Fall 2014.

Berry, John M. *The Great Influenza: The Story of the Deadliest Pandemic in History.* London: Penguin, 2005.

Billings, John S. "The Relations of Hospitals to Public Health." In *Hospitals, Dispensaries, and Nursing*, edited by Henry Mills Hurd, 1–7. Baltimore: Johns Hopkins University Press, 1894.

Billington, Ray Allen. *The Protestant Crusade, 1800–1860: A Study of the Origins of American Nativism.* Chicago: Quadrangle Books, 1964.

Blasingame, F. J. L. *Digest of Official Actions, 1846–1958.* Chicago: American Medical Association, 1959.

Bluestone, E. M. "Aims and Tendencies of Out-Patient Service." *The Modern Hospital* 26, no. 1 (January 1926): 14–16.

Boas, Ernst P. "Chronic Diseases—a Challenge to the Hospital and to the Community." *The Modern Hospital* 26, no. 2 (February 1926): 138–41.

Bodenheimer, Thomas, and Kevin Grumbach. *Understanding Health Policy: A Clinical Approach.* 4th ed. New York: Lange Medical Books; McGraw-Hill, 2002.

Bodenheimer, Thomas, and Kip Sullivan. "How Large Employers Are Shaping the Health Care Marketplace." *New England Journal of Medicine* 338, no. 14 (April 1998): 1003–8.

Bonner, Thomas Neville. *Becoming a Physician: Medical Education in Britain, France, Germany, and the United States, 1750–1945.* Baltimore: Johns Hopkins University Press, 1995.

Breschi, Louis C. "Health Care Reform and the Catholic Perspective: The Catholic Medical Association." *The Linacre Quarterly* 79, no. 3 (August 2012): 334–37.

Brown, Dorothy M., and Elizabeth McKeown. *The Poor Belong to Us: Catholic Charities and American Welfare.* Cambridge, MA: Harvard University Press, 1997.

Brown, Ray E. "To the Public a Hospital Is a Hospital." *New England Journal of Medicine* 269, no. 12 (September 1963): 610–15.

Budrys, Grace. *Our Unsystematic Health Care System.* 3rd ed. Lanham, MD: Rowman & Littlefield, 2012.

Buhler-Wilkerson, Karen. *No Place Like Home: A History of Nursing and Home Care in the United States.* Baltimore: Johns Hopkins University Press, 2001.

Campion, Frank D. *The AMA and U.S. Health Policy Since 1940*. Chicago: Chicago Review Press, 1984.

Canfield, Phillip R. "Family Medicine: An Historical Perspective." *Journal of Medical Education* 51, no. 11 (November 1976): 904–11.

Carey, Ann. *Sisters in Crisis, Revisited: From Unraveling to Reform and Renewal*. San Francisco: Ignatius Press, 1997.

Carlson, Heather L. "Freedom at Risk: The Implications of City of Boerne v. Flores on the Merger of Catholic and Non-Catholic Hospitals." *Saint Louis University Public Law Review* 17, no. 1 (1997): 157–81.

Carter, Ruth C. "Cincinnatians and Cholera: Attitudes Toward the Epidemics of 1832 and 1849." *Queen City Heritage* 50 (Fall 1992): 32–48.

Casterline, Gail Farr. "St. Joseph's and St. Mary's: The Origins of Catholic Hospitals in Philadelphia." *The Pennsylvania Magazine of History and Biography* 108, no. 3 (1984): 289–314.

Castle, A. C. "A Common-Sense Talk About 'Ship Fever.'" *The Boston Medical and Surgical Journal*, March 1849, 290–97.

Catholic Health Association. "Ministerial Juridic Person: The Growing Role for Laity in Canonical Sponsorship of Catholic Health Care." *Health Progress* 95, no. 5 (September–October): 60–63.

Caulfield, Philip A. "History of Providence Hospital, 1861–1961." *Records of the Columbia Historical Society* 60/62 (1960/1962): 231–49.

Cavico, Frank J., and Nancy M. Cavico. "The Nursing Profession in the 1990's: Negligence and Malpractice Liability." *Cleveland State Law Review* 43, no. 4 (1995): 557–626.

Cetina, Judith G. "In Times of Immigration." In *Pioneer Healers: The History of Women Religious in American Health Care*, edited by Ursula Stepsis, CSA, and Dolores Liptak, RSM, 86–117. New York: Crossroad, 1989.

Charpy, Elisabeth. "A Challenge to Napoleon: The Defiance of the Daughters of Charity." *Vincentian Heritage Journal* 30, no. 2 (Spring 2011): 47–89.

Coburn, Carol K. "Ahead of Its Time . . . or, Right on Time? The Role of the Sister Formation Conference for American Women Religious." *American Catholic Studies* 126, no. 3 (Fall 2015): 25–44.

Coburn, Carol K. "Crossing Boundaries and Cultural Barriers: Catholic Sisters, Social Justice, and Transnationalism." *American Catholic Studies* 132, no. 1 (2021): 1–28.

Coburn, Carol K., and Martha Smith. *Spirited Lives: How Nuns Shaped Catholic Culture and American Life, 1836–1920*. Chapell Hill: University of North Carolina Press, 1999.

"Colored Women as Nurses." *The Modern Hospital* 26, no. 2 (February 1926): 144–45.

"The Committee on the Costs of Medical Care Presents Its Final Report." *The Milbank Memorial Fund Quarterly Bulletin* 11, no. 1 (January 1933): 21–30.

Coreil, Bernice, DC. "CHA's Vision of a Redesigned Healthcare System." *Health Progress*, May 1993, 12–14.

Cornely, Paul B. "Trend in Racial Integration in Hospitals in the United States." *Journal of the National Medical Association* 49, no. 1 (1957): 8–10.

Coste, Pierre, CM. *The Life and Works of St. Vincent de Paul.* Translated by Joseph Leonard, CM. Brooklyn: New City Press, 1987.

Crosby, Molly Caldwell. *The American Plague: The Untold Story of Yellow Fever, the Epidemic That Shaped Our History*. New York: Berkley Books, 2006.

Cumming, H. S. "Developing a Community Health Program." *The Modern Hospital* 26, no. 1 (January 1926): 1–5.

Cumming, Kate. *Kate: The Journal of a Confederate Nurse.* Edited by Richard Barksdale Harwell. Baton Rouge: Louisiana State University Press, 1998.

Cummings, Kathleen Sprows. *A Saint of Our Own: How the Quest for a Holy Hero Helped Catholics Become American*. Chapel Hill: University of North Carolina Press, 2019.

Cunningham, H. H. *Doctors in Grey: The Confederate Medical Service.* Baton Rouge: Louisiana State University Press, 1960.

"Dallas Hospital Admits Five Negro Physicians to Staff." *Journal of the National Medical Association* 46, no. 5 (September 1954): 367, 370.

Daly, Walter J. "The Black Cholera Comes to the Central Valley of America in the 19th Century—1832, 1849, and Later." *Transactions of the American Clinical and Climatological Association* 119 (2008): 143–53.

Daniels, Roger. *Coming to America: A History of Immigration and Ethnicity in American Life*. 2nd ed. New York: HarperCollins, 2002.

"Daughters of Charity Mull National System." *Modern Healthcare*, December 1985. https://www.modernhealthcare.com.

Davis, Belinda, ed. "Message from Sr. Teresa George, DC." *Faith Afire*, Winter 2025, 1–28.

Davis, Michael M. "The Boom in Dispensary Work—Its Growth and Development." *The Modern Hospital* 3, no. 2 (August 1914): 85–88.

Davis, Michael M. "'Clinic' or 'Dispensary'—Which?" *The Modern Hospital* 26, no. 2 (February 1926): 119–20.

Davis, Michael M. "Dispensary Progress in 1922." *The Modern Hospital* 20, no. 1 (January 1923): 49–50.

Davis, Michael M. "Dispensary Progress in 1924." *The Modern Hospital* 24, no. 1 (January 1925): 26–27.

de Lavergnée, Matthieu Brejon. *The Streets as a Cloister: History of the Daughters of Charity*. Hyde Park, NY: New City Press, 2020.

Desmond, Humphrey J. *The Know-Nothing Party.* Washington, DC: New Century Press, 1905.

Desselberger, U. "Emerging and Re-Emerging Infectious Diseases." *Journal of Infection* 40 (January 2000): 3–15.

Devine, Shauna. *Learning from the Wounded: The Civil War and the Rise of American Medical Science.* Chapel Hill: University of North Carolina Press, 2014.

DiChristina, Wendy Dunne. "'So Sue Me': Medical Professionals Should Support Strengthening Title VI Anti-Discrimination Laws." *Voices in Bioethics* 7 (2021). https://journals.library.columbia.edu.

Dirvin, Joseph I. *Louise de Marillac of the Ladies and Daughters of Charity.* New York: Farrar, Straus & Giroux, 1970.

"The Disturbance at the Charity Hospital." *New Orleans Medical and Surgical Journal* 19, no. 8 (February 1892): 613–16.

Dock, Lavinia L. *History of American Red Cross Nursing.* New York: Macmillan, 1922.

Dolan, Jay P., R. Scott Appleby, Patricia Byrne, and Debra Campbell. *Transforming Parish Ministry: The Changing Roles of Catholic Clergy, Laity, and Women Religious.* New York: Crossroad, 1989.

Dries, Angelyn. "Living in Ambiguity: A Paradigm Shift Experienced by the Sister Formation Movement." *The Catholic Historical Review* 79, no. 3 (July 1993): 478–87.

Duffy, John. *The Sanitarians: A History of American Public Health.* Urbana: University of Illinois Press, 1992.

Eccard, Walther T. "A Revolution in White—New Approaches in Treating Nurses as Professionals." *Vanderbilt Law Review* 50, no. 4 (May 1977): 839–79.

Endres, David J., and William B. Kurtz, eds. *Soldiers of the Cross, the Authoritative Text: The Heroism of Catholic Chaplains and Sisters in the American Civil War.* Notre Dame, IN: University of Notre Dame Press, 2019.

Engler, Eric S., Stephen L. Jones, and Andrew H. Van de Ven. "Organizing Healthcare for Changing Markets: The Case of Ascension." *Journal of Organization Design* 2, no. 3 (December 2013): 3–15.

"The Epidemic Fever in Ireland." *The Boston Medical and Surgical Journal* 41, no. 20 (December 1849): 389–93.

Falk, I. S. "Medical Care in the USA—1932–1972: Problems, Proposals and Programs from the Committee on the Costs of Medical Care to the Committee for National Health Insurance." *The Milbank Memorial Fund Quarterly, Health and Society* 51, no. 1 (Winter 1973): 1–32.

Fenner, Gertrude, DC. "The Daughters of Charity in the Spanish-American War." *Vincentian Heritage Journal* 8, no. 2 (Fall 1987): 141–64.

Fessler, Pam. *Carville's Cure: Leprosy, Stigma, and the Fight for Justice.* New York: Liveright, 2020.

"The Final Report of the Committee on the Costs of Medical Care." *New England Journal of Medicine* 207, no. 22 (December 1932): 996–97.

"'Final Report' of the Committee on the Costs of Medical Care." *California and Western Medicine* 37, no. 6 (December 1932): 395–400.

Fincher, Jack. "America's Deadly Rendezvous with the 'Spanish Lady.'" *Smithsonian Magazine* 19, no. 10 (January 1989): 130–45.

Fishbein, Morris. "History of the American Medical Association: By Leaps and Bounds." *JAMA* 133, no. 9 (March 1947): 605–13.

Fishbein, Morris. "Present-Day Trends of Private Practice in the United States." *JAMA* 98, no. 24 (June 1932): 2039–45.

Flexner, Simon, and James Thomas Flexner. *William Henry Welch and the Heroic Age of American Medicine*. Baltimore: Johns Hopkins University Press, 1941.

Flint, Austin. "Original Communications." *Buffalo Medical Journal and Monthly Review* 5, no. 6 (November 1849): 313–15.

Flinton, Margaret. "Louise de Marillac: Social Aspects of Her Work." Vincentian Digital Books, 1992. https://via.library.depaul.edu.

Fossier, A. E. *The Charity Hospital of Louisiana*. New Orleans: American Printing Co., 1923.

Freidson, Eliot. *Profession of Medicine: A Study of the Sociology of Applied Knowledge*. New York: Dodd, Mead & Company, 1973.

Fuechtmann, Thomas G. "'There Is Great Charity, But . . .': Vincent de Paul and the Organization of Charity." *Vincentian Heritage Journal* 26, no. 1 (2005): 43–63.

Gabow, Patricia A. *The Catholic Church and Its Hospitals: A Marriage Made in Heaven?* Washington, DC: American Association for Physician Leadership, 2023.

Gallagher, Gary, Stephen Engle, Robert Krick, and Joseph Glatthaar. *Civil War: Fort Sumter to Appomattox*. Oxford: Osprey, 2014.

Gamble, Vanessa Northington. *Making a Place for Ourselves: The Black Hospital Movement, 1920–1945*. New York: Oxford University Press, 1995.

Garceau, Oliver. *The Political Life of the American Medical Association*. Cambridge, MA: Harvard University Press, 1941.

Gaynes, Robert P. *Germ Theory: Medical Pioneers in Infectious Diseases*. Washington, DC: ASM Press, 2011.

Geary, Laurence. "Epidemic Diseases of the Great Famine." *History Ireland* 4, no. 1 (Spring 1996): 27–32.

Gerber, David A. *The Making of an American Pluralism: Buffalo, New York, 1825–60*. Urbana: University of Illinois Press, 1989.

Gerhard, W. W. "Gerhard on Typhus Fever." *The Boston Medical and Surgical Journal* 17, no. 3 (August 1837): 37–39.

Giesberg, Judith Ann. *Civil War Sisterhood: The U.S. Sanitary Commission and Women's Politics in Transition.* Boston: Northeastern University Press, 2000.

Gleeson, David T. *The Irish in the South, 1815–1877.* Chapel Hill: University of North Carolina Press, 2001.

Goffman, Erving. *Asylums: Essays on the Social Situation of Mental Patients and Other Inmates.* New York: Anchor Books, 1961.

Gold, Rachel Benson. "Advocates Work to Preserve Reproductive Health Care Access When Hospitals Merge." *Guttmacher Policy Review* 3, no. 2 (2000). https://www.guttmacher.org.

Goldsmith, Cynthia S., and Sara E. Miller. "Modern Uses of Electron Microscopy for Detection of Viruses." *Clinical Microbial Review* 22, no. 4 (2009): 552–63.

Gottemoeller, Doris, RSM. "Challenges for Sponsorship Today." *Health Progress* 103, no. 3 (Summer 2022): 13–16.

Gottlieb, Scott. "The Clintonian Roots of Obamacare." *National Affairs* 64 (Summer 2015): 53–59.

Graf, Mercedes H. "Women Nurses in the Spanish-American War." *Minerva: Quarterly Report on Women and the Military* 19, no. 1 (2001). https://go.gale.com.

Griffin, Leslie C. "The Catholic Bishops vs. the Contraceptive Mandate." *Religions* 6, no. 4 (2015): 1411–32.

Gunn, T. Jeremy. "Religious Freedom and Laïcité: A Comparison of the United States and France." *BYU Law Review* 2004, no. 2 (Summer 2004): 419–506.

Gunnell, Kriston Ashton. "Daughters of Charity: Women, Religious Mission, and Hospital Care in Los Angeles, 1856–1927." Vincentian Digital Books, 2013. https://via.library.depaul.edu.

Haller, Charles R. *Across the Atlantic and Beyond: The Migration of German and Swiss Immigrants to America.* Bowie, MD: Heritage Books, 1993.

Hamel, Ron. "The Ethical and Religious Directives: Looking Back to Move Forward." *Health Progress*, November–December 2019, 64–71.

Hannefin, Daniel. *Daughters of the Church: A Popular History of the Daughters of Charity in the United States 1809–1987.* Vincentian Digital Books, 1989. https://via.library.depaul.edu.

Hasstedt, Kinsey. "Abortion Coverage Under the Affordable Care Act: Advancing Transparency, Ensuring Choice and Facilitating Access." *Guttmacher Policy Review* 18, no. 1 (April 2015). https://www.guttmacher.org.

Henrietta, Sister. "A Famous New Orleans Hospital: The Charity Hospital of Louisiana at New Orleans." *American Journal of Nursing* 39, no. 3 (March 1939): 249–56.

Hernandez, S. Robert, and Arnold D. Kaluzny. "Hospital Closure: A Review of Current and Proposed Research." *Health Services Research* 18, no. 3 (Fall 1983): 419–36.

Hickey, Daniel. *Local Hospitals in Ancien Régime France: Rationalization, Resistance, Renewal, 1530–1789*. Montreal: McGill-Queen's University Press, 1997.

Hilde, Libra R. *Worth a Dozen Men: Women and Nursing in the Civil War South*. Charlottesville: University of Virginia Press, 2012.

Hoss, Mary Ann Keogh, and Kevin S. Decker. "When All Roads Lead to Rome: The Catholic Hospital Dilemma Impacts Entire U.S. Healthcare System." *Open Journal of Leadership* 2, no. 4 (2013): 106–9.

Hoy, Suellen. *Good Hearts: Catholic Sisters in Chicago's Past*. Urbana: University of Illinois Press, 2006.

Infante, Maria Angeles, DC. "The Daughters of Charity in the History of Military Health Care and in the History of Nursing." *Anales* 123, no. 4 (July–August 2015): 327–43.

"It's Time to Take Our Medicine: An Interview with Sister Carol Keehan, DC." *U.S. Catholic*. 75, no. 5 (May 2010): 18–23.

Jensen, Gail A., Michael A. Morrisey, Shannon Gaffney, and Derek K. Liston. "The New Dominance of Managed Care: Insurance Trends in the 1990s" *Health Affairs* 16, no. 1 (January–February 1997): 125–36.

Johnson, Haynes, and David S. Broder. *The System: The American Way of Politics at the Breaking Point*. Boston: Little, Brown, 1997.

Johnson, Mary, SNDdeN, Patricia Wittberg, SC, and Mary L. Gautier. *New Generations of Catholic Sisters: The Challenge of Diversity*. New York: Oxford University Press, 2014.

Johnson, Peter Leo. *Daughters of Charity in Milwaukee, 1846–1946*. Milwaukee: Daughters of Charity, St. Mary's Hospital, 1946.

Jones, Colin. *The Charitable Imperative: Hospitals and Nursing in Ancien Régime and Revolutionary France*. London: Routledge, 1989.

Jones, Colin. *Charity and Beinfaisance: The Treatment of the Poor in the Montpellier Region, 1740–1815*. Cambridge: Cambridge University Press, 1982.

Jones, Colin. "Sisters of Charity and the Ailing Poor." *Social History of Medicine* 2, no. 3 (December 1989): 339–48.

Kalisch, Philip A. "Heroines of '98: Female Army Nurses in the Spanish-American War." *Nursing Research* 24, no. 6 (November–December 1975): 411–29.

Kauffman, Christopher J. *A Commitment to Healthcare: Celebrating 75 Years of the Catholic Health Association of the United States*. St. Louis: Catholic Health Association of the United States, 1990.

Kauffman, Christopher J. *Ministry and Meaning: A Religious History of Catholic Health Care in the United States*. New York: Crossroad, 1995.

Kellhofer, Jason M. "The Misperception and Misapplication of the First Amendment in the American Pluralistic System: Mergers Between Catholic and Non-

Catholic Healthcare Systems." *Journal of Law and Health* 16, no. 1 (2002): 103–43.

Kendall, John. *History of New Orleans*. Chicago: Lewis, 1922.

Kisacky, Jeanne. *Rise of the Modern Hospital: An Architectural History of Health and Healing, 1870–1940*. Pittsburgh: University of Pittsburgh Press, 2017.

Koehlinger, Amy L. *The New Nuns: Racial Justice and Religious Reform in the 1960s*. Cambridge, MA: Harvard University Press, 2007.

Kotar, S. L., and J. E. Gessler. *Yellow Fever: A Worldwide History*. Jefferson, NC: McFarland & Company, 2017.

Kraman, Carlan, OSF. "Women Religious in Health Care: The Early Years." In *Pioneer Healers: The History of Women Religious in American Health*, edited by Ursula Stepsis, CSA, and Dolores Liptak, RSM, 15–38. New York: Crossroad, 1989.

Kraut, Alan M. *Silent Travelers: Germs, Genes, and the "Immigrant Menace."* New York: Basic Books, 1994.

Kronenfeld, Jennie Jacobs. *The Changing Federal Role in U.S. Health Care Policy*. Westport, CT: Praeger, 1997.

Kuhns, Elizabeth. *The Habit: A History of the Clothing of Catholic Nuns*. New York: Doubleday, 2005.

Kurtz, William B. *Excommunicated from the Union: How the Civil War Created a Separate Catholic America*. New York: Fordham University Press, 2016.

Lambert, Alexander. "Tentative Standards in Organization and Management of Out-Patient Departments." *The Modern Hospital* 20, no. 2 (February 1923): 192–96.

Lambert, Samuel W. "The Real Significance of the Dispensary in Hospital Practice." *The Modern Hospital* 19, no. 4 (October 1922): 281–82.

Libster, Martha M., and Sister Betty Ann McNeil, DC. *Enlightened Charity: The Holistic Nursing Care, Education, and Advices Concerning the Sick of Sister Matilda Coskery, 1799–1870*. West Lafayette, IN: Golden Apple Publications, 2009.

Lomas, Arthur J. "As It Was in the Beginning: A History of the University Hospital." *Bulletin of the School of Medicine, University of Maryland* (1939): 186–92.

Longest, Beaufort B., Jr., Jonathon S. Rakich, and Kurt Darr. *Managing Health Organizations and Systems*. 4th ed. Baltimore: Health Professions Press, 2000.

Maher, Mary Denis, CSA. *To Bind Up the Wounds: Catholic Sister Nurses in the U.S. Civil War*. Baton Rouge: Louisiana State University Press, 1989.

Marmor, Theodore R. *Understanding Health Care Reform*. New Haven, CT: Yale University Press, 1994.

Massey, Mary Elizabeth. *Women in the Civil War*. Lincoln: University of Nebraska Press, 1966.

Mayes, Rick, and Robert A. Berenson. *Medicare Prospective Payment and the Shaping of U.S. Health Care*. Baltimore: Johns Hopkins University Press, 2006.

McCann, Mary Agnes. *The History of Mother Seton's Daughters, the Sisters of Charity of Cincinnati, Ohio, 1809–1917*. Vol. 1. London: Longmans, Green and Co., 1917.

McCauley, Bernadette. *Who Shall Take Care of Our Sick? Roman Catholic Sisters and the Development of Catholic Hospitals in New York City*. Baltimore: Johns Hopkins University Press, 2005.

McCormack, Arthur. "The Nun in the World." *The Furrow* 14, no. 12 (December 1963): 744–50.

McGarvie, Mark D. "Creating Roles for Religion and Philanthropy in a Secular Nation: The Dartmouth College Case and the Design of Civil Society in the Early Republic." *Journal of College and University Law* 25, no. 3 (Winter 1999): 527–68.

McGaugh, Scott. *Surgeon in Blue: Jonathan Letterman, the Civil War Doctor Who Pioneered Battlefield Care*. New York: Arcade, 2013.

McGuinness, Margaret M. *Called to Serve: A History of Nuns in America*. New York: New York University Press, 2013.

McNeil, Betty Ann, DC, ed. *Balm of Hope: Charity Afire Impels Daughters of Charity to Civil War Nursing*. Chicago: DePaul University Vincentian Studies Institute, 2015.

McNeil, D., and R. Williams. "Wide Range of Causes Found for Hospital Closure." *Hospitals* 52, no. 23 (1978): 76–81.

McQueary, Carl R. *Daughters of Charity Community Health Ministries*. Austin, TX: Seton Family of Hospitals, 2011.

Medical News. "Abandon Internship: Establish New 'Primary Physicians,' Commission Urges." *JAMA* 197, no. 13 (September 1966): 37–38.

Mehta, Nirav J., Rajal N. Mehta, and Ijaz A. Khan. "Austin Flint: Clinician, Teacher, and Visionary." *Texas Heart Institute Journal* 27, no. 4 (2000): 386–89.

Meyers, Bertrande, DC. *The Education of Sisters: A Plan for Integrating the Religious, Social, Cultural and Professional Training of Sisters*. New York: Sheed and Ward, 1941.

Meyers, Bertrande, DC. "The Place of Religious in Social Work." In *Gleanings: Sister Bertrande Meyers, Daughter of Charity: An Anthology of Published Articles and Addresses*, edited by Beatrice Brown, DC, 54–72. Hicksville, NY: Exposition Press, 1976.

Meyers, Bertrande, DC. *Sisters for the 21st Century*. New York: Sheed and Ward, 1965.

Mickey, Robert W. "Dr. StrangeRove; or, How Conservatives Learned to Stop Worrying and Love Community Health Centers." In *The Health Care "Safety Net" in a Post-Reform World*, edited by Mark A. Hall and Sara Rosenbaum, 21–66. New Brunswick, NJ: Rutgers University Press, 2012.

Moore, Barbara A., CSJ. "Sponsorship Transformation at Ascension Health." *Health Progress* 88, no. 1 (January–February 2007): 26–28.

Morens, David M. "Commentary: Cholera Conundrums and Proto-Epidemiologic Puzzles. The Confusing Epidemic World of John Lea and John Snow." *International Journal of Epidemiology* 42, no. 1 (February 2013): 43–52.

Morrow, Diane Batts. *Persons of Color and Religious at the Same Time: The Oblate Sisters of Providence, 1828–1860.* Chapel Hill: University of North Carolina Press, 2002.

Mullner, Ross, Calvin S. Byre, and Joseph D. Kubal. "Closed U.S. Community Hospitals, 1972–1978: Prospectives and Trends." *Social Science and Medicine* 14, no. 4 (December 1980): 355–60.

Neal, Marie Augusta SNDdeN. *Catholic Sisters in Transition: From the 1960s to the 1980s.* Wilmington, DE: Michael Glazier, 1984.

Nelson, Leonard J., III. "God and Woman in the Catholic Hospital." *Journal of Legislation* 31, no. 1 (2004): 69–128.

Nelson, Sioban. *Say Little, Do Much: Nursing, Nuns, and Hospitals in the Nineteenth Century.* Philadelphia: University of Pennsylvania Press, 2001.

Newman, Mark. "The Catholic Church in Arkansas and Desegregation, 1946–1988." *The Arkansas Historical Quarterly* 66, no. 3 (2007): 293–319.

Newman, Mark. "'Racial Discrimination Can in No Way Be Justified': The Vatican and Desegregation in the South, 1946–1968." *Journal of American Studies* 56, no. 5 (2022): 665–98.

"News from the Field." *Woodstock Letters* 11, no. 4 (March 1, 1949): 549.

Nightingale, Florence. *Notes on Hospitals.* 3rd ed. London: Longman, Green, Longman, Roberts & Green, 1863.

Numbers, Ronald L. *Almost Persuaded: American Physicians and Compulsory Health Insurance, 1912–1920.* Baltimore: Johns Hopkins University Press, 1978.

Nygren, David A., CM. "Effective Governance in Complex Systems." *Health Progress* 82, no. 4 (July–August 2001): 41–45.

Oates, Mary J. *The Catholic Philanthropic Tradition in America.* Bloomington: Indiana University Press, 1995.

O'Donnell, Catherine. *Elizabeth Seton: American Saint.* Ithaca, NY: Cornell University Press, 2018.

O'Donnell, Hugh F., CM. "Vincent de Paul: His Life and Way." In *Vincent de Paul and Louise de Marillac: Rules, Conference, and Writings*, edited by Frances Ryan, DC, and John E. Rybolt, CM, 13–38. New York: Paulist Press, 1995.

O'Driscoll, M. Felicity. "Political Nativism in Buffalo, 1830–1860." *Records of the American Catholic Historical Society of Philadelphia* 48, no. 3 (September 1937): 279–319.

O'Grady, John. *Catholic Charities in the United States: History and Problems.* National Washington, DC: Conference of Catholic Charities, 1930.

O'Melinn, Liam Seamus. "Neither Contract nor Concession: The Public Personality of the Corporation." *George Washington Law Review* 74, no. 2 (2006): 201–59.

O'Rourke, Kevin D., OP, Thomas Kopfen-Steiner, STD, and Ron Hamel. "A Summary of the Development of the Ethical and Religious Directives for Catholic Health Care Services." *Health Progress* 82, no. 6 (December 2001): 18–21.

Osborne, William. "The Church and the Negro: A Crisis in Leadership." *Cross Currents* 15, no. 2 (1965): 129–50.

O'Toole, G. J. A. *The Spanish War: An American Epic—1898.* New York: W. W. Norton, 1984.

Ouimette, David S., and David E. Rencher. "Irish Emigration and Immigration to North America." *The BYU Family Historian* 6 (Fall 2007): 20–30.

Patel, Kant, and Mark E. Rushefsky. *Health Care Politics and Policy in America.* 2nd ed. Armonk, NY: M. E. Sharpe, 1999.

Peck, Sr. Theresa. "Accounting for Charity Care on a Systemwide Basis." *Health Progress* 69, no. 5 (June 1988): 50–52.

Pfanz, Donald C. *Clara Barton's Civil War: Between Bullet and Hospital.* Yardley, PA: Westholme, 2018.

"Points and Principles of Out-Patient Building Illustrated by Four Recently Constructed Clinics Associated with Medical Schools." *The Modern Hospital* 26, no. 3 (March 1926): 223–27.

Polak, John Osborn. "Relation of the Dispensary to the Community." *The Modern Hospital* 26, no. 2 (February 1926): 153–56.

Porter, Michael E., and Elizabeth Olmstead Teisberg. *Redefining Health Care: Creating Value-Based Competition on Results.* Boston: Harvard Business School Press, 2006.

Powell, John A., and Stephen Menendian. "Beyond Public/Private: Understanding Excessive Corporate Prerogative." *Kentucky Law Journal* 100, no. 1 (2011–2012): 43–124.

Pyle, Geoffrey F. "The Diffusion of Cholera in the United States in the Nineteenth Century." *Geographical Analysis* 1 (1969): 59–75.

Quinn, John F. "Expecting the Impossible? Abolitionist Appeals to the Irish in Antebellum America." *The New England Quarterly* 82, no. 4 (December 2009): 667–710.

Rabinowitz, Howard N. "From Exclusion to Segregation: Health and Welfare Services for Southern Blacks, 1865–1890." *Social Service Review* 48, no. 3 (September 1974): 327–54.

Rada, James, Jr. *Battlefield Angels: The Daughters of Charity as Civil War Nurses.* Gettysburg, PA: Legacy, 2011.

Rapley, Elizabeth. *The Dévotes: Women and Church in Seventeenth-Century France.* Montreal: McGill-Queen's University Press, 1990.

Rappaport, Jordan. "U.S. Urban Decline and Growth, 1950 to 2000." *Federal Reserve Bank of Kansas City Economic Review,* Third Quarter 2003, 15–44.

"Report of the Superintendents of the Poor of Erie County, for the Year Ending Oct. 1, 1849." *Buffalo Medical Journal and Monthly Review of Medical and Surgical Science* 5, no. 7 (December 1849): 424–28.

"Report of the Typhoid Fever Board—War with Spain." *JAMA* 44, no. 11 (March 1905): 877.

Reverby, Susan M. *Ordered to Care: The Dilemma of American Nursing, 1850–1945.* Cambridge: Cambridge University Press, 1987.

"Review of M. Louis's Researches upon Typhoid Fever." *The Boston Medical and Surgical Journal* 40, no. 11 (April 1849): 209–16.

Rice, Mitchell F., and Woodrow Jones, Jr. *Public Policy and the Black Hospital: From Slavery to Segregation to Integration.* Westport, CT: Greenwood Press, 1994.

Richardson, Jean. *A History of the Sisters of Charity Hospital, Buffalo, New York, 1848–1900.* Lewiston, NY: Edwin Mellen Press, 2005.

Risse, Guenter B. *Mending Bodies, Saving Souls: A History of Hospitals.* New York: Oxford University Press, 1999.

Robinson, James C. *The Corporate Practice of Medicine: Competition and Innovation in Health Care.* Berkeley: University of California Press, 1999.

Roemer, Milton I. *Ambulatory Health Services in America: Past, Present, and Future.* Rockville, MD: Aspen Systems Corporation, 1981.

Rosen, George. *The Structure of American Medical Practice, 1875–1941,* edited by Charles E. Rosenberg. Philadelphia: University of Pennsylvania Press, 1983.

Rosenberg, Charles E. *The Care of Strangers: The Rise of America's Hospital System.* Baltimore: Johns Hopkins University Press, 1987.

Rosenberg, Charles E. *The Cholera Years: The United States in 1832, 1849, and 1866.* Chicago: University of Chicago Press, 1987.

Rosenberg, Charles E. "From Almshouse to Hospital: The Shaping of Philadelphia General Hospital." *The Milbank Memorial Fund Quarterly* 60, no. 1 (1982): 108–54.

Rosenberg, Charles E. "Social Class and Medical Care in Nineteenth Century America: The Rise and Fall of the Dispensary." *Journal of the History of Medicine and Allied Sciences* 29, no. 1 (January 1974): 32–54.

Ross, Joseph S. "The Committee on the Costs of Medical Care and the History of Health Insurance in the United States." *Einstein Quarterly Journal of Biology and Medicine* 19 (2002): 129–34.

Ross, Robert R. N., and Deanne E. B. Ross. *Walking to New Orleans: Ethics and the Concept of Participatory Design in Post-Disaster Reconstruction*. Eugene, OR: Wipf and Stock, 2008.

Rucker, Tinsley White. "Fanning the Embers." *Family Medicine and Community Health* 7, no. 3 (August 2019): 1–4.

Rutkow, Ira. *Bleeding Blue and Grey: Civil War Surgery and the Evolution of American Medicine*. Mechanicsburg, PA: Stackpole Books, 2005.

Ryan, Francis, DC, and John E. Rybolt, CM, eds. *Vincent de Paul and Louise de Marillac: Rules, Conference, and Writings*. New York: Paulist Press, 1995.

Rybolt, John E., CM. "The Congregation of the Mission in the United States: An Historical Survey." *Vincentiana* 45, no. 3 (2001): 129–37.

Rybolt, John E., CM. "Growth of the Constitutions of the Daughters of Charity." 2010. https://works.bepress.com.

Rybolt, John E., CM. "Joseph Rosati, CM (1789–1843): Pioneer American Bishop." *Vincentiana* 48, no. 6 (2004): 394–403.

Sager, Alan. "Urban Hospital Closings in the Face of Racial Change." *Health Law Project Library Bulletin* 5, no. 6 (June 1980): 169–81.

Sager, Alan. "Why Urban Voluntary Hospitals Close." *Health Services Research* 18, no. 3 (Fall 1983): 451–81.

Salganicoff, Alina, Adara Beamesderfer, Nisha Kurani, and Laurie Sobel. "Coverage for Abortion Services and the ACA." *KFF Issue Brief*, September 19, 2014. https://www.kff.org.

Salvaggio, John. *New Orleans' Charity Hospital: A Story of Physicians, Politics, and Poverty*. Baton Rouge: Louisiana State University Press, 1992.

Scally, Sr. Anthony. "Two Nuns and Old Thad Stevens." *Biography* 5, no. 1 (1982): 66–73.

Schneider, Mary L. "American Sisters and the Roots of Change: The 1950s." *U.S. Catholic Historian* 7, no. 1 (Winter 1988): 55–72.

Schroeder-Lein, Gleena R. *The Encyclopedia of Civil War Medicine*. Armonk, NY: M. E. Sharpe, 2008.

Schultz, Jane E. *Women at the Front: Hospital Workers in Civil War America*. Chapel Hill: University of North Carolina Press, 2004.

Schwitalla, Alphonse S. "Basic Considerations in Minority Report of Committee on the Costs of Medical Care." *JAMA* 100, no. 12 (March 1933): 863–67.

Schwitalla, Alphonse S. "Catholic Viewpoints: With Reference to a National Health Program and the Wagner-Murray Bill." *The Linacre Quarterly* 12, no. 2 (April 1944): 24–34.

Seem, Ralph B. "Organization of the Dispensary of Johns Hopkins Hospital." *The Modern Hospital* 3 (1914): 33–35.

Senn, Nicholas. *Medical-Surgical Aspects of the Spanish American War*. Chicago: American Medical Association, 1900.

Shadid, Michael. *A Doctor for the People*. New York: Vanguard Press, 1939.

Shanahan, Robert J., SJ. *The History of the Catholic Hospital Association, 1950–1965*. St. Louis: Catholic Hospital Association, 1965.

Shi, Leiyu, and Douglas A. Singh. *Essentials of the U.S. Health Care System*. 4th ed. Burlington, MA: Jones & Bartlett Learning, 2017.

Singer, Lawrence E., and Elizabeth J. Lantz. "The Coming Millenium: Enduring Issues Confronting Catholic Health Care." *Annals of Health Law* 8, no. 1 (1999): 299–330.

Smith, Brian. "Form Follows Function: The Evolution of Mission Integration in U.S. Catholic Health Care." *Health Progress*, March–April 2020, 51–60.

Smith, David Barton. "Population Ecology and the Racial Integration of Hospitals and Nursing Homes in the United States." *The Milbank Quarterly* 68, no. 4 (1990): 561–96.

Smith, David Barton. "Racial Disparities in Care: The Concealed Legacy of a Divided System." *Sexually Transmitted Diseases* 33, no. 7 suppl. (July 2006): S65–69.

Smith, David Barton. "The Racial Integration of Medical and Nursing Associations in the United States." *Hospital and Health Services Administration* 37, no. 3 (1992): 387–401.

"Specialism in Medicine." *New England Journal of Medicine* 143, no. 15 (1900): 379–80.

Starr, Paul. *The Social Transformation of American Medicine: The Rise of a Sovereign Profession and the Making of a Vast Industry*. New York: Basic Books, 1982.

Stepsis, Ursula, CSA, and Dolores Liptak, RSM, eds. *Pioneer Healers: The History of Women Religious in American Health*. New York: Crossroad, 1989.

Stevens, Rosemary. *American Medicine and the Public Interest: A History of Specialization*. Berkeley: University of California Press, 1998.

Stevens, Rosemary. *In Sickness and in Wealth: American Hospitals in the Twentieth Century*. New York: Basic Books, 1989.

Stewart, George C., Jr. *Marvels of Charity: History of American Sisters and Nuns*. Huntington, IN: Our Sunday Visitor Publishing Division, 1994.

Stone, Judith F. "Anticlericals and *Bonnes Soeurs*: The Rhetoric of the 1901 Law of Associations." *French Historical Studies* 23, no. 1 (Winter 2000): 103–28.

Strum, Harvey. "To Feed the Hungry: Rochester and Irish Famine Relief." *Rochester History* 68, no. 3 (Summer 2006): 1–22.

Suenens, Leon Joseph Cardinal. *The Nun in the World: Religious and the Apostolate.* Westminster, MD: Newman Press, 1963.

Sullivan, Louise, DC. "Louise de Marillac: A Spiritual Portrait." In *Vincent de Paul and Louise de Marillac: Rules, Conference, and Writings*, edited by Frances Ryan, DC, and John E. Rybolt, CM, 39–64. New York: Paulist Press, 1995.

Sulmasy, Daniel P. "Can Medical Schools Be Catholic?" *Health Progress* 84, no. 4 (July–August 2003): 10–13, 50.

Sultz, Harry A., and Kristina M. Young. *Health Care USA: Understanding Its Organization and Delivery*. 2nd ed. Gaithersburg, MD: Aspen, 1999.

Taeuber, Karl E., and Alma F. Taeuber. *Negroes in Cities: Residential Segregation and Neighborhood Change*. Chicago: Aldine, 1965.

Tieman, Jeff. "Quite a Moment." *Health Progress*, May–June 2010, 4–5.

Torrens, Paul R., and Donna G. Yedvab. "Variations Among Emergency Room Patients: A Comparison of Four Hospitals in New York City." *Medical Care* 8, no. 1 (1970): 60–75.

Tourscher, Francis E. "Work of the Sisters During the Epidemic of Influenza, October, 1918." *Records of the American Catholic Historical Society of Philadelphia* 30, no. 3 (1919): 193–226.

US Conference of Catholic Bishops. *Ethical and Religious Directives for Catholic Health Care Services*. 6th ed. 2018. https://www.usccb.org.

Varon, Elizabeth R. *Armies of Deliverance: A New History of the Civil War*. Oxford: Oxford University Press, 2019.

Walker, Alice H. "Social Service Problems in the Hospital." *The Modern Hospital* 20, no. 3 (March 1923): 264–65.

Wall, Barbra Mann. *American Catholic Hospitals: A Century of Changing Markets and Missions.* New Brunswick, NJ: Rutgers University Press, 2016.

Wall, Barbra Mann. "Catholic Sister Nurses in Selma, Alabama, 1940–1972." *Advances in Nursing Science* 32, no. 1 (2009): 91–102.

Wall, Barbra Mann. "Conflict and Compromise: Catholic Public Hospital Partnerships." *Nursing Historical Review* 18 (2010): 100–17.

Wall, Barbra Mann. "'Definite Lines of Influence': Catholic Sisters and Nurse Training Schools, 1890–1920." *Nursing Research* 50, no. 5 (September–October 2001): 314–21.

Wall, Barbra Mann. "Science and Ritual: The Hospital as Medical and Sacred Space." *Nursing History Review* 11 (2003): 51–68.

Wall, Barbra Mann. "Textual Analysis as a Method for Historians of Nursing." *Nursing History Review* 14, no. 1 (2006): 227–42.

Wall, Barbra Mann. *Unlikely Entrepreneurs: Catholic Sisters and the Hospital Marketplace, 1865–1925*. Columbus: Ohio State University Press, 2005.

Washington, Harriet A., Robert B. Baker, Ololade Olakanmi, Todd L. Savitt, Elizabeth A. Jacobs, Eddie Hoover, and Matthew K. Wynia. "Segregation, Civil Rights, and Health Disparities: The Legacy of African American Physicians and Organized Medicine, 1910–1968." *Journal of the National Medical Association* 101, no. 6 (2009): 513–27.

Watson, William. "The Sisters of Charity, the 1832 Cholera Epidemic in Philadelphia and Duffy's Cut." *Philadelphia Catholicism* 27, no. 4 (Fall 2009): 1–16.

Weiss, John H. "Origins of the French Welfare State: Poor Relief in the Third Republic, 1871–1914." *French Historical Studies* 13, no. 1 (Spring 1983): 47–66.

Weissert, Carol, and William Weissert. *Governing Health: The Politics of Health Policy*. Baltimore: Johns Hopkins University Press, 1996.

Weitzman, Louis G. *One Hundred Years of Catholic Charities in the District of Columbia*. Washington, DC: Catholic University of America, 1931.

Wildes, Kevin W., SJ. "A Memo from the Central Office: The 'Ethical and Religious Directives for Catholic Health Care Services.'" *Kennedy Institute of Ethics Journal* 5, no. 2 (1995): 133–39.

Williams, Harold A. *History of the Hibernian Society of Baltimore*. Baltimore: Hibernian Society of Baltimore, 1957.

Wisner, Elizabeth. "The Howard Association of New Orleans." *Social Service Review* 41, no. 4 (December 1967): 411–18.

Wittberg, Patricia. "Declining Institutional Sponsorship and Religious Orders: A Study of Reverse Impacts." *Sociology of Religion* 61, no. 3 (2000): 315–24.

Wittberg, Patricia. *The Rise and Fall of Catholic Religious Orders: A Social Movement Perspective.* Albany: State University of New York Press, 1994.

Wormeley, Katharine Prescott. *The United States Sanitary Commission: A Sketch of Its Purposes and Its Work*. Boston: Little, Brown, 1868.

Wuerl, Donald W. "Catholic Health Ministry in Transition." *Health Progress*, May–June 1999, 14–16.

Wurdock, Stephanie M. "Doctors, Dioceses, and Decisions: Examining the Impact of the Catholic Hospital System and Federal Conscience Clauses on Medical Education." *Journal of Environmental and Public Health Law* 6, no. 2 (Spring 2012): 179–214.

Zall, Richard J. "Maintaining Health Care in the Inner City: Title VI and Hospital Relocations." *New York University Law Review* 55 (May 1980): 271–302.

Zerr, Sheila Rankin. "Beyond the Bricks and Mortar: The Role of Residences in Opening Doors to Nursing Education and Practice." *Canadian Bulletin of Medical History* 23, no.1 (Spring 2006): 209–18.

Zwierlein, Frederick J. "Catholic Beginnings in the Diocese of Rochester." *The Catholic Historical Review* 1, no. 3 (October 1915): 282–98.

Zwierlein, Frederick J. "Know Nothingism in Rochester, N.Y." *United States Catholic Historical Society Records and Studies* 14 (1912): 20–69.

Studies and Reports

Catholic Health Association. *No Room in the Marketplace: Health Care of the Poor.* St. Louis: Catholic Health Association, 1986.

Catholic Health Association. *Setting Relationships Right: A Working Proposal for Systemic Healthcare Reform.* St. Louis: Catholic Health Association, 1992.

Davis, Michael M., and Anna Mann Richardson. *New Clinics for Old: A Study of Clinics Unattached to Hospitals in New York City.* New York: Committee on Dispensary Development of the United Hospital Fund of New York, 1927.

Gibson, Campbell. *Population of the 100 Largest Cities and Other Urban Places in the United States: 1790 to 1990.* Washington, DC: US Government Printing Office, 1998.

Goldsmith, Jeff., Lawton R. Burns, Aditi Sen, and Trevor Goldsmith. *Integrated Delivery Networks: In Search of Benefits and Market Effects.* Washington, DC: National Academy of Social Insurance, 2015.

National Center for Health Statistics. *Health, United States, 2004, with Chartbook on Trends in the Health of Americans.* Hyattsville, MD: National Center for Health Statistics, 2004.

Office of Attorney General Martha Coakley. *Statement of the Attorney General as to the Caritas Christi Transaction.* Boston: Office of Attorney General Martha Coakley, 2010.

Office of Senator Edward J. Markey. *The Steward Health Care Report: How Corporate Greed Hurt Patients, Health Workers, and Communities.* Washington, DC: Office of Senator Edward J. Markey, 2024.

Reed, Walter, Victor C. Vaughan, and Edward O. Shakespeare. *Report on the Origin and Spread of Typhoid Fever in U.S. Military Camps During the Spanish War of 1898.* Washington, DC: US Government Printing Office, 1904.

United States Commission Appointed by the President to Investigate the Conduct of the War Department in the War with Spain. *Report of the Commission Appointed by the President to Investigate the Conduct of the War Department in the War with Spain* (Dodge Commission Report). Washington, DC: US Government Printing Office, 1899.

United States Commission on Civil Rights. *Title VI, One Year After: A Survey of Desegregation of Health and Welfare Services in the South.* Washington, DC: US Government Printing Office, 1966.

United States Conference of Catholic Bishops. *Ethical and Religious Directives for Catholic Health Care Services.* 6th ed. Washinton, DC: United States Conference of Catholic Bishops, 2018.

United States Conference of Catholic Bishops, Committee on Domestic Justice and Human Development. "Letters from the Most Reverend Frank J. Dewane to the United States House of Representatives and the United States Senate." January 18, 2017. https://www.usccb.org.

United States Congress, House. "Providence Hospital." *Congressional Record,* June 6, 1961.

United States Congress, Senate. *1980 Census of Population and Housing.* July 1983.

United States Congress, Senate Subcommittee of the Committee on Education and Labor. 76th Cong., 1st sess., May 25–26 and 1 June, 1939.

United States Department of Commerce, Bureau of the Census. *Hospitals and Dispensaries, 1923.* Washington, DC: US Government Printing Office, 1925.

United States Department of Commerce, Bureau of the Census, Population Division. *1980 Census of Population and Housing.* Washington, DC: US Government Printing Office, 1983.

United States Department of Health, Education, and Welfare. *Compliance with Antidiscrimination Provision of the Civil Rights Act by Hospitals and Other Facilities Under Medicare and Medicaid.* Report to the Committee on the Judiciary, House of Representatives, by the Comptroller General of the United States. Washington, DC: General Accounting Office, 1972.

United States Department of the Interior, National Park Service. *DePaul Hospital Complex Historic District.* NPS Form 10-900, OMB Control No. 1024-0018. 2023.

Wilson, Elizabeth W. *Compulsory Health Insurance.* Studies in Individual and Collective Security 3. New York: National Industrial Conference Board, 1947.

Unpublished Sources

Flynn, George Quitman. "Franklin D. Roosevelt and American Catholicism, 1932–1936." PhD dissertation, Louisiana State University, 1966.

Nako, Elizabeth D. "Nuns in the Newsroom: The Sisters of Marillac College and U.S. Sisters' Involvement in Social Justice Reform." *History and Classics Undergraduate Theses,* 2014. Providence College Digital Commons. https://digitalcommons.providence.edu.

Rubin, Michael H. "Immigration, Quotas and Its Impact on Medical Education." PhD dissertation, Wake Forest University, 2013.

Court Cases

Bradfield v. Roberts, 175 U.S. 291 (1899).
Brown v. Board of Education, 347 U.S. 483 (1954).
Frederick County Com'rs v. Sisters of Charity of St. Joseph, 48 Md. 34 (1878).
Goldfarb v. Virginia State Bar, 421 U.S. 773 (1975).
Griswald v. Connecticut, 381 U.S. 479 (1965).
Little Sisters of the Poor Saints Peter and Paul Home v. Pennsylvania, 140 S.Ct. 2367 (2020).
National Federation of Independent Business v. Sebelius, 567 U.S. 519 (2012).
Roe v. Wade, 410 U.S. 113 (1973).
St. Anges Hospital of City of Baltimore, Inc. v. Riddick, 748 F.Supp. 319 (D. Md., 1990).
Taylor v. St. Vincent's Hospital, 369 F.Supp. 948 (D. Mont., 1973).
Trustees of Dartmouth College v. Woodward, 17 U.S. (4 Wheat) 518 (1819).
United States v. American Medical Ass'n, 317 U.S. 519 (1943).
United States v. Oregon State Medical Society, 343 U.S. 326 (1952).

INDEX

Note: Page numbers in *italics* refer to figures and numbers in **bold** refer to tables.

CARL F. AMERINGER is a former Maryland assistant attorney general and professor of health policy and politics at three different universities.

www.ingramcontent.com/pod-product-compliance
Lightning Source LLC
LaVergne TN
LVHW011810200926
848484LV00005B/1130
* 9 7 8 0 2 6 8 2 1 1 3 8 7 *